CW01260967

# Preface

While it has been known for close to 100 years that the pituitary gland regulates growth and for almost 60 years that human growth hormone (GH) stimulates growth in GH-deficient children, our knowledge about GH function and GH-deficient states continues to grow. Both basic science and clinical research have contributed to our understanding about GH, although the interactions between various systems are complex, and some mechanisms remain unclear. The goal of this book is to provide up-to-date information to the clinical endocrinologist on GH function and what occurs in GH deficiency.

After the Introduction, the book is divided into three parts. The first describes the mechanisms of human GH secretion and action. Growth hormone structure and function are explained, along with various important regulators of GH secretion, including sex steroids and thyroid hormone. Additionally, insight into how undernutrition, inflammation, and catabolic illness affect GH secretion is discussed; as well as how the opposite state, obesity, affects GH function and testing. Included in this part are the metabolic effects of GH on body composition and on cardiovascular risk factors.

The second part deals with the diagnosis of GH deficiency, both in children and in adults. It describes both the tests that can be utilized and their interpretation and points out the challenges faced in using these studies to make a diagnosis. A chapter is devoted to magnetic resonance imaging of the pituitary gland.

The third part explains various etiologies of GH deficiency, from molecular mechanisms to cranial radiation to traumatic brain injury, as well as syndromes associated with GH deficiency where the molecular defect is less clear.

The definition of "GH deficiency" remains a challenge. This book should guide clinicians in understanding their patients' underlying pathology. In the future, additional insights into the hypothalamic-pituitary-GH axis and GH signaling, plus newer technologies (e.g., whole exome sequencing) to determine molecular defects, may help us better determine which individuals have a defect in the GH signaling pathway and which individuals do not.

Boston, MA, USA                                                                                           Laurie Cohen

# Abbreviations

| | |
|---|---|
| aa | Amino acid |
| BPS | Branching point site or branch point sequence |
| cAMP | Cyclic adenosine monophosphate |
| CHT | Compound heterozygous |
| CRH | Corticotropin-releasing hormone |
| CSS | Cryptic splice site |
| D1 | Type 1 5′-deiodinase |
| D2 | Type 2 5′-deiodinase |
| D3 | Type 3 5′-deiodinase |
| ERK | Extracellular signal-regulated kinases |
| ESE | Exonic splice enhancer |
| GH | Growth hormone |
| GHD | Growth hormone deficiency |
| GHRH | Growth hormone-releasing hormone |
| GHRHR | Growth hormone-releasing hormone receptor |
| GHRP | Growth hormone-releasing peptides |
| GHRP-2 | Growth hormone-releasing peptide-2 |
| GHRP-6 | Growth hormone-releasing peptide-6 |
| GHS | Growth hormone secretagogues |
| HGMD | Human Gene Mutation Database |
| HGVS | Human Genome Variation Society |
| HM | Homozygous |
| HT | Heterozygous |
| IGF-I | Insulin-like growth factor-1 |
| IGHD | Isolated growth hormone deficiency |
| ISE | Intronic splice enhancer |
| LCR | Locus control region |
| PKC | Protein kinase C |
| RTH | Resistance to thyroid hormone |
| SDS | Standard deviation score |
| SP | Signal peptide |

| | |
|---|---|
| T1DM | Type 1 diabetes mellitus |
| T3 | Triiodothyronine |
| T4 | Thyroxine |
| TR | Thyroid hormone receptor |
| TRE | Thyroid response element |
| TRH | Thyrotropin-releasing hormone |

# Contents

1 **Introduction: Discovery of Growth Hormone and Synthesis of Recombinant Human Growth Hormone**.......................... 1
Laurie E. Cohen

**Part I  Mechanisms of Human Growth Hormone Secretion and Action**

2 **Growth Hormone Physiology**................................................................ 7
Philippe Backeljauw and Vivian Hwa

3 **Sex Steroids and Growth Hormone Secretion**...................................... 21
Diane E.J. Stafford

4 **The Influence of Thyroid Hormone on Growth Hormone Secretion and Action**.................................................................. 29
Angela M. Leung and Gregory A. Brent

5 **Undernutrition, Inflammation and Catabolic Illness, and Growth Hormone Secretion**........................................... 47
Charumathi Baskaran and Madhusmita Misra

6 **Obesity and Growth Hormone Secretion**............................................. 63
Takara L. Stanley

7 **Metabolic Benefits of Growth Hormone Therapy** ............................. 79
Roberto Lanes

**Part II  Diagnosis of Human Growth Hormone Deficiency**

8 **Laboratory Diagnosis of Growth Hormone Deficiency in Children**................................................................................ 95
Constantin Polychronakos

9 **Laboratory Diagnosis of Growth Hormone Deficiency in Adults**................................................................................. 109
Kevin C.J. Yuen

10 **Pituitary Gland Imaging** ..................................................................... 123
Natascia Di Iorgi, Giovanni Morana, Flavia Napoli, Andrea Rossi, and Mohamad Maghnie

**Part III Etiologies of Human Growth Hormone Deficiency**

11 **Growth Hormone-Releasing Hormone Receptor and Growth Hormone Gene Abnormalities** ......................................... 149
Jan M. Wit, Monique Losekoot, and Gerhard Baumann

12 **Combined Pituitary Hormone Deficiency**............................................. 177
Frédéric Castinetti and Thierry Brue

13 **Cranial Radiation and Growth Hormone Deficiency** ......................... 195
Wassim Chemaitilly

14 **Traumatic Brain Injury and Growth Hormone Deficiency** ................ 205
Erick Richmond and Alan D. Rogol

15 **Syndromes Associated with Growth Hormone Deficiency**................... 213
Sara A. DiVall

**Index**............................................................................................................... 223

# Contributors

**Philippe Backeljauw, MD** Division of Pediatric Endocrinology/Center for Growth Disorders, Cincinnati Children's Hospital Medical Center, Cincinnati, OH, USA

**Charumathi Baskaran, MD** Harvard Medical School, Boston, MA, USA

Pediatric Endocrine Unit, Massachusetts General Hospital, Boston, MA, USA

**Gerhard Baumann, MD** Division of Endocrinology, Metabolism and Molecular Medicine, Northwestern University Feinberg School of Medicine, Chicago, IL, USA

**Gregory A. Brent, MD** Departments of Medicine and Physiology, David Geffen School of Medicine at UCLA, VA Greater Los Angeles Healthcare System, Los Angeles, CA, USA

**Thierry Brue, MD, PhD** Aix-Marseille Université, CNRS, Centre de Recherche en Neurobiologie et Neurophysiologie de Marseille CRN2M UMR 7286, Marseille, France

APHM, Hôpital Conception Adultes, Service d'Endocrinologie, Diabète et Maladies Métaboliques, Marseille, France

Centre de Référence des Maladies Rares d'Origine Hypophysaire DEFHY, Marseille, France

**Frédéric Castinetti, MD, PhD** Aix-Marseille Université, CNRS, Centre de Recherche en Neurobiologie et Neurophysiologie de Marseille CRN2M UMR 7286, Marseille, France

APHM, Hôpital Conception Adultes, Service d'Endocrinologie, Diabète et Maladies Métaboliques, Marseille, France

Centre de Référence des Maladies Rares d'Origine Hypophysaire DEFHY, Marseille, France

**Wassim Chemaitilly, MD** Division of Endocrinology, Department of Pediatric Medicine, MS-737, St. Jude Children's Research Hospital, Memphis, TN, USA

**Laurie E. Cohen, MD** Division of Endocrinology, Boston Children's Hospital, Harvard Medical School, Boston, MA, USA

**Sara A. DiVall, MD** Pediatric Endocrinology, Seattle Children's Hospital, Seattle, WA, USA

**Vivian Hwa, PhD** Division of Pediatric Endocrinology/Center for Growth Disorders, Cincinnati Children's Hospital Medical Center, Cincinnati, OH, USA

**Natascia Di Iorgi, MD** Department of Pediatrics, IRCCS Giannina Gaslini, University of Genova, Genoa, Italy

**Roberto Lanes, MD** Pediatric Endocrine Unit, Hospital de Clinicas Caracas, Caracas, Venezuela

**Angela M. Leung, MD, MSc** Division of Endocrinology, Department of Medicine, David Geffen School of Medicine at UCLA, VA Greater Los Angeles Healthcare System, Los Angeles, CA, USA

**Monique Losekoot, PhD** Department of Clinical Genetics, Leiden University Medical Center, Leiden, The Netherlands

**Mohamad Maghnie, MD, PhD** Department of Pediatrics, IRCCS Giannina Gaslini, University of Genova, Genoa, Italy

**Madhusmita Misra, MD, MPH** Harvard Medical School, Boston, MA, USA

Pediatric Endocrine Unit, Massachusetts General Hospital, Boston, MA, USA

**Giovanni Morana, MD** Department of Pediatric Neuroradiology, Instituto Giannina Gaslini, Genoa, Italy

**Flavia Napoli, MD** Department of Pediatrics, IRCCS Giannina Gaslini, University of Genova, Genoa, Italy

**Constantin Polychronakos, MD** Departments of Paediatrics and Human Genetics, Child Health and Human Development, The McGill University Health Centre, Montreal, QC, Canada

**Erick Richmond, MD** Pediatric Endocrinology, National Children's Hospital, San José, Costa Rica

**Alan D. Rogol, MD, PhD** Pediatric Endocrinology, University of Virginia, Charlottesville, VA, USA

**Andrea Rossi, MD** Department of Pediatric Neuroradiology, Instituto Giannina Gaslini, Genoa, Italy

**Diane E.J. Stafford, MD** Division of Endocrinology, Boston Children's Hospital, Harvard Medical School, Boston, MA, USA

**Takara L. Stanley, MD** Pediatric Endocrine Unit, Massachusetts General Hospital for Children and Harvard Medical School, Boston, MA, USA

**Jan M. Wit, MD, PhD** Department of Pediatrics, Leiden University Medical Center, Leiden, The Netherlands

**Kevin C.J. Yuen, MD, FRCP (UK)** Swedish Pituitary Center, Swedish Neuroscience Institute, Seattle, WA, USA

# Chapter 1
# Introduction: Discovery of Growth Hormone and Synthesis of Recombinant Human Growth Hormone

Laurie E. Cohen

The most famous likely growth hormone (GH)-deficient individual was Charles S. Stratton (born February 4, 1838), nicknamed General Tom Thumb by P.T. Barnum who discovered him at age of 10. He was born to parents of normal height who were first cousins. His birth weight was nine and a half pounds, and he grew steadily until age 18 months. Thereafter, he grew poorly and had delayed puberty, growing several inches in his late twenties; he achieved an adult height of only 3 ft 2 in. He married Lavinia Warren Bump (born October 31, 1842) on February 10, 1863, in a highly publicized affair. Ms. Bump had grown normally until age 1 year but then only slowly, until cessation of growth at age 10 years and achieving an adult height of 2 ft 8 in. Her parents were third cousins of normal height. Due to their proportionate short stature, normal birth length and weight, growth retardation starting late in the first year of life, normal intelligence, and normal sexual development, it is assumed that both Stratton and Bump had autosomal recessive growth hormone deficiency (GHD) [1, 2].

In the nineteenth century, individuals with growth stunting were defined as "dwarfs" if disproportionate and as "midgets" if proportionate. At the turn of the nineteenth to twentieth centuries, an English physician, Hastings Gilford, created the term "ateliosis" to describe those with normal proportions and subdivided them into "sexual" (displayed normal sexual development) and "asexual" (did not display normal sexual development) [2].

While it was determined in 1922 that the pituitary gland regulates growth, GH was not isolated until 1944, and human GH was not isolated until 1956. Attempts to use GH to promote growth began in 1932, but success did not occur until 1958 when human GH was utilized. Cadaveric human GH was used until 1985, when Creutzfeldt–Jakob

---

L.E. Cohen (✉)
Division of Endocrinology, Boston Children's Hospital, Harvard Medical School, Boston, MA, USA
e-mail: laurie.cohen@childrens.harvard.edu

© Springer International Publishing Switzerland 2016
L.E. Cohen (ed.), *Growth Hormone Deficiency*,
DOI 10.1007/978-3-319-28038-7_1

disease, a neurodegenerative disorder caused by prions, was diagnosed in recipients of cadaveric GH. From 1985 to present, recombinant human GH has been utilized [3].

The following are the seminal events that shaped our knowledge and understanding of GH and GH therapy in the United States (USA), with parallel events in therapy occurring worldwide [2–7]:

1922—Evans and Long determined that the pituitary gland regulates growth, as injection of bovine pituitary extract into normal rats caused excess growth.

1927—Smith demonstrated that a substance in the pituitary is responsible for growth, as hypophysectomy of rats led to cessation of growth and implantation of pituitary tissue into these rats resulted in return of growth.

1932—Engelbach attempted to treat children with pituitary GH. From then until close to the next 30 years, no success was reported (now known to be due to species specificity of GH).

1943—Evans et al. reported the first bioassay for pituitary GH based on the width of proximal tibial epiphyseal cartilage in hypophysectomized rats.

1944—Li and Evans reported the isolation of bovine (ox) GH.

1945—Koneff and Li showed that chronic treatment of rats with pituitary GH caused gigantism.

1951—Raben and Westermeyer reported the isolation and purification of porcine GH.

1956–1957—Three different laboratories purified GH from monkey and human pituitaries using different extraction methods (Li and Papkoff, Wilhelmi, and Raben).

1957—Knobil et al. determined that the effects of GH are species specific, as bovine GH had no effect, while monkey GH had anabolic effects in hypophysectomized rhesus monkeys.

1957—Beck et al. demonstrated the metabolic effectiveness of human GH in a boy.

1957—Salmon and Daughaday determined that the actions of GH are mediated through a factor, which they named sulfation factor, later renamed somatomedin. Subsequently, somatomedin was found to be "insulin-like" and renamed insulin-like growth factor-I (IGF-I).

1958—Raben reported the effectiveness of human GH on growth promotion in a boy with GHD.

1961—The National Institutes of Health established the National Pituitary Agency (NPA) to collect pituitary glands in the USA to organize and guide the collection, extraction, and distribution of human GH to counter the black market that had arisen. Other countries established similar agencies.

1963—Berson and Yalow's group created a radioimmunoassay (RIA) to measure GH.

1966—McKusick's group used RIA to determine a marked deficiency of GH in the blood of "dwarfs with sexual ateliosis" [8].

1969—Li's group announced the complete structure of human GH, revised in 1971, and by others in 1973.

1970—Li and Yamashiro reported the synthesis of human GH.

1973—Guillemin and coworkers reported a hypothalamic polypeptide that inhibits GH, later named somatostatin.
1976—Commercial human pituitary GH entered the US market.
1977—Furlanetto et al. created a RIA to measure human IGF-I.
1978—Rinderknecht and Humbel reported the complete amino acid sequence of human IGF-I.
1979—Genentech decided to produce recombinant GH by inserting the human *GH* gene into the bacteria *Escherichia coli*.
1980—The *GH* gene was mapped to human chromosome 17.
1981—The first Genentech trials of recombinant human GH in children with GHD were initiated.
1982—Two groups identified a GH-releasing factor from pancreatic tumors, later designated growth hormone-releasing hormone (GHRH).
1985—Four young adults, who had received NPA GH in the 1960s, were diagnosed with Creutzfeldt–Jakob disease (a neurodegenerative disease caused by prions), and the distribution and use of human GH in the USA were halted. Other cases of Creutzfeldt–Jakob disease were noted throughout the world.
1985—The US Food and Drug Administration (FDA) approved the use of Genentech's biosynthetic GH for treating children with GHD.

Between 1963 and 1985, most of the GH treatment in the USA was supervised by the NPA. During that 22-year period, about 7700 children in the USA and 27,000 worldwide with severe childhood GHD were treated with cadaveric human GH [6]. Because of the limited supply of GH, children could not be treated continuously and there was often a height cap (152 cm, 5 ft). In 1984, the last year of its distribution, 2450 children were receiving NPA GH and 600–800 were receiving commercial GH in the USA [5]. In 1985 at the time of the US FDA approval of the first biosynthetic GH, 10,000–15,000 children in the USA were estimated to suffer from GH deficiency [9]. With the production of recombinant human GH, GH availability has markedly increased, and indications for many non-GH-deficient conditions have

**Table 1.1** Indications for growth hormone therapy and year of approval by the US Food and Drug Administration [6]

| Condition | Year |
|---|---|
| Childhood growth hormone deficiency | 1985 |
| Chronic renal insufficiency | 1993 |
| Adult growth hormone deficiency | 1996 |
| AIDS wasting | 1996 |
| Turner syndrome | 1997 |
| Prader–Willi syndrome | 2000 |
| Small for gestational age | 2001 |
| Idiopathic short stature | 2003 |
| Short bowel syndrome | 2003 |
| *Short stature homeobox-containing (SHOX) gene deficiency* | 2006 |
| Noonan syndrome | 2007 |

been approved (see Table 1.1, not discussed in this book). In 2006, it was predicted that more than 40,000 children in the USA qualified for GH therapy [10].

## References

1. The Loving Lilliputians; Warren-Thumbiana. Marriage of General Tom Thumb and the Queen of Beauty. Who they are, what they have done, where they came from, where they are going. Their courtship and wedding ceremonies, presents, crowds of people. The Reception the Serenade. 1863.http://www.nytimes.com/1863/02/11/news/loving-lilliputians-warren-thumbiana-marriage-general-tom-thumb-queen-beauty-who.html?pagewanted=all. Accessed 26 Sept 2015.
2. McKusick VA, Rimoin DL. General Tom Thumb and other midgets. Sci Am. 1967;217:102–6.
3. Lindholm J. Growth hormone: historical notes. Pituitary. 2006;9:5–10.
4. Gupta V. Adult growth hormone deficiency. Indian J Endocrinol Metab. 2011;15 Suppl 3:S197–202.
5. Frasier SD. The not-so-good old days: working with pituitary growth hormone in North America, 1956 to 1985. J Pediatr. 1997;131:S1–4.
6. Ayyar VS. History of growth hormone therapy. Indian J Endocrinol Metab. 2011;15 Suppl 3:S162–5.
7. Cronin MJ. Pioneering recombinant growth hormone manufacturing: pounds produced per mile of height. J Pediatr. 1997;131:S5–7.
8. Rimoin DL, Merimee TJ, McKusick VA. Sexual ateliotic dwarfism: a recessively inherited isolated deficiency of growth hormone. Trans Assoc Am Phys. 1966;79:297–311.
9. FDA Approves Genentech's Drug to Treat Children's Growth Disorder. 1985. http://www.gene.com/media/press-releases/4235/1985-10-18/fda-approves-genentechs-drug-to-treat-ch. Accessed 4 April 2015.
10. Lee JM, Davis MM, Clark SJ, Hofer TP, Kemper AR. Estimated cost-effectiveness of growth hormone therapy for idiopathic short stature. Arch Pediatr Adolesc Med. 2006;160:263–9.

# Part I
# Mechanisms of Human Growth Hormone Secretion and Action

# Chapter 2
# Growth Hormone Physiology

Philippe Backeljauw and Vivian Hwa

## Growth Hormone Biochemistry

### *Introduction*

Human pituitary-derived growth hormone (GH), also known as somatotropin, is encoded by the *GH1* gene, one of the five closely related genes in the 46.8 kb *GH1* locus located on chromosome 17q24.2. The five exon-containing *GH1* gene generates three transcript variants. The transcript variant 1 (NM_000515.4) encodes the largest of the putative GH isoforms, a protein containing 217 amino acid residues (isoform 1). The removal of the signal peptide (residues 1–26) generates a mature GH polypeptide of 191 residues, corresponding to a molecular mass of 22 kiloDalton (kDa). Although this 22 kDa is the predominant human GH found in the circulation (approximately 90 %), smaller GH isoforms have been described [1]. These include a 20 kDa variant from an alternative in-frame splicing event (NM_022559.3) that lacks 14 amino acid residues in the central coding region (residues 32–46) and a 17 kDa isoform lacking residues 1–66. In this section, we will summarize the known chemistry of the predominant 22 kDa GH isoform (amino acid residue numbering will be based on published nomenclature, which excludes the 26-amino-acid signal peptide). We describe how accumulated biochemical knowledge led to the development of human GH antagonists for GH excess in clinical conditions such as acromegaly as well as to the development of formulations of long-acting recombinant human GH (rhGH) for treatment of GH deficiency.

---

P. Backeljauw (✉) • V. Hwa
Division of Pediatric Endocrinology/Center for Growth Disorders, Cincinnati Children's Hospital Medical Center, 3333 Burnet Ave, Rm T5.272, Cincinnati, OH 45229, USA
e-mail: philippe.backeljauw@cchmc.org; vivian.hwa@cchmc.org

© Springer International Publishing Switzerland 2016
L.E. Cohen (ed.), *Growth Hormone Deficiency*,
DOI 10.1007/978-3-319-28038-7_2

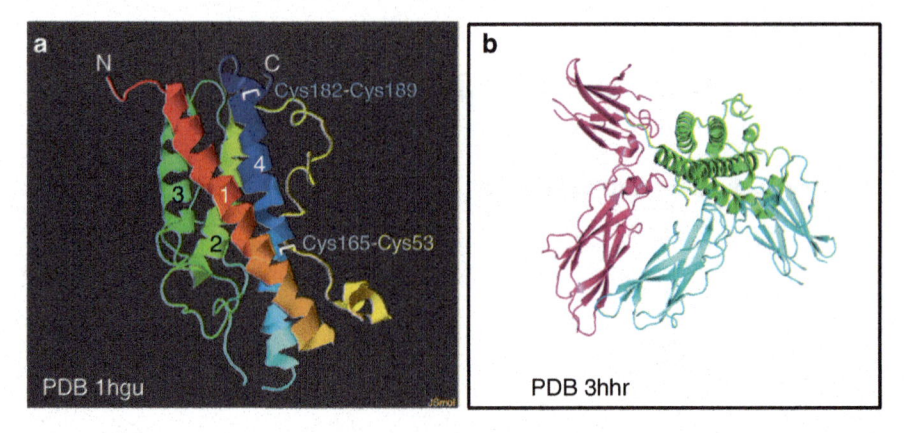

**Fig. 2.1** Model of the human growth hormone. Crystal structure analyses indicate GH is a four-helical bundle protein. (**a**) The four helices are numbered (PDB 1hgu; [4]), with N-terminal and C-terminus indicated. *Yellow*, loop connecting helix 1 to helix 2. *Light blue*, part of loop connecting helix 3 to helix 4. The two disulfide linkages are depicted. (**b**) Crystal structure of GH in complex with the dimeric extracellular domain of the GH receptor (PDB 3hhr; [3])

## Growth Hormone Structure

The 22 kDa GH polypeptide has the three-dimensional fold of a four-helical bundle protein, a configuration shared with other cytokines such as prolactin, erythropoietin, and many interleukins [2]. Crystal structure analyses indicate the first two helices are parallel to each other and antiparallel to the remaining two helices, with long connecting loops between the first two helices and second two helices [3, 4] (Fig. 2.1). Of the two disulfide bonds, one links the N-terminal and C-terminal regions (Cys53-Cys165). The second disulfide bond is located at the C-terminus (Cys182-Cys189, Fig. 2.1a). Human GH also carries two zinc ($Zn^{2+}$)-binding sites, identified at residues His44 and Glu200. The binding of $Zn^{2+}$ is critical for facilitating GH dimerization and aggregation in the secretory granule biogenesis, which occurs in the anterior pituitary. This is an important GH storage mechanism that permits rapid release of GH in response to appropriate stimulation without necessitating de novo protein synthesis [5].

The 22 kDa GH initiates its growth-promoting and metabolic activities by interacting with the cell-surface GH receptor (GHR, Fig. 2.1b), a homo-dimeric single-pass transmembrane receptor belonging to the type 1 cytokine receptor superfamily. It was initially proposed that the binding of GH induced dimerization of monomeric GHR polypeptides. More recent evidence supports preformation of the dimeric GHR independent of GH binding, followed by subsequent binding of one molecule of GH and inducing GHR conformational and rotation changes that activate the GHR signaling cascades [6]. Extensive in vitro mutagenesis and crystal structure analyses reveal two essential sites within the GH protein which interact with each monomer of the dimeric GHR [3, 7–10]. Site 1 was identified as the high-affinity GHR binding site, with interacting residues in the connecting loop between helices

1 and 2 (residues 41–72) and in the carboxyl region of helix 4 (residues 167–175). Site 2 interactions involve the NH2-terminus (residues 1–16) and helix 3 (residues 103–119) [3, 9, 10]. Remarkably, up to a 400-fold change in Site 1 affinity of GH-GHR did not significantly impact biological response, suggesting that human GH, unlike other mammalian GH, is highly efficient at forming GH-GHR complexes [11, 12]. Of note, the extracellular domain of human GHR can be proteolytically cleaved to circulate as a monomeric GH binding protein (GHBP), and binds circulating GH in a 1:1 ratio, an association which could serve as a dynamic reservoir for bound and free GH [13].

While the GHR is the cognate receptor for human GH, GH can also bind to the prolactin receptor (PRLR), albeit with considerably lower affinity. High affinity is achieved only in the presence of $Zn^{2+}$, which is chelated in the binding interface [14, 15]. Physiological implications of this remain unclear.

## *Human Growth Hormone Analogs: Antagonistic Effects*

In the course of elucidating residues within human GH important for binding and inducing GHR biological activities, a glycine 120 to arginine (Gly120Arg) amino acid exchange in helix 3 was found to abolish site 2 binding capacity without affecting site 1 binding functions [9, 11, 16]. This observation, first recognized in bovine GH [17, 18], suggested Gly120Arg acted as a competitive antagonist for GH signaling. Indeed, substitution of Gly120 with any amino acid but alanine antagonized GHR activation [19]. This was a crucial observation that has led to the development of the GHR antagonist B2036-PEG (pegvisomant, hGH-Gly120Lys variant) to counteract pathological GH excess in clinical conditions such as acromegaly [19, 20]. Additional modifications introduced into pegvisomant included eight amino acid substitutions at site 1 to enhance receptor binding, and incorporation of four to five polyethylene-glycol (PEG) modifiers, which prolonged the half-life of the GH variant from 20 to 30 min to about 90 h, reduced immunogenicity, and reduced interactions with GHBP as well [20, 21]. Pegvisomant is currently available worldwide for the indication of GH excess/acromegaly and is presently being considered for cancer indications and diabetes-induced end-organ damage [20].

## *Modifying Human GH: Toward Long-Acting rhGH Therapy*

Recombinant hGH therapy has been available since the mid-1980s for an increasing number of clinical indications, including GH deficiency, idiopathic short stature, small-for-gestational-age (SGA) children not showing adequate postnatal catch-up growth, as well as for genetic conditions such as Noonan, Prader-Willi, and Turner syndromes. The rapid proteolysis and clearance of rhGH, however, necessitate daily subcutaneous injection, which often results in compliance and treatment adherence issues [22]. These concerns have driven interest in developing long-acting rhGH compounds. Based on accumulated understanding of GH biochemistry, a variety of formulations have been generated and tested. Some of these formulations have since been abandoned due to unexpected adverse effects. One such formulation was derived from PEGylation, which prolonged the in vivo mean half-life of rhGH as was observed with pegvisomant. Unlike with pegvisomant, the PEGylated GH had safety and efficacy issues: it induced lipoatrophy at the site of injection. This was reported for 13 out of 105 treated GH-deficient adults [23]. In addition, reduced efficacy was determined when readout of once-weekly insulin-like growth factor-I (IGF-I) response profiles was not reached (hGH PEGylated at glutamine 141) [24], and PEG-containing vacuoles were discovered in epithelial cells of the choroid plexus of treated monkeys (GH analog PEGylated at substituted residue 35) [25]. A number of other formulations, however, have passed safety surveillance and are currently in clinical trials [25]. These include prodrug formulations such as GH fused to carriers with self-cleavage properties (ACP-001) [25] and GH carrying a single-point mutation in the backbone to which a side chain with terminal fatty acids (with non-covalent albumin-binding properties) has been attached (NNC0195-0092) [26]. Formulations based on GH fusion protein technology undergoing clinical trials include human serum albumin fused to the N-terminus of GH (TV-1106) [25, 27], long hydrophilic sequences of amino acids (XTEN) added to the N- and C- terminus of GH (VRS-317) [28], and (e) carboxyl-terminal peptide (CTP, 28 carboxyl-terminal residues of human chorionic gonadotropin) added to the N- and C-terminus of GH (MOD-4023) [29]. Altogether, the manipulation of GH, based on its chemistry and function, has allowed for the expansion of the therapeutic options for a variety of clinical indications.

## The Regulation of Growth Hormone Secretion

### *Introduction: Stimulatory [S] and Inhibitory [I] Influences*

Growth hormone secretion occurs predominantly according to an intermittent or pulsatile pattern rather than through continuous release. This is the case both during childhood and in adult life [30]. On a day-to-day basis, more GH will be secreted during the early to mid-adolescence years: about 700 μg/day, almost double the secretion measured in adulthood (approximately 400 μg/day) [31]. Because of the pulsatile pattern of GH secretion, GH concentrations are usually low (<0.2 μg/L) when measured in serum of healthy individuals (except in neonates or young infants). This episodic nature of GH secretion, and the regulation of it by a variety of other hormones and particular physiologic conditions, is further linked to the notion that GH not only plays an important role in statural growth, but is also of great importance in a variety of nongrowth-related biological processes, e.g., the intermediary metabolism. Growth hormone therefore has many sites of action, consistent with its variety of physiological effects: the bone and the growth plate,

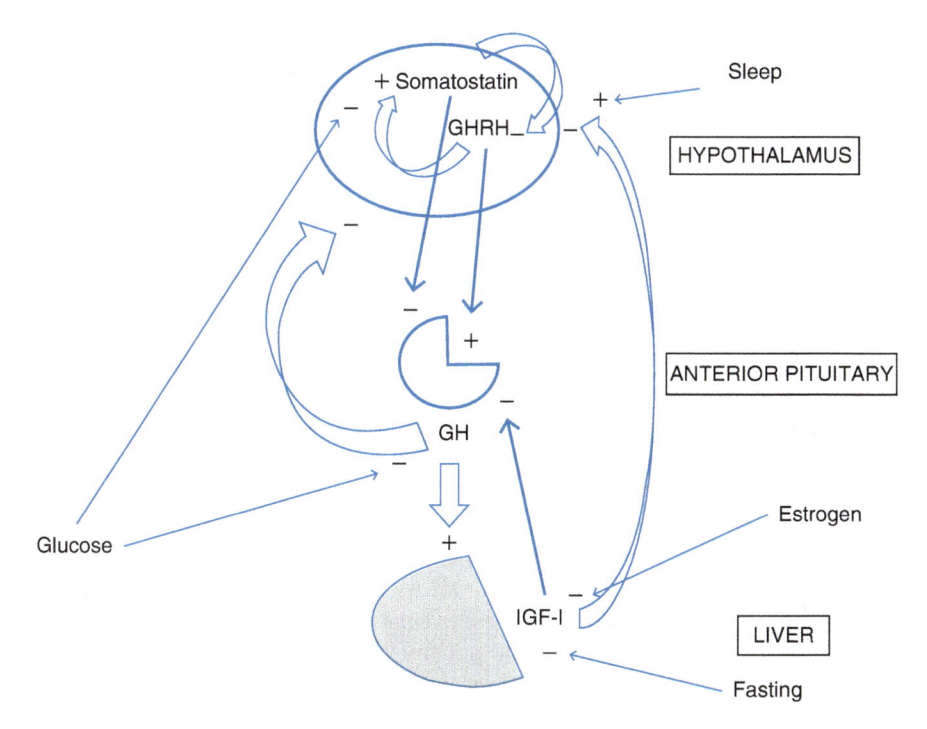

Fig. 2.2 Simplified schematic representation of the regulation of GH secretion

muscle, and adipose tissue. As the next couple of paragraphs will illustrate, GH secretion is controlled by many factors/influences that make it one of the more complex-regulated hormones in the body (Fig. 2.2).

## *Growth Hormone-Releasing Hormone (GHRH) [S]*

The episodic GH secretory pulses that occur naturally and can be documented through frequent serum sampling are the result of the interaction between several regulatory peptides. The most important of these are two hypothalamic peptides, GHRH and somatostatin [32]. Growth hormone-releasing hormone, also known as GH-releasing factor (GRF), will bind to its receptor on the anterior pituitary somatotroph cells to stimulate the production of cyclic adenosine monophosphate (cAMP). This will lead to increased GH synthesis and secretion via a complex path of intracellular signaling ultimately resulting in increased *GH* gene transcription [30, 33]. The GHRH receptor (GHRH-R) belongs to the family of the G protein-coupled receptors, and the amino acid sequence of GHRH-R is, in part, similar to receptors for parathyroid hormone and calcitonin, among others [34]. Humans given synthetic exogenous GHRH experience a quick release of GH from the somatotrophs. Growth hormone, synthesized and stored in secretory granules [5], will be released within minutes; peak GH concentrations are reached after about 30 min, and these will be sustained for 1–2 h [35]. Growth hormone-releasing hormone is used in some countries in combination with other GH secretagogues (such as arginine) to test patients for the diagnosis of GH deficiency. Endogenously produced GHRH is very difficult to measure, because dilution affects the peripheral serum concentration of GHRH and does not reflect the hypothalamic GHRH output. To assess the latter, one would need to perform direct portal blood sampling, which is neither recommended nor practically possible. Endogenous GHRH is a 44-amino-acid peptide produced in the arcuate and ventromedial nuclei of the hypothalamus. In humans, this will first occur between 18 and 29 weeks of gestation, which correlates to the beginning of production of GH in the developing fetus [31].

The first real indication that GHRH stimulates GH secretion and is an important regulator of pulsatile GH release came from observations that body growth in young rats is severely affected after damaging their hypothalamus [36]. Additional other animal work then confirmed the role of GHRH secreted by the hypothalamic nuclei in GH secretion; destruction of these nuclei leads to GH reduction, and stimulation of these nuclei leads to GH release [37, 38]. However, it is of interest to note that GHRH was first isolated from extrahypothalamic/extrapituitary (pancreatic) tumor cells in patients with acromegaly and not from human hypothalamic tissue [39]. Many studies in different animal models, and in humans, have unequivocally documented the role of GHRH as a GH pulse generator, but the mechanisms by which this occurs may vary between humans and some of the animal models used. The activity of GHRH is therefore believed to be species specific. Despite these differences, strong correlations are found between the detection of GH pulses and increased pituitary portal blood GHRH concentrations. Furthermore, overnight episodic GH secretory pulses after acute administration of synthetic GHRH become suppressed when humans are treated beforehand with competitive GHRH antagonists [40, 41]. Additional investigations with GHRH-R antagonists in patients given different stimuli for GH secretion (e.g., clonidine, arginine, and insulin) confirmed the importance of GHRH in the regulation of GH secretion: those stimuli still require the action of GHRH to induce increased GH production, which, again, can be inhibited by the administration of GHRH-R antagonists [42].

As already described above, GH secretion is stronger in the childhood and adolescent age range than in adulthood. This age-related change in GH secretion appears to be mediated by GHRH also. Evidence for this comes from studies demonstrating that the somatotroph cells maintain their ability to respond to GHRH, while GH pulse amplitude decreases as one gets older. In addition, through pharmacological approaches, GHRH output was found to be decreased in aging monkeys [43], and similar findings were observed in older men [44]. At all ages, the effect of GHRH on GH secretion is partially blocked by the administration of somatostatin. Somatostatin inhibits GH secretion and controls the GH pulse frequency [45]—see below.

## Ghrelin and GH Secretagogues [S]

A number of synthetic peptides have now been identified that are also capable of stimulating GH secretion. These particular molecules, called GH-releasing peptides (GHRPs) or non-GHRH secretagogues, interact through a receptor that is different from the GHRH-R. This distinct receptor is known as the GH secretagogue receptor and is also a member of the G protein-coupled receptor family. It is strongly expressed in the hypothalamus [46]. Ghrelin has now been identified as the GH secretagogue receptor's endogenous ligand, which is the reason why this receptor has also been named the ghrelin receptor. In fact, it is the intensive study of the GHRPs that indirectly led to the discovery and characterization of both the ghrelin receptor and its ligand, ghrelin [46]. The GH-releasing peptides are analogous to ghrelin, directly stimulate GH release from the pituitary gland, and can promote GH release after stimulation by GHRH [47]. The practical application of the GHRPs is through their ability to stimulate GH release in patients with a functionally intact anterior pituitary gland and as possible therapeutic agents for GH deficiency that is not secondary to pituitary damage. Administration of GHRP, which can be done via the oral route, induces a physiological-like GH pulsatile secretion pattern, in contrast to the single GH peak caused by a subcutaneous GH injection [48].

Ghrelin itself is a peptide hormone primarily expressed in stomach cells and functions as a neuropeptide in the central nervous system. However, ghrelin mRNA has been identified in the hypothalamus also [49]. Small amounts of ghrelin are further expressed at other sites of the gastrointestinal system (bowel, pancreas) and in the kidneys and gonads as well. Ghrelin is a 28-amino acid molecule that circulates in two different forms. The ghrelin that is octanoylated seems to be the ghrelin capable of stimulating GH. Ghrelin may release GH together with GHRH in a more or less synergistic fashion, and mutations of the ghrelin receptor have been implicated as a cause of GH deficiency [50]. Despite all this, it is still not clear what the exact role of ghrelin is in controlling GH release. The other form, encoded by the same gene, is called obestatin; it does not stimulate GH secretion, but plays a role in weight regulation [51]. Ghrelin has many physiologic actions [49]. Ghrelin regulates appetite and is important in energy homeostasis. It controls gastric secretion, affects glucose metabolism and endocrine pancreatic function, and plays a role in gonadal function and behavior as well.

## Other Neurotransmitters and Neuropeptides Influencing GH Secretion [Both S and I]

Many neurotransmitters and neuropeptides play some role in the regulation of GHRH, as well as the regulation of somatostatin (see below), and indirectly in the secretion of GH. They may affect GH secretion in a number of different physiologic

Table 2.1 Neurotransmitters and neuropeptides that alter GH secretion

| |
|---|
| Acetylcholine |
| Calcitonin |
| Corticotropin-releasing hormone (CRH) |
| Dopamine |
| Gamma-aminobutyric acid (GABA) |
| Gastrin |
| Histamine |
| Neuropeptide Y |
| Neurotensin |
| Norepinephrine |
| Serotonin |
| Substance P |
| Thyroid-releasing hormone (TRH) |
| Vasopressin |

and pathologic conditions such as sleep, exercise, physical and emotional stress situations, prolonged fasting, and in response to hypoglycemia. The major neurotransmitters and peptides that affect GH secretion are listed in Table 2.1.

## Somatostatin- or Somatotropin-Inhibiting Factor (SRIF) [I]

Somatostatin, also called somatotropin release-inhibiting factor (SRIF), is a 14-amino-acid molecule (tetradecapeptide) and strong inhibitor to basal, as well as stimulated, GH secretion [52]. Somatostatin achieves this through effects on timing and amplitude of the GH pulses (and not by a direct effect on GH synthesis). Somatostatin is produced by neuroendocrine cells located in the ventromedial nucleus of the hypothalamus. Released somatostatin reaches the anterior pituitary gland through the hypothalamo-portal vascular network, where it inhibits the secretion of GH from the somatotroph cells. At this level, it has a dominant effect over GHRH on GH release. There exists a classic negative feedback mechanism to GH secretion, because somatostatin-secreting neurons respond to increased GH and IGF-I concentrations by increasing somatostatin release and activity. The actions of somatostatin are mediated through specific receptors. Five subtypes of somatostatin receptors are known. The key GH suppressive action of somatostatin is through its binding with somatostatin receptors 2 and 5 [45]. The half-life of somatostatin is approximately 3 min, and it suppresses GH secretion after binding to its receptors via inhibition of adenylate cyclase activity and reducing intracellular calcium. This has been demonstrated after treating somatotroph cells with GHRH and somatostatin together, where the latter blocks the mitogenic effects of GHRH on the somatotrophs [53]. The currently accepted mechanism of the role of somatostatin in GH secretion was determined from the administration of selective somatostatin agonists and antibodies against somatostatin in both animal models and in humans while assessing the effects of these substances on GH secretion [32, 53]. It appears that somatostatin modulates GH release by attenuating the effect of GHRH; GH pulses and the GH concentrations between these pulses are suppressed, whereas the GH pulsatility generation remains unmodified.

Long-acting somatostatin analogs (e.g., octreotide, lanreotide) are small synthetic peptides that mimic the action of somatostatin, have a much longer half-life than naturally occurring endogenous somatostatin, and thus have strong GH suppressive effects. They are used for the treatment of GH hypersecretion, as found in acromegaly patients [54].

## *Effect of Sleep on GH Secretion [S]*

Sleep also appears to influence the secretory pattern of GH, and a sleep-associated increase in GH secretion has been documented in both animal models and humans. The exact mechanism for this sleep-related increase in GH release is not known. Growth hormone-releasing hormone may play an important role, because nighttime GH secretion is attenuated after administration of GHRH antagonists [55]. However, additional regulatory factors, such as hypothalamic somatostatin or ghrelin, may also contribute. On a day-to-day basis, an irregular and intermittent pattern of GH secretion can be observed soon after the onset of slow-wave sleep (during stages 3 and 4 of the sleep cycle); this is also when maximum GH concentrations are achieved. The sleep-associated GH pulses are more pronounced in children and adolescents and decrease with increasing age. The nighttime increase in GH secretion accounts for a large fraction of GH secretory output in males, whereas in females, the nocturnal GH bursts only make up a fraction of total daily GH secretion [56].

## *Effect of Nutrition on GH Secretion [Both S and I]*

Different aspects of nutrition influence GH secretion and involve carbohydrates, as well as proteins and lipids. These nutritional influences vary between fasting versus fed conditions and are different in overweight/obese versus lean individuals.

*Hypoglycemia*: This causes an acute rise in GH secretion that is dependent both on the severity of the hypoglycemia as well as the rate of glucose decline. Insulin-induced hypoglycemia has been demonstrated to lead to an acute rise in GH secretion that is secondary to a coincident intracellular glycopenia. This has long been used as part of the assessment of pituitary integrity. For example, this approach to test GH secretion from the pituitary somatotrophs is still used in adults, but seldom in pediatric patients because of the risks associated with hypoglycemia [57].

*Hyperglycemia*: This causes suppression of GH secretion. In controlled settings, administration of a fixed amount of glucose, as during an oral glucose tolerance test, is used to assess an individual's ability to suppress serum GH concentrations.

Lack of suppression of GH below a certain cutoff during an oral glucose tolerance test is diagnostic for acromegaly, although there is some debate on what this cutoff should be (≤1 µg/L versus ≤ 0.4 µg/L depending on the sensitivity of the GH assay used and whether one is looking at confirming the diagnosis of acromegaly versus defining cure after therapeutic intervention) [58].

Fasting tends to result in increased GH secretion, whereas fatty acid elevation causes inhibition of GH release. The elevated free fatty acids probably increase somatostatin tone, because GHRH-induced GH secretion is found to be attenuated in the setting of free fatty acid elevation. Acute administration of amino acids leads to GH release (arginine infusion is a commonly used provocative agent in GH deficiency testing protocols), as is the ingestion of a meal rich in protein content.

*Obesity (see Chap. 6 for more detail)*: This is associated with overall decreased GH secretion and GH concentrations, mainly due to a decreased number of GH secretory pulses. The amount of adipose tissue (visceral fat in particular) is correlated with the degree of GH suppression [59]. Several mechanisms may be at play here, including an effect of free fatty acids on the somatotroph cells or an increase in basal somatostatin tonicity.

## *Insulin-Like Growth Factor I (IGF-I) [I]*

GH secretion is also under negative feedback control from the insulin-like growth factors, and receptors for these peptides have been identified on pituitary cells. Insulin-like growth factor I may inhibit GH secretion either directly at the level of the pituitary gland or indirectly at the level of the hypothalamus (Fig. 2.2). Although the exact mechanism is not completely known, studies have clearly shown that IGF-I infusion leads to both decreased GH pulse amplitude and lower GH concentrations in serum [60]. Furthermore, there also appears to be a difference in how males and females respond to the negative feedback of IGF-I (selective suppression of GHRH in females only). In contrast, patients with severe GH resistance or GH insensitivity generate little IGF-I and will have significantly elevated GH concentrations, which will decrease when recombinant human IGF-I is administered to them via subcutaneous injection. On top of this classic negative feedback mechanism affecting GH secretion, the two main regulators of GH secretion (GHRH and somatostatin) also inhibit their own secretion and thereby provide an alternative feedback loop system important for acute GH release.

## *Sex Steroids [S] (see Chap. 3 for more detail)*

Growth hormone secretion is also influenced by the sex steroids. Although the exact regulatory interactions between estrogens and androgens and GH are still to be fully elucidated, in general terms, one can state that puberty is associated with increased

GH production and consequently increased GH and IGF-I in serum. The effect of sex steroids on GH secretion is also different in males versus females, as already described above during the discussion of the sexual dimorphism of GHRH's effects on GH secretion. Some of the difficulties in elucidating the exact interplay of sex steroids and GH secretion are due to [1] the fact that the effects of sex steroids in certain animal models are quite different than in humans and [2] the fact that sex steroids have direct effects on IGF-I production by other organs such as the liver, which by itself also alters GH secretion by changes in the negative feedback resulting from this. Exogenous androgen administration in boys with delayed sexual maturation leads to increased IGF-I concentrations, related to increased pulse amplitude of GH secretion without change in pulse frequency [61]. This effect may be first mediated through conversion of the (aromatizable) androgens to estrogens, because when non-aromatizable androgens are given, no changes in the GH pulse amplitude are observed. Additional work employing sex steroid blocking agents further confirmed that the increase in GH secretion during puberty is related to increased estrogen concentrations. Finally, the GH response to GHRH is stronger in females than in males.

## *Summary*

From the above notes, it is evident that GH secretion occurs in a pulsatile manner and that many other hormones and neuropeptides interact to alter GH pulsatility. The main regulators of GH secretion are GHRH and somatostatin, but other peptides, such as IGF-I, also have an important role. Between the GH pulses, and in the normal physiologic state, GH concentrations are usually below the lower limit of conventional assays (<0.2 µg/L). Growth hormone pulses occur mostly at night, with the onset of slow-wave sleep, are more common in younger men (up to 12 per day), are more common during the puberty years, and occur less often in older individuals. Although much is known about the regulation of GH secretion and the interactions between the GH-IGF-I axis and peptides such as GHRH and somatostatin, more investigation is needed to decipher the biological role of the pulsatile nature of GH secretion and its implications in both healthy and pathological conditions.

## References

1. Lewis UJ, Sinha YN, Lewis GP. Structure and properties of members of the hGH family: a review. Endocr J. 2000;47(Suppl):S1–8.
2. Mott HR, Campbell ID. Four-helix bundle growth factors and their receptors: protein-protein interactions. Curr Opin Struct Biol. 1995;5:114–21.
3. de Vos AM, Ultsch M, Kossiakoff AA. Human growth hormone and extracellular domain of its receptor: crystal structure of the complex. Science. 1992;255:306–12.

4. Chantalat L, Jones ND, Korber F, Navaza J, Pavlovsky AG. The crystal-structure of wild-type growth-hormone at 2.5 Angstrom resolution. Protein Pept Lett. 1995;2:333–40.
5. Cunningham BC, Mulkerrin MG, Wells JA. Dimerization of human growth hormone by zinc. Science. 1991;253:545–8.
6. Brown RJ, Adams JJ, Pelekanos RA, Wan Y, Mckinstry WJ, Palethorpe K, Seeber RM, Monks TA, Eidne KA, Parker MW, Waters MJ. Model for growth hormone receptor activation based on subunit rotation within a receptor dimer. Nat Struct Mol Biol. 2005;12:814–21.
7. Ultsch M, de Vos AM, Kossiakoff AA. Crystals of the complex between human growth hormone and the extracellular domain of its receptor. J Mol Biol. 1991;222:865–8.
8. Cunningham BC, Ultsch M, De Vos AM, Mulkerrin MG, Clauser KR, Wells JA. Dimerization of the extracellular domain of the human growth hormone receptor by a single hormone molecule. Science. 1991;254:821–5.
9. Sundstrom M, Lundqvist T, Rodin J, Giebel LB, Milligan D, Norstedt G. Crystal structure of an antagonist mutant of human growth hormone, G120R, in complex with its receptor at 2.9 A resolution. J Biol Chem. 1996;271:32197–203.
10. Behncken SN, Waters MJ. Molecular recognition events involved in the activation of the growth hormone receptor by growth hormone. J Mol Recognit. 1999;12:355–62.
11. Fuh G, Cunningham BC, Fukunaga R, Nagata S, Goeddel DV, Wells JA. Rational design of potent antagonists to the human growth hormone receptor. Science. 1992;256:1677–80.
12. Pearce Jr KH, Cunningham BC, Fuh G, Teeri T, Wells JA. Growth hormone binding affinity for its receptor surpasses the requirements for cellular activity. Biochemistry. 1999;38:81–9.
13. Baumann G, Lowman HB, Mercado M, Wells JA. The stoichiometry of growth hormone-binding protein complexes in human plasma: comparison with cell surface receptors. J Clin Endocrinol Metab. 1994;78:1113–8.
14. Cunningham BC, Bass S, Fuh G, Wells JA. Zinc mediation of the binding of human growth hormone to the human prolactin receptor. Science. 1990;250:1709–12.
15. Cunningham BC, Henner DJ, Wells JA. Engineering human prolactin to bind to the human growth hormone receptor. Science. 1990;247:1461–5.
16. Chen WY, Chen NY, Yun J, Wagner TE, Kopchick JJ. In vitro and in vivo studies of antagonistic effects of human growth hormone analogs. J Biol Chem. 1994;269:15892–7.
17. Chen WY, Wight DC, Mehta BV, Wagner TE, Kopchick JJ. Glycine 119 of bovine growth hormone is critical for growth-promoting activity. Mol Endocrinol. 1991;5:1845–52.
18. Chen WY, Wight DC, Chen NY, Coleman TA, Wagner TE, Kopchick JJ. Mutations in the third alpha-helix of bovine growth hormone dramatically affect its intracellular distribution in vitro and growth enhancement in transgenic mice. J Biol Chem. 1991;266:2252–8.
19. Kopchick JJ, Parkinson C, Stevens EC, Trainer PJ. Growth hormone receptor antagonists: discovery, development, and use in patients with acromegaly. Endocr Rev. 2002;23:623–46.
20. Kopchick JJ. Lessons learned from studies with the growth hormone receptor. 2015 Jun 3. pii: S1096-6374(15)30005-8. doi:10.1016/j.ghir. 2015.06.003 [epub ahead of print].
21. Ross RJ, Leung KC, Maamra M, Bennett W, Doyle N, Waters MJ, Ho KK. Binding and functional studies with the growth hormone receptor antagonist, B2036-PEG (pegvisomant), reveal effects of pegylation and evidence that it binds to a receptor dimer. J Clin Endocrinol Metab. 2001;86:1716–23.
22. Rosenfeld RG, Bakker B. Compliance and persistence in pediatric and adult patients receiving growth hormone therapy. Endocr Pract. 2008;14:143–54.
23. Touraine P, D'Souza GA, Kourides I, Abs R, Barclay P, Xie R, Pico A, Torres-Vela E, Ekman B, Group GHLS. Lipoatrophy in GH deficient patients treated with a long-acting pegylated GH. Eur J Endocrinol. 2009;161:533–40.
24. de Schepper J, Rasmussen MH, Gucev Z, Eliakim A, Battelino T. Long-acting pegylated human GH in children with GH deficiency: a single-dose, dose-escalation trial investigating safety, tolerability, pharmacokinetics and pharmacodynamics. Eur J Endocrinol. 2011;165:401–9.
25. Hoybye C, Cohen P, Hoffman AR, Ross R, Biller BM, Christiansin JS, Frowth Hormone Research Society. Status of long-acting growth hormone preparations - 2015. Growth Horm IGF Res 2015. Oct; 25(5): 201–206.

26. Rasmussen MH, Olsen MW, Alifrangis L, Klim S, Suntum M. A reversible albumin-binding growth hormone derivative is well tolerated and possesses a potential once-weekly treatment profile. J Clin Endocrinol Metab. 2014;99:E1819–29.
27. Osborn BL, Sekut L, Corcoran M, Poortman C, Sturm B, Chen G, Mather D, Lin HL, Parry TJ. Albutropin: a growth hormone-albumin fusion with improved pharmacokinetics and pharmacodynamics in rats and monkeys. Eur J Pharmacol. 2002;456:149–58.
28. Cleland JL, Geething NC, Moore JA, Rogers BC, Spink BJ, Wang CW, Alters SE, Stemmer WP, Schellenberger V. A novel long-acting human growth hormone fusion protein (VRS-317): enhanced in vivo potency and half-life. J Pharm Sci. 2012;101:2744–54.
29. Fares F, Guy R, Bar-Ilan A, Felikman Y, Fima E. Designing a long-acting human growth hormone (hGH) by fusing the carboxyl-terminal peptide of human chorionic gonadotropin beta-subunit to the coding sequence of hGH. Endocrinology. 2010;151:4410–7.
30. Barinaga M, Yamonoto G, Rivier C, Vale W, Evans R, Rosenfeld MG. Transcriptional regulation of growth hormone gene expression by growth hormone-releasing factor. Nature. 1983;306:84–5.
31. Burgess R, Lunyak V, Rosenfeld M. Signaling and transcriptional control of pituitary development. Curr Opin Genet Dev. 2002;12:534–9.
32. Goldenberg N, Barkan A. Factors regulating growth hormone secretion in humans. Endocrinol Metab Clin North Am. 2007;36:37–55.
33. Mayo KE, Godfrey PA, Suhr ST, Kulik DJ, Rahal JO. Growth hormone-releasing hormone: synthesis and signaling. Recent Prog Horm Res. 1995;50:35–73.
34. Mayo KE. Molecular cloning and expression of a pituitary-specific receptor for growth hormone-releasing hormone. Mol Endocrinol. 1992;6:1734–44.
35. Vance ML, Kaiser DL, Martha Jr PM, Furlanetto R, Rivier J, Vale W, Thorner MO. Lack of in vivo somatotroph desensitization or depletion after 14 days of continuous growth hormone (GH)-releasing hormone administration in normal men and a GH-deficient boy. J Clin Endocrinol Metab. 1989;68:22–8.
36. Abrams RL, Parker ML, Blanco S, Reichlin S, Daughaday WH. Hypothalamic regulation of growth hormone secretion. Endocrinology. 1966;78:605–13.
37. Frohman LA, Bernardis LL. Growth hormone and insulin levels in weanling rats with ventromedial hypothalamic lesions. Endocrinology. 1968;82:1125–32.
38. Frohman LA, Nernardis LL, Kant KJ. Hypothalamic stimulation of growth hormone secretion. Science. 1968;162:580–2.
39. Thorner MO, Perryman RL, Cronin MJ, Rogol AD, Draznin M, Johanson A, Vale W, Horvath E, Kovacs K. Somatotroph hyperplasia. Successful treatment of acromegaly by removal of a pancreatic islet tumor secreting a growth hormone-releasing factor. J Clin Invest. 1982;70:965–77.
40. Jaffe CA, Friberg RD, Barkan AL. Suppression of growth hormone (GH) secretion by a selective GH-releasing hormone (GHRH) antagonist. Direct evidence for involvement of endogenous GHRH in the generation of GH pulses. J Clin Invest. 1993;92:695–701.
41. Jaffe CA, Ho PJ, Demott-Friberg R, Bowers CY, Barkan AL. Effects of a prolonged growth hormone (GH)-releasing peptide infusion on pulsatile GH secretion in normal men. J Clin Endocrinol Metab. 1993;77:1641–7.
42. Jaffe CA, DeMott-Friberg R, Barkan AL. Endogenous growth hormone (GH)-releasing hormone is required for GH responses to pharmacological stimuli. J Clin Invest. 1996;97:934–40.
43. Nakamura S, Mizuno M, Katakami H, Gore AC, Terasawa E. Aging-related changes in in vivo release of growth hormone-releasing hormone and somatostatin from the stalk-median eminence in female rhesus monkeys (*Macaca mulatta*). J Clin Endocrinol Metab. 2003;88:827–33.
44. Russell-Aulet M, Dimaraki EV, Jaffe CA, DeMott-Friberg R, Barkan AL. Aging-related growth hormone (GH) decrease is a selective hypothalamic GH-releasing hormone pulse amplitude mediated phenomenon. J Gerontol Ser A Biol Med Sci. 2001;56:M124–9.
45. Turner JP, Tannenbaum GS. In vivo evidence of a positive role for somatostatin to optimize pulsatile growth hormone secretion. Am J Physiol. 1995;269:E683–90.

46. Smith RG, Palyha OC, Feighner SD, Tan CP, McKee KK, Hreniuk DL, Yang L, Morriello G, Nargund R, Patchett AA, Howard AD. Growth hormone releasing substances: types and their receptors. Horm Res. 1999;51 Suppl 3:1–8.
47. Bowers CY, Sartor AO, Reynolds GA, Badger TM. On the actions of the growth hormone-releasing hexapeptide, GHRP. Endocrinology. 1991;128:2027–35.
48. Smith RG, Van der Ploeg LH, Howard AD, Feighner SD, Cheng K, Hickey GJ, Wyvratt Jr MJ, Fisher MH, Nargund RP, Patchett AA. Peptidomimetic regulation of growth hormone secretion. Endocr Rev. 1997;18:621–45.
49. Muccioli G, Tschop M, Papotti M, Deghenghi R, Heiman M, Ghigo E. Neuroendocrine and peripheral activities of ghrelin: implications in metabolism and obesity. Eur J Pharmacol. 2002;440:235–54.
50. Pantel J, Legendre M, Nivot S, Morisset S, Vie-Luton MP, le Bouc Y, Epelbaum J, Amselem S. Recessive isolated growth hormone deficiency and mutations in the ghrelin receptor. J Clin Endocrinol Metab. 2009;94:4334–41.
51. Zhang JV, Ren PG, Avsian-Kretchmer O, Luo CW, Rauch R, Klein C, Hsueh AJ. Obestatin, a peptide encoded by the ghrelin gene, opposes ghrelin's effects on food intake. Science. 2005;310:996–9.
52. Dimaraki EV, Jaffe CA, Bowers CY, Marbach P, Barkan AL. Pulsatile and nocturnal growth hormone secretions in men do not require periodic declines of somatostatin. Am J Physiol Endocrinol Metab. 2003;285:E163–70.
53. Ben-Shlomo A, Melmed S. Pituitary somatostatin receptor signaling. Trends Endocrinol Metab. 2010;21:123–33.
54. Korytnaya E, Barkan A. Pharmacological treatment of acromegaly: its place in the overall therapeutic approach. J Neuro-Oncol. 2014;117:415–20.
55. Jessup SK, Malow BA, Symons KV, Barkan AL. Blockade of endogenous growth hormone-releasing hormone receptors dissociates nocturnal growth hormone secretion and slow-wave sleep. Eur J Endocrinol. 2004;151:561–6.
56. Jaffe CA, Ocampo-Lim B, Guo W, Krueger K, Sugahara I, DeMott-Friberg R, Bermann M, Barkan AL. Regulatory mechanisms of growth hormone secretion are sexually dimorphic. J Clin Invest. 1998;102:153–64.
57. Molitch ME, Clemmons DR, Malozowski S, Merriam GR, Vance ML, Endocrine S. Evaluation and treatment of adult growth hormone deficiency: an Endocrine Society clinical practice guideline. J Clin Endocrinol Metab. 2011;96:1587–609.
58. Carmichael JD, Bonert VS, Mirocha JM, Melmed S. The utility of oral glucose tolerance testing for diagnosis and assessment of treatment outcomes in 166 patients with acromegaly. J Clin Endocrinol Metab. 2009;94:523–7.
59. Clasey JL, Weltman A, Patrie J, Weltman JY, Pezzoli S, Bouchard C, Thorner MO, Hartman ML. Abdominal visceral fat and fasting insulin are important predictors of 24-hour GH release independent of age, gender, and other physiological factors. J Clin Endocrinol Metab. 2001;86:3845–52.
60. Ceda GP, Davis RG, Rosenfeld RG, Hoffman AR. The growth hormone (GH)-releasing hormone (GHRH)-GH-somatomedin axis: evidence for rapid inhibition of GHRH-elicited GH release by insulin-like growth factors I and II. Endocrinology. 1987;120:1658–62.
61. Martha Jr PM, Rogol AD, Veldhuis JD, Kerrigan JR, Goodman DW, Blizzard RM. Alterations in the pulsatile properties of circulating growth hormone concentrations during puberty in boys. J Clin Endocrinol Metab. 1989;69:563–70.

# Chapter 3
# Sex Steroids and Growth Hormone Secretion

Diane E.J. Stafford

## Introduction

The influence of sex steroids on growth is obvious to anyone who has witnessed the progression of a child to adulthood. With the onset of puberty and increases in sex steroids, boys and girls exhibit the development of secondary sexual characteristics, but also a significant increase in growth velocity. While it is reasonable to assume that sex steroids cause growth acceleration due to influence on growth hormone (GH) secretion and action, the mechanisms of these interactions are complex, and some remain elusive.

## Sex Steroids and Growth Hormone-Releasing Hormone/ Somatostatin Secretion

Growth hormone secretion from the hypothalamus is largely controlled by the opposing influences of stimulatory growth hormone-releasing hormone (GHRH) and inhibitory somatostatin. The interplay between these neuropeptides is presumed to determine patterns of GH secretion by the pituitary. Studies in a variety of species, including humans, reveal sexual dimorphism in GH secretion related to pulse frequency and GH peaks. In rats, males have high, regular, infrequent GH pulses with low basal levels between pulses. Females have a higher baseline GH level with irregular and more frequent low-amplitude pulses [1]. Studies in the rat have concluded that this difference in secretory patterns may account for sexual differences

---

D.E.J. Stafford (✉)
Division of Endocrinology, Boston Children's Hospital, Harvard Medical School,
300 Longwood Ave, Boston, MA 02115-5724, USA
e-mail: diane.stafford@childrens.harvard.edu

in body growth [1]. Tannenbaum and others have proposed a model in which gender differences in the pattern of GHRH and somatostatin signaling to the pituitary result in these variations in pulse frequency and amplitude [2] with phasic cycles of GHRH and somatostatin resulting in regular GH pulsatility and inhibition in males. Indeed, gender-related differences have been found in gene expression of GHRH and somatostatin, with male rats having higher mRNA levels of both of these neuropeptides [3]. Clifton et al. [4] have shown that somatostatin mRNA levels are increased by the binding of testosterone to androgen receptors on somatostatin neurons in the periventricular nucleus, though the effects of testosterone on GHRH neurons is likely indirect.

## Childhood Growth and Gender Influences

In the prepubertal phases of growth, gender and sex steroids play little role in determining growth. Children with hypogonadism (with normal karyotype) have normal prepubertal growth [5], and there is a significant overlap in patterns of growth between boys and girls before puberty. Gender does not appear to influence GH secretion in prepubertal children; there is no relationship between a child's gender and peripheral GH levels or amount secreted [6, 7].

While there is speculation that low, prepubertal levels of gonadal sex steroids may affect normal prepubertal GH physiology, common laboratory methodology is unable to measure sex steroids at the necessary levels. However, using an ultrasensitive bioreceptor assay for estradiol (detection limit 100-fold lower than conventional assays), Klein et al. found that prepubertal girls had eightfold higher levels of estradiol than boys, suggestive of a difference in production of sex steroids prior to puberty. The authors of this study hypothesize that this may explain the earlier timing of puberty and growth spurt in girls [8].

## Effects of Sex Steroids on Pubertal Growth and GH Secretion

The growth spurt is one of the hallmarks of adolescence. The timing of the pubertal growth spurt and the maximal growth velocity during this phase of development are different in boys and girls. The increase in growth velocity in girls typically occurs early in puberty with a peak growth velocity averaging 8 cm/year and occurring at 11 to 12 years of age. Boys have an increase in growth velocity relatively later in puberty with maximal growth velocity occurring at 13 to 14 years of age and peaking at 9 cm/year on average. The increase in GH secretion noted in puberty demonstrates a sexually dimorphic pattern that parallels these changes in growth velocity with the increase occurring early in puberty for girls (Tanner stage II breast development) and later in boys (Tanner stage IV genitalia) [9].

The relationship between increases in testosterone and changes in GH secretion has been investigated by several groups, though the methods used have varied. In a study of normal, healthy boys at various stages of pubertal development, Kerrigan and Rogel demonstrated that endogenous GH levels rise during mid- to late puberty, apparently due to increased pulse amplitude [10]. Perry et al. demonstrated that pulsatile GH increases, along with a threefold increase in serum insulin-like growth factor-I (IGF-I) levels, through puberty [9]. When studied over a 24 h period with frequent blood sampling, prepubertal boys had lower 24 h GH concentrations when compared with sexually mature boys of the same age. Prepubertal boys treated with exogenous testosterone exhibited a marked increase in total GH output with this effect resulting from an increase in pulse amplitude rather than pulse frequency [11].

Tanner and colleagues demonstrated the independent and additive contributions of GH and gonadal steroids to the adolescent growth spurt by studying GH-deficient children, some of whom also had gonadotropin deficiency [12]. Subsequent studies demonstrated that gonadal steroids are necessary, but not sufficient for appropriate pubertal growth. In GH-deficient patients, sex steroid supplementation alone did not augment height velocity unless administered with concomitant GH [13]. Inversely, GH therapy alone will not result in an appropriate increase in growth rate without accompanying administration of sex steroids [14]. Boys and girls with Laron syndrome (IGF-I deficiency) do not have a discernible pubertal growth spurt, implying that stimulation of growth through testosterone and estrogen is mediated through the GH-IGF-I axis [15].

Multiple studies have shown that administration of testosterone causes an increase in GH secretion. In prepubertal and peri-pubertal boys, administration of testosterone in physiologic and pharmacologic doses increases spontaneous and stimulated GH secretion [16–18]. The effect of testosterone appears to be mediated through aromatization to estrogen, rather than direct effects on the androgen receptor. This is suggested by studies demonstrating that administration of tamoxifen, an estrogen receptor antagonist, to prepubertal boys causes decreased GH production [19]. In addition, other studies demonstrate a lack of effect of the non-aromatizable androgen, dihydrotestosterone (DHT), on GH production [20].

While studies on the direct effects of estrogen on GH secretion are less numerous, the relationship can be demonstrated by the use of estradiol for "priming" prior to GH stimulation testing. Estrogen exposure has been shown to improve the specificity of these tests in the diagnosis of GH deficiency. Administration of β-estradiol for 2 days prior to GH stimulation testing increases the GH response in children with normal GH secretion and allows improved differentiation from those with GH deficiency (see Chap. 8) [21, 22].

## Sex Steroids and IGF-I

In addition to effects on GH secretion from the pituitary, sex steroids exert effects on downstream activity of GH. IGF-I, produced by the liver, is the mediator of the anabolic effects of GH. As the liver is also responsive to sex steroids, it is a potential site for regulatory interactions between GH and sex steroids. Coutant et al. showed that increases in sex steroids, GH, and IGF-I concentrations are associated with progression through puberty. In addition, IGF-I response to GH administration increased during puberty, suggesting that increased sex steroids result in increased sensitivity to GH [23].

Studies in boys with GH deficiency due to hypopituitarism reveal that administration of testosterone alone causes minimal increase in IGF-I, but that concomitant administration of GH causes a greater than threefold increase [24]. Similar results are found with administration of βHCG to GH-deficient boys [25]. βHCG causes an increase in gonadal testosterone production through cross-reactivity with the LH receptor. In men with hypopituitarism, while GH therapy increased IGF-I levels, this was enhanced by coadministration of testosterone [26]. These studies indicate that testosterone does not directly regulate circulating IGF-I levels, but enhances IGF-I response to GH.

The relationship between estrogen and hepatic IGF-I production appears to be more complex. Estrogen appears to have a biphasic effect on IGF-I secretion. Low doses of exogenous estrogen enhance IGF-I generation, and high doses decrease IGF-I [27–33]. Estrogen is metabolized by the hepatic cytochrome system. Elevated estrogen concentrations in the portal system impair hepatic IGF-I production and increase GH binding protein, resulting in a blunting of GH action [34]. In girls with tall stature, high doses of oral estrogen reduced IGF-I levels [35]. In girls with delayed puberty, administration of oral 17β-estradiol revealed reduced IGF-I response to GH administration [23].

Transdermal estrogen is not metabolized in the liver and, therefore, may have a different effect on IGF-I production, but results remain unclear. One study revealed that GH administration to women with hypopituitarism elevates IGF-I to a higher degree with transdermal estrogen compared with oral treatment [36]. However, other studies have shown that estrogen inhibits hepatic IGF-I production in a dose-dependent manner regardless of route of administration [34]. As a result, while some argue for the use of transdermal estrogen for replacement, it is unclear if this has a distinct advantage with regard to IGF-I production. The effects of endogenous estradiol on IGF-I production also remain unclear.

The divergent actions of estrogen and testosterone on IGF-I production suggests that while the estrogen receptor may mediate the neurosecretory effects of testosterone, the peripheral effects may be mediated through the androgen receptor [37].

## Effects on the Bone and Epiphyseal Fusion

In addition to exerting effects through hepatic IGF-I production, GH also has direct effects on the bone at the level of the growth plate, increasing local IGF-I production and recruitment of resting zone chondrocytes [38]. Androgen and estrogen receptors have been demonstrated in the human growth plate with no gender variation. Studies imply a direct stimulatory effect of androgens on growth plate cartilage, possibly by promoting local IGF-I synthesis and increasing IGF-I receptor expression [38]. The use of high-dose estrogen in girls with tall stature results in rapid reduction of growth velocity, but with only modest decreases in IGF-I levels, implying direct non-GH-dependent effect on the epiphysis [39]. The active role of estrogen on epiphyseal closure has been elucidated by patients with rare genetic syndromes. Patients with inactivating mutations of either estrogen receptor α or the aromatase gene have a lack of pubertal growth spurt and tall stature due to lack of epiphyseal fusion. This suggests that estrogen is responsible for the growth spurt seen in pubertal development and growth plate closure at the end of adolescence in both sexes [40, 41].

## Conclusion

In this chapter, the complex interaction between sex steroids and the GH axis were reviewed. While it is clear that there are interactions at many levels and much has been learned about their nature, questions remain. Among this is the nature of the sexual dimorphisms resulting in the common variation in height between men and women. Hopefully, with continued use of "natural experiments" to elucidate mechanisms of action and improvements in assays and other experimental techniques, these questions can be answered in the future.

## References

1. Jansson J-O, Eden S, Isaksson O. Sexual dimorphism in the control of growth hormone secretion. Endocr Rev. 1985;2(6):128–50.
2. Tannenbaum G. Hypothalamic control mechanisms of sexually dimorphic growth hormone secretory patterns in the rat. In: Veldhuis JD, Giustina A, editors. Sex-steroid interactions with growth hormone, Serono Symposia USA; 1999. p. 133–143.
3. Argent J, Chowen JC, Zeitler P, Clifton DK, Steiner RA. Sexual dimorphism of growth hormone-releasing hormone and somatostatin gene expression in the hypothalamus of the rat during development. Endocrinology. 1991;5(128):2369–75.
4. Clifton DK, Steiner RA. Sex differences in growth hormone-releasing hormone (GHRH) and somatostatin neurons. In: Veldhuis JD, Giustina A, editors. Sex-steroid interactions with growth hormone, serono symposia USA; 1999. p. 144–152.
5. Campos SP, MacGillivray MH. Sex steroids do not influence somatic growth in childhood. Am J Dis Child. 1989;143:942.
6. Albertsson-Wikland K, Rosberg S. Analyses of 24-hour growth hormone profiles in children: relation to growth. J Clin Endocrinol Metab. 1988;67:493.
7. Zadik Z, Chalew SA, McCarter Jr RJ, Meistas M, Kowarski AA. The influence of age on the 24-hour integrated concentration of growth hormone in normal individuals. J Clin Endocrinol Metab. 1985;60:513.
8. Klein KO, Baron J, Colli MJ, McDonnell DP, Cutler GB. Estrogen levels in childhood determined by an ultrasensitive recombinant cell bioassay. J Clin Invest. 1994;94:2475–80.
9. Perry RJ, Farquharson C, Ahmed SF. The role of sex steroids in controlling pubertal growth. Clin Endo. 2008;68(208):4–15.
10. Kerrigan JR, Rogol AD. The impact of gonadal steroid hormone action on growth hormone secretion during childhood and adolescence. Endocr Rev. 1992;2(13):281–98.

11. Mauras N, Blizzard RM, Link K, Johnson ML, Rogol AD, Veldhuis JD. Augmentation of GH secretion during puberty: evidence for a pulse amplitude-modulated phenomenon. J Clin Endocrinol Metab. 1987;64:596–601.
12. Tanner JM, Whitehouse RH, Hughes PCR, Carter BS. Relative importance of growth hormone and sex steroids for the growth at puberty of trunk length, limb length, and muscle width in growth hormone-deficient children. J Pediatr. 1976;89:1000.
13. Aynsley-Green A, Zachmann M, Prader A. Interrelation of the therapeutic effects of growth hormone and testosterone on growth in hypopituitarism. J Pediatr. 1976;89:992.
14. Van Dop C, Burstein S, Conte F, Grumbach M. Isolated gonadotropin deficiency in boys: clinical characteristics and growth. J Pediatr. 1987;111:684.
15. Laron Z, Lilos P, Klinger B. Growth curves for Laron syndrome. Arch Dis Child. 1993;68:768–70.
16. Guistina A, Scalvini T, Tassi C, Desenzani P, Poiesi C, Wehrenberg WB, Rogol AD, Veldhuis JD. Maturation of the regulation of growth hormone secretion in young males with hypogonadotropic hypogonadism pharmacologically exposed to progressive increments in serum testosterone. J Clin Endocrinol Metab. 1997;82:1210–9.
17. Loche S, Caloa A, Cappa M, Beloone J, Aimaretti G, Farello G, Faedda A, Lombardi G, Deghenghi R, Chigo E. The growth hormone response to hexarelin in children: reproducibility and effect on sex steroids. J Clin Endocrinol Metab. 1997;82:861–4.
18. Keenan BS, Richards GE, Ponder SW, Dallas JS, Nagamani M, Smith ER. Androgen-stimulated pubertal growth: the effects of testosterone and dihydrotestosterone on growth hormone and insulin-like growth factor-I in the treatment of short stature and delayed puberty. J Clin Endocrinol Metab. 1993;76:996–1001.
19. Metzger DL, Kerrigan JR. Estrogen receptor blockade with tamoxifen diminishes GH secretion in boys: evidence for a stimulatory role of endogenous estrogen during male adolescence. J Clin Endocrinol Metab. 1994;79:513–8.
20. Metzger DL, Rogol AD. Disparate effects of testosterone and dihydrotestosterone therapy on growth hormone secretion in boys with constitutional delay of growth and adolescence. Abstract 552. Proceedings of the 76th annual meeting endocrine society. Anaheim, 1994.
21. Martinez AS, Domene HM, Ropelato MG, Jasper HG, Pennisi PA, Escobar ME, Heinrich JJ. Estrogen priming effect on growth hormone (GH) provocative test: a useful tool for the diagnosis of GH deficiency. J Clin Endocrinol Metab. 2000;85(11):4168–72.
22. Marin G, Domené HM, Barnes KM, Blackwell BJ, Cassorla FG, Cutler Jr GB. The effects of estrogen priming and puberty on the growth hormone response to standardized treadmill exercise and arginine-insulin in normal girls and boys. J Clin Endocrinol Metab. 1994;79(2):537–41.
23. Coutant R, de Casson FB, Rouleau S, Douay O, Mathieu E, Gatelais F, Bouhours-Nouet N, Voinot C, Audran M, Limal JM. Divergent effect of endogenous and exogenous sex steroids on the insulin-like growth factor I response to growth hormone in short normal adolescents. J Clin Endocrinol Metab. 2004;89:6185–92.
24. Mauras N, Rini A, Welch S, Sager B, Murphy SP. Synergistic effects of testosterone and growth hormone on protein metabolism and body composition in prepubertal boys. Metabolism. 2003;52:964–9.
25. Saggese G, Cesaretti G, Franchi G, Startari I. Testosterone-induced increase of insulin-like growth factor I levels depends upon normal levels of growth hormone. Eur J Endocrinol. 1996;135:211–5.
26. Gibney J, Wolthers T, Johannsson G, Umpleby AM, Ho KK. Growth hormone and testosterone interact positively to enhance protein and energy metabolism in hypopituitary men. Am J Physiol Endocrinol Metab. 2005;289:E266–71.
27. Wiedemann E, Schwartz E, Frantz AG. Acute and chronic estrogen effects upon serum somatomedin activity, growth hormone and prolactin in man. J Clin Endocrinol Metab. 1976;42:942.
28. Rosenfield RL, Furlanetto R, Bock D. Relationship of somatomedin-C concentrations to pubertal changes. J Pediatrics. 1983;103:723.

29. Ross JL, Cassorla FG, Skerda MC, Valk IM, Loriaux DL, Cutler GB. A preliminary study of the effect of estrogen dose on growth in Turner's syndrome. N Engl J Med. 1983;309:1104.
30. Cutler L, Van Vliet G, Conte FA, Kaplan SL, Brumbach MM. Somatomedin-C levels in children and adolescents with gonadal dysgenesis: differences from age-matched normal females and effect of chronic replacement therapy. J Clin Endocrinol Metab. 1985;60:1087.
31. Clemmons DR, Underwood LE, Ridgway EC, Kliman B, Kjellberg RN, Van Wyk JJ. Estradiol treatment of acromegaly, reduction of immunoreactive somatomedin C and improvement of metabolic status. Am J Med. 1980;69:571.
32. Copeland KC, Johnson DM, Kuehl TJ, Castracane VD. Estrogen stimulates growth hormone and somatomedin-C in castrate and intake female baboons. J Clin Endocrinol Metab. 1984;58:698.
33. Meyer WJ, Furlanetto RW, Walker PA. The effect of sex steroids on radioimmunoassayable plasma somatomedin C concentrations. J Clin Endocrinolo Metab. 1982;55:1184.
34. Leung KC, Johannsson G, Leong GM, Ho KKY. Estrogen regulation of growth hormone action. Endocr Rev. 2004;25(6):693–721.
35. Rooman RP, De Beeck LO, Martin M, van Doorn J, Mohan S, Du Caju MV. Ethinylestradiol and testosterone have divergent effects on circulating IGF system components in adolescents with constitutional tall stature. Eur J Endocrinol. 2005;152:597–604.
36. Wolthers T, Hoffman DM, Nugent AG, Duncan MW, Umpleby M, Ho KK. Oral estrogen antagonizes the metabolic actions of growth hormone in growth hormone-deficient women. Am J Physiol Endocrinol Metab. 2001;281:E1191–6.
37. Meinhardt UJ, Ho KKY. Modulation of growth hormone action by sex steroids. Clin Endocrinol. 2006;65:413–22.
38. Krohn K, Haffner D, Hugel U, Himmele R, Klaus G, Mehls O, Schaefer F. 1,25 (OH) 2D3 and dihydrotestosterone interact to regulate proliferation and differentiation of epiphyseal chondrocytes. Calcif Tissue Int. 2003;73:400–10.
39. Svan H, Ritzen EM, Hall K, Johansson L. Estrogen treatment of tall girls: dose dependency of effects on subsequent growth and IGF-I levels in blood. Acta Paediatr Scand. 1991;80:328–32.
40. Smith EP, Boyd J, Frank GR, Takahashi H, Cohen RM, Specker B, Williams TC, Lubahn DB, Korach KS. Estrogen resistance caused by a mutation in the estrogen-receptor gene in a man. New England J Med. 1994;331:1056–61.
41. Morishima A, Grumbach MM, Simpson ER, Fisher C, Qin K. Aromatase deficiency in male and female siblings caused by a novel mutation and the physiological role of estrogens. J Clin Endocrinol Metab. 1995;80:3689–98.

# Chapter 4
# The Influence of Thyroid Hormone on Growth Hormone Secretion and Action

Angela M. Leung and Gregory A. Brent

## Introduction

Thyroid hormone and growth hormone (GH) are essential for normal growth [1]. There are multiple levels where these two pathways intersect, both in the regulation of secretion and in sites of action, especially the bone. Deficiencies of thyroid hormone and GH can occur together, such as in individuals with pituitary or hypothalamic disease. The more common clinical scenario, however, is the impact of isolated thyroid hormone deficiency on GH secretion and action. Thyroid hormone is important for GH stimulation of insulin-like growth factor-I (IGF-I) in the liver, although less is known about the mechanism of this action. We will examine the impact of thyroid hormone on GH secretion and action in in vitro models, in animal models, and in humans [2]. Although thyroid hormone may impact GH secretion and action across the lifespan, its effects are most significant during the intense period of somatic and linear growth in childhood [3], which will be the focus of this review.

---

A.M. Leung (✉)
Division of Endocrinology, Department of Medicine, David Geffen
School of Medicine at UCLA, VA Greater Los Angeles Healthcare System,
11301 Wilshire Blvd, Los Angeles, CA 90073, USA
e-mail: amleung@mednet.ucla.edu

G.A. Brent
Departments of Medicine and Physiology, David Geffen School
of Medicine at UCLA, VA Greater Los Angeles Healthcare System,
11301 Wilshire Blvd, Los Angeles, CA 90073, USA
e-mail: gbrent@mednet.ucla.edu

# Molecular Studies of Thyroid Hormone Regulation of Growth Hormone Expression

## *Thyroid Hormone Receptor and Gene Regulation*

Thyroid hormone action is mediated predominantly by the thyroid hormone nuclear receptor (TR) which is coded by two genes α and β, TRα and TRβ [4, 5] (Fig. 4.1a). Thyroid hormone also acts through nonnuclear pathways, and a membrane receptor has been identified, although this pathway has not yet been linked to GH secretion or action [4, 5]. The two TR isoforms, α and β, differ in expression developmentally, among different tissues, and even within areas of a given tissue, such as the heart and brain. In general, TRα is expressed first and is the predominant isoform in the cerebral cortex [6]. TRβ is crucial in sensory development, including the cochlea and retina. The predominant TR isoforms in the anterior pituitary and hypothalamus are TRβ1 and the TRβ alternative splice product, TRβ2. TRβ1 is the isoform that mediates T3-mediated negative regulation of the thyrotropin-releasing hormone (TRH) and thyroid-stimulating hormone (TSH) genes [5, 7]. TR resides predominantly in the nucleus and, for most thyroid hormone-mediated nuclear signaling, forms a heterodimer with the retinoid-X-receptor (RXR), and then binds to a specific DNA sequence, the thyroid hormone response element (TRE), located in the 5′-flanking region of most thyroid hormone-regulated genes [5] (Fig. 4.1b). For positively regulated genes, the unliganded TR/RXR heterodimer binds to a nuclear corepressor, such as nuclear receptor corepressor (NCoR), and this promotes chromatin deacetylation and inhibits gene transcription. Binding of triiodothyronine (T3) to the receptor disrupts interaction with the corepressor and promotes binding of the coactivator, which then recruits factors that promote chromatin acetylation and gene transcription. Negative regulation by thyroid hormone, as in the case for the regulation of TSH and TRH, is more complex but involves ligand-dependent recruitment of corepressors [7]. Corepressors, such as NCoR, control thyroid hormone sensitivity and the set point of the hypothalamic-pituitary-thyroid axis by modulating feedback inhibition from circulating thyroxine (T4) and T3 [8]. The DNA sequences that bind TR to confer negative regulation are more diverse than those that confer positive regulation and likely mediate negative regulation by virtue of the negative response element configuration, as well as the location of the response element in the gene [9].

The first fully characterized native TRE was in the 5′-flanking region of the rat GH gene [10]. In vitro studies showed significant T3 induction of this element, corresponding to in vivo studies showing the dependence of thyroid hormone for normal GH synthesis and release in the rat. Subsequent studies in other species, including mice, showed similar sites with T3 induction, but the rat *GH* gene TRE had the most robust T3 response of any of those identified in GH genes [11]. Evaluation of the analogous TRE in the human *GH* gene showed more complex regulation with modest T3 induction, compared to the TRE in the rat *GH* gene, and some studies reported a negative TRE. Although the influence of thyroid hormone

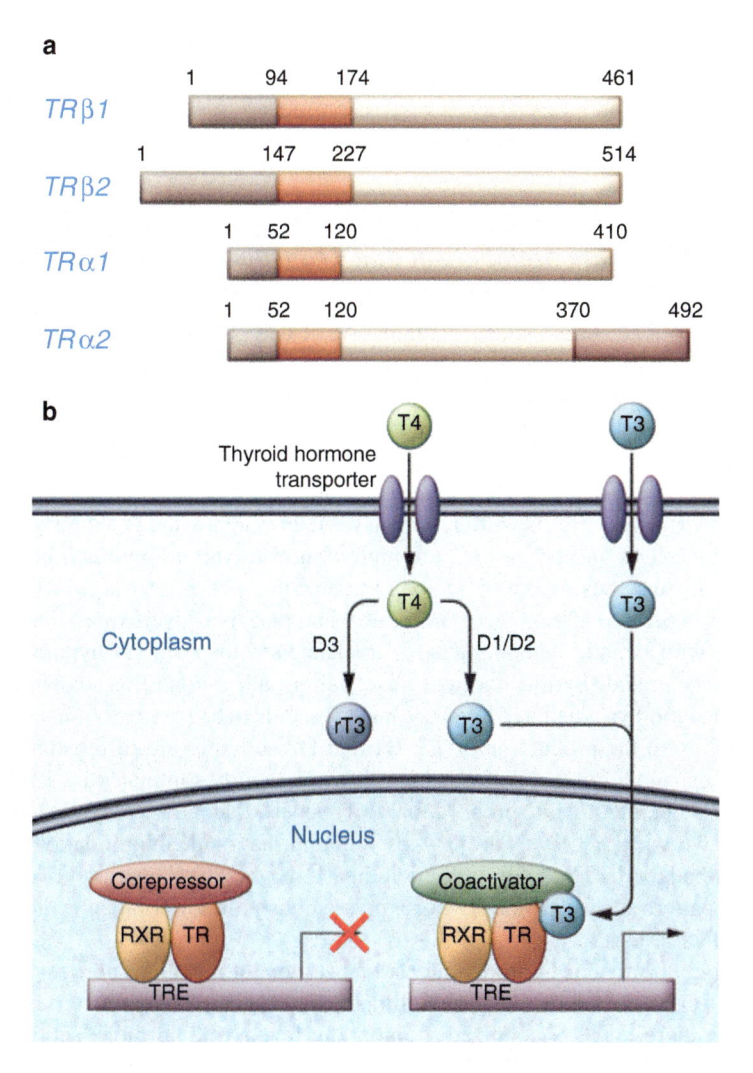

4 The Influence of Thyroid Hormone on Growth Hormone Secretion and Action 31

**Fig. 4.1** Nuclear action of thyroid hormone. (**a**) The *TR* gene has two major isoforms, *TRβ* and *TRα*; the structures of *TRα1* and *TRα2* (non-T3 binding) and *TRβ1* and *TRβ2* are shown. (**b**) Circulating T4 is converted locally in some tissues by membrane-bound D2 to the active form, T3. D3 converts T3 to the inactive rT3. In specific tissues, such as the brain, transporters such as MCT8 transport T4 and T3 into the cell. Unliganded TR heterodimerizes with RXR and binds to a TRE and then to a corepressor, such as NCoR or SMRT, repressing gene expression. T3 binding to the ligand-binding domain results in movement of the carboxy-terminal helix 12, disruption of corepressor binding, and promotion of coactivator binding, which then leads to recruitment of polymerase III and initiation of gene transcription (From Brent GA J Clin Invest 2012;122:3035–43)

on *GH* gene regulation in humans is clear from clinical studies (see below), it is likely that mechanisms in addition to transcriptional regulation are important. Additional regulators of *GH* gene expression include glucocorticoids and cAMP, which augment basal expression and T3 responsiveness [11].

## Thyroid Hormone Metabolism and Transport

Thyroid hormone action, such as stimulation of *GH* gene expression, is also regulated at the level of ligand activation, as well as thyroid hormone transporters in specific tissues [12–14]. Thyroid hormone is secreted from the thyroid gland primarily in the inactive form, T4, and must be activated by the 5′-deiodinase enzymes, D1 or D2, to the active form, T3 [12]. The deiodinase enzymes have different subcellular localizations, with D1 expressed on the cell membrane and D2 expressed intracellularly. There is also differential tissue expression with D1 expressed at high levels in the liver and D2 in high concentration in the brain, pituitary, brown adipose tissue, and muscle. The 5′-deiodinase enzyme, D3, inactivates T4 to reverse T3 and is expressed at high levels in the skin and placenta. Overexpression of D3 in children with hepatic hemangiomas is associated with profound hypothyroidism due to accelerated thyroid hormone inactivation and a condition known as consumptive hypothyroidism [15]. In humans, D2 seems to be the predominant enzyme contributing to the production of T3. D1 and D2 activities are differentially regulated by thyroid hormone. *D1* gene expression is directly stimulated by T3, and the levels of D1 expression are proportional to T3 levels. In contrast to D1, D2 becomes more active when T3 levels are low, by a ubiquitination/deubiquitination process. As described for the TR isoforms, the deiodinase enzymes also have a developmental-specific pattern of expression. D3 is expressed early in development, followed by D2 and then D1.

Thyroid hormone is hydrophobic, and most thought that it did not require transporters to cross the cell membrane. Cellular thyroid hormone transporters, however, are being increasingly recognized as important for thyroid hormone action in specific tissues, although the role of tissue transporters differs in human and rodent models. The thyroid hormone transporters, MCT8 and OATP1C1, are important for thyroid hormone action in the brain but not required for action in the liver [13, 14]. In mouse models, inactivation of both genes is required to see a robust neurological phenotype [16]. In humans, however, mutations of the *MCT8* gene alone have been identified as the underlying defect in the Allan-Herndon-Dudley syndrome, which is associated with profound intellectual disability, spasticity, and delayed development [17]. Individuals with Allan-Herndon-Dudley syndrome have a pattern of thyroid studies with a low serum T4 concentration and an elevated T3. MCT8 is required for secretion of T4 from the thyroid, so affected individuals have a low T4. Since T4 feedback to the pituitary and hypothalamus requires transport and is impaired, the serum TSH is usually in the upper normal range or elevated. Affected individuals are hypermetabolic due to the elevated serum T3 levels, and these metabolic and nutrition issues likely secondarily influence growth [18]. Delayed growth is part of the syndrome, although specific assessment of the GH axis has not been reported and many other factors likely contribute to growth impairment.

## In Vitro and Animal Models of Thyroid Hormone and Growth Hormone Regulation

### Thyroid Hormone and Regulation of GH Secretion

Thyroid hormone modulates GH secretion and action at the levels of both the hypothalamus and pituitary gland [19]. The effects of thyroid hormone on GH production and secretion are variable in different species, likely due to a range of additional regulatory factors that influence gene expression. These include the regulatory region in the genes that confer thyroid hormone responsiveness, as well as other species-specific factors that modulate GH secretion, such as cAMP and cortisol (Table 4.1) [11, 34, 35].

Table 4.1 Thyroid hormone regulation of growth hormone secretion and action in vitro and in animal models

| Target of thyroid hormone regulation | Effect | References |
| --- | --- | --- |
| *GHRH* gene expression | Increases with thyroid hormone | [20] |
| *GH* gene expression | Increases with thyroid hormone (especially in rodent models) | [21, 22] |
| *GH receptor* gene expression | Increases with thyroid hormone | [23] |
| Hepatic expression of the *GH receptor* | Increases with T3 replacement in thyroidectomized sheep fetuses | [24, 25] |
| Serum GH concentrations | Increases with T3 replacement in thyroidectomized sheep fetuses | [25] |
| Growth plate | Thyroid hormone mediates growth plate chondrocyte proliferation and terminal differentiation | [26] |
| | Senescent in hypothyroid young mice | [27, 28] |
| *IGF-I* gene transcription | Increases with T3 | [29] |
| Plasma IGF-I concentrations | Increases with T4 replacement in hypophysectomized fetal pigs | [30] |
| Bone growth | Decreases in hypophysectomized fetal sheep (seen as shorter limbs and long bones and delayed osseous maturation) | [31] |
| | Skeletal dysplasia and impaired bone maturation in mice with mutations of thyroid hormone receptor α and β | [32, 33] |

The requirement of thyroid hormone for GH production and secretion in rats is observed at postnatal days 5–10 [36, 37]. GH levels are first detectable in the serum at postnatal days 18–19 [38]. In rats that are made hypothyroid for 4 weeks, pituitary GH concentrations are only about 1 % that of controls [21]. The decline of GH levels is progressive and can continue up to 90 days following thyroidectomy [39]. The population of somatotrophs in the rat pituitary falls from 40 % of the cell population to <5 % in the 2–3 weeks after thyroid hormone deprivation [40]. Hypothyroid rats show a compensatory increase in hypothalamic growth hormone-releasing hormone (GHRH) mRNA levels [41]. The increase in hypothalamic GHRH gene expression is thought to be an indirect effect of the reduction in GH, rather than from reduction of thyroid hormone. Hypothyroidism is associated with reduced GH, which results in reduced negative feedback to GHRH and an increase in GHRH secretion, consistent with GH providing negative feedback to GHRH [21]. The reduction of GH secretion in response to GHRH is consistent with reduced levels of somatotrophs and pituitary GH mRNA levels [42].

Thyroid hormone has a role in both the pulsatile and induced GH secretion in rats [43]. In a mild state of hypothyroidism in rats, GH secretory pulsatility changes from a pattern of low frequency, high amplitude to a pattern of high frequency, low amplitude [44]. Some investigators have suggested that in the hypothyroid newborn rat, the lack of thyroid hormone may affect pituitary somatotroph function prior to GHRH secretion [45].

Adequate iodine nutrition is required for the production of thyroid hormone. Rats with a modest reduction in iodine intake, however, compensate with an increase in TSH and D2 expression, preferentially secreting triiodothyronine (T3) to maintain euthyroidism, and thus GH secretion is not affected [46]. Iodine deficiency of sufficient magnitude and duration to produce reduced serum T4, however, would then be associated with reduced GH, as is seen in hypothyroidism.

IGF-I is regulated by and mediates GH levels, and an inhibition of IGF-I release has been demonstrated in hypothyroid rats [47]. In the fetal and neonatal rat, high circulating GH concentrations are observed, a time of relative pituitary resistance to IGF-I feedback; in an in vitro model, this was reversed with the addition of T3 [38]. Administration of thyroxine to hypophysectomized or thyroidectomized rats results in an increase in serum IGF-I levels, and treatment with both T4 and GH produces an even greater increase [35].

## *Thyroid Hormone and Response to Stimulation of GH Secretion*

The role of thyroid hormone in GH secretion has been studied both with pharmacologic stimulatory agents, as well as physiologic stimulation of GH, including direct and indirect stimulatory pathways.
1. TRH

    TRH induces secretion of GH in hypothyroidism, likely due to the presence of TRH receptors on somatotrophs, which have increased expression when thyroid hormone levels are low [48]. Addition of TRH to cultured rat pituitary cells results in a significant increase in both GH and TSH concentrations [49]. Injection of TRH in euthyroid control rats increases serum GH and TSH concentrations [50], while hypothyroid rats show an exaggerated elevation of GH and TSH concentrations [50]. Low thyroid levels are associated with enhanced GH response to TRH, and in hyperthyroid rats, the GH and TSH responses after TRH administration are significantly inhibited [50].

In chickens and other avian species, but not in mammals [51], TRH is similarly somatotropic and an important contributor to GH secretion [52, 53]. Regulatory feedback is achieved by the action of thyroid hormone. T3 directly inhibits the secretion of pituitary GH release in birds [54]. Glucocorticoids also play an important role, and interactions between the increased concentrations of glucocorticoid and T3 prior to hatching in chickens also regulate *GHRH receptor* gene expression [20] and GH secretion [55]. These effects in chickens, however, are in contrast to the findings in mammals, where thyroid hormone directly stimulates *GH* gene transcription, and thyroid hormone deprivation reduces GH synthesis and release [54].

2. GHRP-6, Clonidine, and GHRH

Thyroid hormone deprivation impairs the response of GH to the stimulatory actions of clonidine, GHRH [35, 56, 57], and growth hormone-releasing peptide-6 (GHRP-6). GHRP-6 is a synthetic molecule which stimulates GH release. In a study of 11 patients with primary hypothyroidism, GHRP-6 administration resulted in a higher GH response, compared to that from GHRH [58]. The stimulus for GH release by GHRP-6 and GHRH may be regulated through distinct mechanisms.

Thyroid hormone may not influence the physiologic neonatal GH surge that is observed in response to GHRH. Ezzat and colleagues reported that GHRH treatment of primary pituitary cell cultures from 2- to 12-day-old neonatal rats stimulated GH secretion by fivefold [38]. These effects were independent of the presence of T3 and inhibited only minimally (20 %) by IGF-I. In contrast, adult rat pituitary cells showed a 70 % inhibition of GH secretion by IGF-I, thus suggesting that the neonatal surge of GH may, in part, be affected by IGF-I resistance and relative thyroid hormone deficiency, as detected by the developing somatotroph. Ignacio and colleagues showed that in rats, there is an approximately 60 % increase of D1 activity and a corresponding sixfold higher concentration of GH immediately following exercise [59].

In hypothyroid rats, T3 induces changes in the cellular distribution of GH and plays a role in the regulation of polyadenylation of GH mRNA [60]. The administration of T3 to hypothyroid rats results in a significant increase of the DNA synthesis of somatotrophs after 2–5 days and restoration of the normal somatotroph population after 5–10 days [35], resulting in the gradual normalization of pituitary GH stores and serum GH concentrations [61]. However, pharmacologic doses of T3 injected into euthyroid rats do not further increase pituitary GH content, and similarly, the GH response to GHRH is not augmented in hyperthyroid rats [35]. The addition of T3 to normal human (18–22 weeks gestation) and monkey fetal pituitary cells decreases basal GH secretion and attenuates the responses to GHRH [62]. Conversely, there is a reduction of both GHRH mRNA and peptide levels among hyperthyroid rats [42].

## *Thyroid Hormone, Growth Hormone, and Bone Development*

Thyroid hormone receptor isoforms and thyroid hormone play an important role in bone development and growth [29]. These findings are primarily based on rodent models with TR isoform deletions and mutations, although many of the findings have been supported by the evaluation of individuals with thyroid hormone receptor gene mutations [5]. The bone manifestations in congenital hypothyroidism include delayed epiphyseal closure and widely spaced cranial sutures. Even in promptly treated congenital hypothyroidism, this is seen in infants with the most severe thyroid hormone deficiency at birth. In the adult, thyroid hormone excess is associated with loss of bone density and osteoporosis, indicating retained sensitivity to the actions of thyroid hormone. During development, thyroid hormone acts on chondrocytes and growth plate cartilage. Thyroid hormone also acts directly on osteoclasts and osteoblasts. Thyroid hormone directly stimulates IGF-I transcription and stimulates expression of the binding proteins IGFBP-2 and IGFBP-4, which is a likely pathway of thyroid hormone and GH interactions.

## Thyroid Hormone and Growth Hormone in Clinical Studies

### *Thyroid Hormone and GH Stimulators*

1. Exercise is a potent stimulator of GH secretion in humans. Acute activation of the thyroid D1 is seen with physical exercise [63] and may enhance the rise of GH following exertion. Puberty is a strong inducer of the GH response to exercise in normal subjects [64].

2. Food Restriction and Obesity
   Starvation and obesity have opposing physiologic effects and have been studied as models for thyroid hormone regulation of GH secretion. In thyroidectomized rats, which are exposed to less food intake than control animals, there is a reduction in the nuclear T3 content and T3 receptor occupancy. Following T3 replacement, nuclear T3 content is restored and there is an increase in pituitary GH [65]. In contrast, in obesity models, basal GH levels are low, although IGF-I levels are normal, and there is an impaired response of GH to GHRH [66]. GH response levels after TRH injection are higher among subclinically hypothyroid obese individuals, compared to euthyroid obese individuals [67].

3. Type 1 Diabetes Mellitus

   In patients with type 1 diabetes mellitus (T1DM), there is a paradoxically increased GH response to TRH [68]. In a study of 13 patients with T1DM, this increase was observed in 7 individuals and was blocked by corticotropin-releasing hormone (CRH) administration [69]. In contrast, CRH had no effect on TSH response, thus suggesting that there may be distinct components in the neuroregulatory pathways of GH and TSH secretion [69]. Other studies demonstrate that the administration of insulin attenuates the stimulatory effect of T3 on GH mRNA levels, perhaps through mediation at the transcriptional and posttranscriptional levels [70].

4. Acute Illness

   During critical illness, there is a suppression of D1 activity and increase of D3 activity, the latter of which is jointly regulated by the somatotropic and thyrotropic axes [71]. Administration of growth hormone-releasing peptide-2 (GHRP-2) and TRH reactivates the GH and TSH axes, thereby increasing T4 to T3 conversion [72]. In a study of 14 patients with a mean critical illness duration of $40 \pm 28$ (SD) days, infusion of GHRP-2 and TRH for 5 days resulted in increased anabolic effects (seen as increase osteocalcin and leptin levels) and decreased protein degradation (as measured by urea/creatinine ratios), suggesting that this novel tropic endocrine strategy reactivated the blunted secretions of GH and TSH during protracted critical illness [73]. A study of 12 hypothyroid patients who were administered exogenous GH showed decreased IGF-I concentrations in 11 of the study samples, which was suggested to be due to either reduced GH secretion or as a direct effect from impaired thyroid hormone production [74]. The effects of thyroid hormone deprivation may be reversible upon thyroid hormone replacement in the short-term setting, as administration of thyroid hormone augments the GH response to GH-releasing factor (i.e., GHRH) in patients with primary hypothyroidism [75].

## *Resistance to Thyroid Hormone TRα and TRβ and Growth*

Resistance to thyroid hormone (RTH) syndromes provide clinical models for the understanding of the effects of thyroid hormone regulation on GH production and secretion [5, 13]. The genetic defects of RTH are ascribed to mutations of TRβ and, as has been described more recently, also TRα [5]. The significant difference in phenotype between the two types of RTH is likely due to both the differences in the TR isoform and also the difference in the thyroid hormone levels in the two conditions. Interestingly, reduced growth and short stature have been reported in individuals with either TRβ or TRα mutations [5, 76].

Since RTH-TRβ impairs TH feedback to the pituitary, which is mediated by TRβ, TSH and thyroid hormone levels are elevated. This may partially compensate for the mutant TR. In RTH-TRα, feedback response to the pituitary is normal, TSH and T4 levels are normal, and the hypothyroid phenotype is more pronounced, since there is no opportunity to compensate for the mutant receptor by increased thyroid hormone levels.

Individuals with RTH are characterized by decreased end-organ responsiveness to elevated serum T3 concentrations, which occur with impairment of TSH suppression. The phenotypes of the RTH syndromes are variable, and manifestations include short stature and delayed bone growth in RTHβ. The original kindred had stippled epiphyses and winged scapulae. The effects on growth, however, are not to the same extent as the deficits seen with thyroid hormone deficiency. In contrast to the classic RTH-TRβ, the identification of families with mutations in the TRα gene shows individuals with delayed growth and skeletal abnormalities as a central feature. Although rare, these individuals generally have normal thyroid function since thyroid hormone feedback at the pituitary is mediated by TRβ, which functions normally. They typically have a low normal serum T4, high normal T3 (perhaps due to reduced D3 activity and conversion to rT3), and normal TSH concentrations. Since thyroid hormone levels do not increase to compensate for reduced tissue sensitivity, TRβ-specific actions are reduced. Growth retardation affects the lower segment more than the upper segment, so there is growth retardation with relatively short limbs, hands, and feet with a long thoracic span [77]. Other manifestations include delayed bone maturation and skeletal dysplasia, constipation, intellectual disability, relatively macrocephaly, and round/puffy facial features. Treatment of these patients with thyroid hormone was associated with improved lipid profile, enhanced IGF-I, and improved growth, but there was no improvement of cognitive or motor deficits [78].

## Clinical Effects of Thyroid Hormone Treatment of Hypothyroidism on GH Secretion and Growth

The reduced GH secretion observed in hypothyroidism normalizes following the administration of thyroid hormone in both man and rats [40]. Thyroid hormones increase GH, GHRH receptor, and GH secretagogue receptor mRNA levels [23] and the rate of *GH* gene transcription [35]. Clinical studies confirm that hypothyroid individuals demonstrate a blunted GH response to GHRH that is correctable with thyroid hormone replacement [79]. In a case report of three children with untreated primary hypothyroidism, pituitary hyperplasia and decreased GH secretion were observed but improved after initiation of thyroid hormone treatment [80]. Another study reported 12 children with congenital hypothyroidism who received appropriate treatment with thyroid replacement hormone and showed no abnormalities of GH concentrations following TRH stimulation [81].

In a study of 15 children with neglected congenital hypothyroidism from Egypt, a range of parameters were followed after levothyroxine replacement was begun [82]. The children had growth acceleration from a height standard deviation score (SDS) from −4.3 to −2.7, an increase in peak GH to clonidine, and a peak IGF-I response to GH. Ultimately, T4 replacement produced significant but incomplete catch-up growth and only partial recovery.

Given the rapid identification and treatment of congenital hypothyroidism through neonatal screening and earlier diagnosis of hypothyroidism in children and adults, the impact of prolonged hypothyroidism on growth is fortunately not easily studied. One study looked at long-term growth in children with prepubertal severe hypothyroidism (18 girls and 6 boys) whose heights at diagnosis were 4.04 (girls) and 3.15 (boys) SDs below the mean normal height for their ages [83]. During the first 18 months of thyroid hormone therapy, they experienced rapid growth, whether or not they were undergoing puberty, but their adult height was significantly below predicted midparental height or their pre-illness standard deviation score for height. The reduction in adult height was significantly correlated to the duration of untreated hypothyroidism, with the onset based on the bone age at time of diagnosis. Although catch-up growth was seen in this group, it was not sufficient to compensate for the loss of growth during the period of hypothyroidism. These patients had severe hypothyroidism, total serum T4 of 1.0 in girls and 1.3 µg/dl in boys (normal 5–12 µg/dl) and mean serum TSH concentrations of 506 mIU/ml in the girls and 551 mIU/ml in the boys. It is unlikely that this magnitude or duration of hypothyroidism is common now, as children are tested for thyroid functional disorders earlier, but this study shows that prolonged severe hypothyroidism can be associated with deficits of adult height (Table 4.2).

## Effects of GH Replacement on Serum Thyroid Function

Although the most significant clinical scenario is the impact of altered thyroid status on GH secretion and growth, alterations of serum thyroid function have been observed in GH-deficient states. In a study of 800 children with short stature suspected of having GH deficiency, abnormalities of serum thyroid hormone function tests were helpful in corroborating the diagnosis when GH stimulation test results were inconclusive [94]. In another study, prepubertal children with short stature and decreased GH concentrations, but normal GH responses to provocative testing, showed no differences in TSH secretory patterns and of thyroid hormone levels, compared to children with short stature and normal baseline GH concentrations [95].

GH replacement therapy in children with GH deficiency results in decreased serum-free T4 concentrations and increased serum T3 levels, likely due to increased peripheral conversion of T4 to T3 [96]. GH replacement in GH-deficient individuals is positively correlated with thyroid hormone receptor TRα mRNA levels and negatively with TRβ mRNA levels, suggesting that basal mRNA levels may be helpful in determining sensitivity to GH treatment [97].

**Table 4.2** Thyroid hormone regulation of growth hormone action in humans

| Type of thyroid dysfunction | Growth outcome | References |
|---|---|---|
| Endemic cretinism | Retarded bone maturation | [84] |
| Congenital hypothyroidism | Permanent height loss in four patients with delayed thyroid hormone treatment | [85] |
| | Normal height in patients diagnosed by conventional screening and treated with thyroid hormone replacement | [86–88] |
| Juvenile-acquired hypothyroidism | Failure to attain normal midparental adult height, correlated with duration of hypothyroidism before thyroid hormone replacement | [83] |
| | Decreased predicted adult height in severe acquired juvenile hypothyroidism is correctable with GH and GnRH agonist therapies | [89] |
| *Prop-1* gene mutation[a] | Normal linear growth following replacement of GH and thyroid hormone | [90] |
| *Pit-1* gene mutation[a] | Near-normal linear growth following replacements of GH and thyroid hormone | [91] |
| Resistance to thyroid hormone (TRβ) | Stippled epiphyses and winged scapula in the original kindred, reduced bone density, reduced height relative to prediction from parental height | [92, 93] |
| Resistance to thyroid hormone (TRα) | Growth retardation affects the lower segment more than the upper segment, so there are relatively short limbs, hands, and feet with a long thoracic span. Delayed bone maturation, skeletal dysplasia, macrocephaly, reduced height relative to prediction from parental height | [92, 93] |

[a]Genes involved in pituitary development, in which mutation lead to TSH deficiency, among other pituitary hormone deficits

## Conclusion

Normal GH synthesis and secretion requires thyroid hormone, and regulation occurs at multiple levels, including the stimulation and action of IGF-I. The early diagnosis and treatment of thyroid hormone deficiency in children is especially important with respect to preserving normal linear growth and bone development. Genetic defects in TR, especially TRα, although likely very rare, represent a new link of thyroid hormone action with growth and display a primary phenotype of delayed linear growth in children. The study of these children is likely to identify additional targets of thyroid hormone in growth.

**Acknowledgments** Supported by NIH K23HD068552 (AML), NIH RO1 DK98576 (GAB), and VA Merit Review (GAB).

# References

1. Brent GA. Regulation of gene expression by thyroid hormones; relation to growth and development. In: Kostyo JL, editor. Hormonal control of growth: handbook of physiology. New York: Oxford University Press; 1999. p. 757–82.
2. Scanlon MF, Issa BG, Dieguez C. Regulation of growth hormone secretion. Horm Res. 1996;46(4–5):149–54.
3. Murray PG, Clayton PE. Endocrine control of growth. Am J Med Genet C Semin Med Genet. 2013;163C(2):76–85.
4. Cheng SY, Leonard JL, Davis PJ. Molecular aspects of thyroid hormone actions. Endocr Rev. 2010;31(2):139–70.
5. Brent GA. Mechanisms of thyroid hormone action. J Clin Invest. 2012;122(9):3035–43.
6. Williams GR. Neurodevelopmental and neurophysiological actions of thyroid hormone. J Neuroendocrinol. 2008;20(6):784–94.
7. Chiamolera MI, Wondisford FE. Minireview: thyrotropin-releasing hormone and the thyroid hormone feedback mechanism. Endocrinology. 2009;150(3):1091–6.
8. Astapova I, Vella KR, Ramadoss P, Holtz KA, Rodwin BA, Liao XH, et al. The nuclear receptor corepressor (NCoR) controls thyroid hormone sensitivity and the set point of the hypothalamic-pituitary-thyroid axis. Mol Endocrinol. 2011;25(2):212–24.
9. Brent GA, Williams GR, Harney JW, Forman BM, Samuels HH, Moore DD, et al. Effects of varying the position of thyroid hormone response elements within the rat growth hormone promoter: implications for positive and negative regulation by 3,5,3′-triiodothyronine. Mol Endocrinol. 1991;5(4):542–8.
10. Koenig RJ, Brent GA, Warne RL, Larsen PR, Moore DD. Thyroid hormone receptor binds to a site in the rat growth hormone promoter required for induction by thyroid hormone. Proc Natl Acad Sci U S A. 1987;84(16):5670–4.
11. Brent GA, Harney JW, Moore DD, Larsen PR. Multihormonal regulation of the human, rat, and bovine growth hormone promoters: differential effects of 3′,5′-cyclic adenosine monophosphate, thyroid hormone, and glucocorticoids. Mol Endocrinol. 1988;2(9):792–8.
12. Gereben B, Zavacki AM, Ribich S, Kim BW, Huang SA, Simonides WS, et al. Cellular and molecular basis of deiodinase-regulated thyroid hormone signaling. Endocr Rev. 2008; 29(7):898–938.
13. Refetoff S, Dumitrescu AM. Syndromes of reduced sensitivity to thyroid hormone: genetic defects in hormone receptors, cell transporters and deiodination. Best Pract Res Clin Endocrinol Metab. 2007;21(2):277–305.
14. Bernal J, Guadaño-Ferraz A, Morte B. Thyroid hormone transporters-functions and clinical implications. Nat Rev Endocrinol. 2015 Dec;11(12):690.
15. Luongo C, Trivisano L, Alfano F, Salvatore D. Type 3 deiodinase and consumptive hypothyroidism: a common mechanism for a rare disease. Front Endocrinol (Lausanne). 2013;4:115.
16. Mayerl S, Müller J, Bauer R, Richert S, Kassmann CM, Darras VM, et al. Transporters MCT8 and OATP1C1 maintain murine brain thyroid hormone homeostasis. J Clin Invest. 2014;124(5):1987–99.
17. Dumitrescu AM, Liao XH, Best TB, Brockmann K, Refetoff S. A novel syndrome combining thyroid and neurological abnormalities is associated with mutations in a monocarboxylate transporter gene. Am J Hum Genet. 2004;74(1):168–75.
18. Verge CF, Konrad D, Cohen M, Di Cosmo C, Dumitrescu AM, Marcinkowski T, et al. Diiodothyropropionic acid (DITPA) in the treatment of MCT8 deficiency. J Clin Endocrinol Metab. 2012;97(12):4515–23.
19. Giustina A, Wehrenberg WB. Influence of thyroid hormones on the regulation of growth hormone secretion. Eur J Endocrinol. 1995;133(6):646–53.
20. Korytko AI, Cuttler L. Thyroid hormone and glucocorticoid regulation of pituitary growth hormone-releasing hormone receptor gene expression. J Endocrinol. 1997;152(2):R13–7.

21. Downs TR, Chomczynski P, Frohman LA. Effects of thyroid hormone deficiency and replacement on rat hypothalamic growth hormone (GH)-releasing hormone gene expression in vivo are mediated by GH. Mol Endocrinol. 1990;4(3):402–8.
22. Martial JA, Seeburg PH, Guenzi D, Goodman HM, Baxter JD. Regulation of growth hormone gene expression: synergistic effects of thyroid and glucocorticoid hormones. Proc Natl Acad Sci U S A. 1977;74(10):4293–5.
23. Kamegai J, Tamura H, Ishii S, Sugihara H, Wakabayashi I. Thyroid hormones regulate pituitary growth hormone secretagogue receptor gene expression. J Neuroendocrinol. 2001;13(3):275–8.
24. Forhead AJ, Li J, Saunders JC, Dauncey MJ, Gilmour RS, Fowden AL. Control of ovine hepatic growth hormone receptor and insulin-like growth factor I by thyroid hormones in utero. Am J Physiol Endocrinol Metab. 2000;278(6):E1166–74.
25. Richards GE, Morrow DA, Thominet JL, Silverman BL, Gluckman PD. The effect of thyroidectomy on growth hormone regulation in the ovine fetus. J Dev Physiol. 1993;19(4):165–9.
26. Wang L, Shao YY, Ballock RT. Thyroid hormone-mediated growth and differentiation of growth plate chondrocytes involves IGF-I modulation of beta-catenin signaling. J Bone Miner Res. 2010;25(5):1138–46.
27. Lui JC, Nilsson O, Baron J. Growth plate senescence and catch-up growth. Endocr Dev. 2011;21:23–9.
28. Endo T, Kobayashi T. Excess TSH causes abnormal skeletal development in young mice with hypothyroidism via suppressive effects on the growth plate. Am J Physiol Endocrinol Metab. 2013;305(5):E660–6.
29. Williams GR. Thyroid hormone actions in cartilage and bone. Eur Thyroid J. 2013;2(1):3–13.
30. Latimer AM, Hausman GJ, McCusker RH, Buonomo FC. The effects of thyroxine on serum and tissue concentrations of insulin-like growth factors (IGF-I and -II) and IGF-binding proteins in the fetal pig. Endocrinology. 1993;133(3):1312–9.
31. Mesiano S, Young IR, Baxter RC, Hintz RL, Browne CA, Thorburn GD. Effect of hypophysectomy with and without thyroxine replacement on growth and circulating concentrations of insulin-like growth factors I and II in the fetal lamb. Endocrinology. 1987;120(5):1821–30.
32. Bassett JH, Boyde A, Zikmund T, Evans H, Croucher PI, Zhu X, et al. Thyroid hormone receptor α mutation causes a severe and thyroxine-resistant skeletal dysplasia in female mice. Endocrinology. 2014;155(9):3699–712.
33. Göthe S, Wang Z, Ng L, Kindblom JM, Barros AC, Ohlsson C, et al. Mice devoid of all known thyroid hormone receptors are viable but exhibit disorders of the pituitary-thyroid axis, growth, and bone maturation. Genes Dev. 1999;13(10):1329–41.
34. Vakili H, Jin Y, Nagy JI, Cattini PA. Transgenic mice expressing the human growth hormone gene provide a model system to study human growth hormone synthesis and secretion in non-tumor-derived pituitary cells: differential effects of dexamethasone and thyroid hormone. Mol Cell Endocrinol. 2011;345(1-2):48–57.
35. Valcavi R, Zini M, Portioli I. Thyroid hormones and growth hormone secretion. J Endocrinol Invest. 1992;15(4):313–30.
36. Kitauchi S, Yamanouchi H, Hirano N, Toné S, Shiino M. Effect of neonatal thyroidectomy on growth hormone secretion in the rat. J Endocrinol. 1998;157(2):245–50.
37. Montes A, Hervás F, Jolin T. Effects of thyroidectomy and thyroxine on plasma growth hormone and insulin levels in rats. Horm Res. 1977;8(3):148–58.
38. Ezzat S, Laks D, Oster J, Melmed S. Growth hormone regulation in primary fetal and neonatal rat pituitary cell cultures: the role of thyroid hormone. Endocrinology. 1991;128(2):937–43.
39. Varela C, Cacicedo L, Fernández G, de los Frailes T, Sánchez Franco F. Influence of hypothyroidism duration on developmental changes in the hypothalamic factors implicated in growth hormone secretion in the male rat. Neuroendocrinology. 1991;54(4):340–5.
40. Tsai JS, Samuels HH. Thyroid hormone action: stimulation of growth hormone and inhibition of prolactin secretion in cultured GH1 cells. Biochem Biophys Res Commun. 1974;59(1):420–8.

41. Root AW, Shulman D, Root J, Diamond F. The interrelationships of thyroid and growth hormones: effect of growth hormone releasing hormone in hypo- and hyperthyroid male rats. Acta Endocrinol Suppl (Copenh). 1986;279:367–75.
42. Jones PM, Burrin JM, Ghatei MA, O'Halloran DJ, Legon S, Bloom SR. The influence of thyroid hormone status on the hypothalamo-hypophyseal growth hormone axis. Endocrinology. 1990;126(3):1374–9.
43. Martin D, Epelbaum J, Bluet-Pajot MT, Prelot M, Kordon C, Durand D. Thyroidectomy abolishes pulsatile growth hormone secretion without affecting hypothalamic somatostatin. Neuroendocrinology. 1985;41(6):476–81.
44. Bruhn TO, McFarlane MB, Deckey JE, Jackson IM. Analysis of pulsatile secretion of thyrotropin and growth hormone in the hypothyroid rat. Endocrinology. 1992;131(6):2615–21.
45. De Gennaro V, Cella SG, Bassetti M, Rizzi R, Cocchi D, Muller EE. Impaired growth hormone secretion in neonatal hypothyroid rats: hypothalamic versus pituitary component. Proc Soc Exp Biol Med. 1988;187(1):99–106.
46. Walker P, Dussault JH. Hypothalamic somatostatin and pituitary and serum growth hormone concentrations during postnatal development in rats exposed chronically to propylthiouracil or a low iodine diet. J Dev Physiol. 1980;2(3):111–7.
47. Chang YJ, Hwu CM, Yeh CC, Wang PS, Wang SW. Effects of subacute hypothyroidism on metabolism and growth-related molecules. Molecules. 2014;19(8):11178–95.
48. Szabo M, Stachura ME, Paleologos N, Bybee DE, Frohman LA. Thyrotropin-releasing hormone stimulates growth hormone release from the anterior pituitary of hypothyroid rats in vitro. Endocrinology. 1984;114(4):1344–51.
49. Welsh JB, Cuttler L, Szabo M. Ontogeny of the in vitro growth hormone stimulatory effect of thyrotropin-releasing hormone in the rat. Endocrinology. 1986;119(5):2368–75.
50. Chihara K, Kato Y, Ohgo S, Iwasaki Y, Maeda K. Effects of hyperthyroidism and hypothyroidism on rat growth hormone release induced by thyrotropin-releasing hormone. Endocrinology. 1976;98(6):1396–400.
51. Kühn ER, Geelissen SM, Van der Geyten S, Darras VM. The release of growth hormone (GH): relation to the thyrotropic- and corticotropic axis in the chicken. Domest Anim Endocrinol. 2005;29(1):43–51.
52. Scanes CG, Denver RJ, Bowen SJ. Effect of thyroid hormones on growth hormone secretion in broiler chickens. Poult Sci. 1986;65(2):384–90.
53. Harvey S, Scanes CG, Klandorf H. Thyrotropin-releasing hormone induces growth hormone secretion in adult hypothyroid fowl. Gen Comp Endocrinol. 1988;69(2):233–7.
54. Denver RJ, Harvey S. Thyroidal inhibition of chicken pituitary growth hormone: alterations in secretion and accumulation of newly synthesized hormone. J Endocrinol. 1991;131(1):39–48.
55. Porter TE, Dean KJ. Regulation of chicken embryonic growth hormone secretion by corticosterone and triiodothyronine: evidence for a negative synergistic response. Endocrine. 2001;14(3):363–8.
56. Martins MC, Knobel M, Medeiros-Neto G. Decreased growth hormone (GH) response to oral clonidine in endemic cretinism: effect of L-T3 therapy. J Endocrinol Invest. 1988;11(7):477–81.
57. Velardo A, Zizzo G, Della Casa L, Coletta F, Pantaleoni M, Marrama P, et al. Effects of thyroid hormone status on the growth hormone responses to clonidine. Exp Clin Endocrinol. 1993;101(4):243–8.
58. Pimentel-Filho FR, Ramos-Dias JC, Ninno FB, Façanha CF, Liberman B, Lengyel AM. Growth hormone responses to GH-releasing peptide (GHRP-6) in hypothyroidism. Clin Endocrinol (Oxf). 1997;46(3):295–300.
59. Ignacio DL, da Silvestre SDH, Cavalcanti-de-Albuquerque JP, Louzada RA, Carvalho DP, Werneck-de-Castro JP. Thyroid hormone and estrogen regulate exercise-induced growth hormone release. PLoS One. 2015;10(4), e0122556.
60. Silva FG, Giannocco G, Santos MF, Nunes MT. Thyroid hormone induction of actin polymerization in somatotrophs of hypothyroid rats: potential repercussions in growth hormone synthesis and secretion. Endocrinology. 2006;147(12):5777–85.

61. Wood DF, Franklyn JA, Docherty K, Ramsden DB, Sheppard MC. The effect of thyroid hormones on growth hormone gene expression in vivo in rats. J Endocrinol. 1987;112(3):459–63.
62. Mulchahey JJ, Di Blasio AM, Jaffe RB. Effects of growth hormone (GH)-releasing hormone and somatostatin on GH secretion from individual human and monkey fetal anterior pituitary cells: modulation by thyroid hormones and glucocorticoids. J Clin Endocrinol Metab. 1988;66(2):395–401.
63. Fortunato RS, Ignácio DL, Padron AS, Peçanha R, Marassi MP, Rosenthal D, et al. The effect of acute exercise session on thyroid hormone economy in rats. J Endocrinol. 2008;198(2):347–53.
64. Marin G, Domené HM, Barnes KM, Blackwell BJ, Cassorla FG, Cutler GB. The effects of estrogen priming and puberty on the growth hormone response to standardized treadmill exercise and arginine-insulin in normal girls and boys. J Clin Endocrinol Metab. 1994;79(2):537–41.
65. Rodriguez M, Rodriguez F, Jolin T. Effect of restricted feeding, fasting, and diabetes on the relationship between thyroid hormone receptor occupancy, growth hormone induction, and inhibition of thyrotropin release in thyroidectomized rats. Endocrinology. 1992;131(4):1612–8.
66. Douyon L, Schteingart DE. Effect of obesity and starvation on thyroid hormone, growth hormone, and cortisol secretion. Endocrinol Metab Clin North Am. 2002;31(1):173–89.
67. Coiro V, Volpi R, Capretti L, Speroni G, Marchesi C, Vescovi PP, et al. Influence of thyroid status on the paradoxical growth hormone response to thyrotropin-releasing hormone in human obesity. Metabolism. 1994;43(4):514–7.
68. Colao A, Merola B, Ferone D, Calabrese MR, Longobardi S, Spaziante R, et al. Effect of corticotrophin-releasing hormone administration on growth hormone levels in acromegaly: in vivo and in vitro studies. Eur J Endocrinol. 1994;131(1):14–9.
69. Barbarino A, Corsello SM, Tofani A, Sciuto R, Della Casa S, Rota CA, et al. Corticotropin-releasing hormone inhibition of paradoxical growth hormone response to thyrotropin-releasing hormone in insulin-dependent diabetics. Metabolism. 1992;41(9):949–53.
70. Prager D, Weber MM, Gebremedhin S, Melmed S. Interaction between insulin and thyroid hormone in rat pituitary tumour cells: insulin attenuates tri-iodothyronine-induced growth hormone mRNA levels. J Endocrinol. 1993;137(1):107–14.
71. Debaveye Y, Ellger B, Mebis L, Van Herck E, Coopmans W, Darras V, et al. Tissue deiodinase activity during prolonged critical illness: effects of exogenous thyrotropin-releasing hormone and its combination with growth hormone-releasing peptide-2. Endocrinology. 2005;146(12):5604–11.
72. Weekers F, Michalaki M, Coopmans W, Van Herck E, Veldhuis JD, Darras VM, et al. Endocrine and metabolic effects of growth hormone (GH) compared with GH-releasing peptide, thyrotropin-releasing hormone, and insulin infusion in a rabbit model of prolonged critical illness. Endocrinology. 2004;145(1):205–13.
73. Van den Berghe G, Wouters P, Weekers F, Mohan S, Baxter RC, Veldhuis JD, et al. Reactivation of pituitary hormone release and metabolic improvement by infusion of growth hormone-releasing peptide and thyrotropin-releasing hormone in patients with protracted critical illness. J Clin Endocrinol Metab. 1999;84(4):1311–23.
74. Chernausek SD, Underwood LE, Utiger RD, Van Wyk JJ. Growth hormone secretion and plasma somatomedin-C in primary hypothyroidism. Clin Endocrinol (Oxf). 1983;19(3):337–44.
75. Valcavi R, Jordan V, Dieguez C, John R, Manicardi E, Portioli I, et al. Growth hormone responses to GRF 1-29 in patients with primary hypothyroidism before and during replacement therapy with thyroxine. Clin Endocrinol (Oxf). 1986;24(6):693–8.
76. Dong Q, Gong CX, Gu Y, Su C. A new mutation in the thyroid hormone receptor gene of a Chinese family with resistance to thyroid hormone. Chin Med J (Engl). 2011;124(12):1835–9.
77. Tylki-Szymańska A, Acuna-Hidalgo R, Krajewska-Walasek M, Lecka-Ambroziak A, Steehouwer M, Gilissen C, et al. Thyroid hormone resistance syndrome due to mutations in the thyroid hormone receptor α gene (THRA). J Med Genet. 2015;52(5):312–6.

78. van Mullem AA, Chrysis D, Eythimiadou A, Chroni E, Tsatsoulis A, de Rijke YB, et al. Clinical phenotype of a new type of thyroid hormone resistance caused by a mutation of the TRα1 receptor: consequences of LT4 treatment. J Clin Endocrinol Metab. 2013;98(7): 3029–38.
79. Williams T, Maxon H, Thorner MO, Frohman LA. Blunted growth hormone (GH) response to GH-releasing hormone in hypothyroidism resolves in the euthyroid state. J Clin Endocrinol Metab. 1985;61(3):454–6.
80. Nishi Y, Hamamoto K, Kajiyama M, Fujita A, Kawamura I, Kagawa Y, et al. Pituitary enlargement, hypertrichosis and blunted growth hormone secretion in primary hypothyroidism. Acta Paediatr Scand. 1989;78(1):136–40.
81. Sack J, Shafrir Y, Urbach D, Amado O. Thyroid-stimulating hormone, prolactin, and growth hormone response to thyrotropin-releasing hormone in treated children with congenital hypothyroidism. Pediatr Res. 1985;19(10):1037–9.
82. Soliman AT, Omar M, El Awwa A, Rizk MM, El Alaily RK, Bedair EM. Linear growth, growth-hormone secretion and IGF-I generation in children with neglected hypothyroidism before and after thyroxine replacement. J Trop Pediatr. 2008;54(5):347–9.
83. Rivkees SA, Bode HH, Crawford JD. Long-term growth in juvenile acquired hypothyroidism: the failure to achieve normal adult stature. N Engl J Med. 1988;318(10):599–602.
84. Je D, Am E, Pa B. Thyroid function in a goiter endemic. V. Mechanism of thyroid failure in the Uele endemic cretins. J Clin Endocrinol Metab. 1963;23:847–60.
85. Boersma B, Otten BJ, Stoelinga GB, Wit JM. Catch-up growth after prolonged hypothyroidism. Eur J Pediatr. 1996;155(5):362–7.
86. Salerno M, Micillo M, Di Maio S, Capalbo D, Ferri P, Lettiero T, et al. Longitudinal growth, sexual maturation and final height in patients with congenital hypothyroidism detected by neonatal screening. Eur J Endocrinol. 2001;145(4):377–83.
87. Morin A, Guimarey L, Apezteguía M, Ansaldi M, Santucci Z. Linear growth in children with congenital hypothyroidism detected by neonatal screening and treated early: a longitudinal study. J Pediatr Endocrinol Metab. 2002;15(7):973–7.
88. Dickerman Z, De Vries L. Prepubertal and pubertal growth, timing and duration of puberty and attained adult height in patients with congenital hypothyroidism (CH) detected by the neonatal screening programme for CH--a longitudinal study. Clin Endocrinol (Oxf). 1997;47(6):649–54.
89. Quintos JB, Salas M. Use of growth hormone and gonadotropin releasing hormone agonist in addition to L-thyroxine to attain normal adult height in two patients with severe Hashimoto's thyroiditis. J Pediatr Endocrinol Metab. 2005;18(5):515–21.
90. Lee JK, Zhu YS, Cordero JJ, Cai LQ, Labour I, Herrera C, et al. Long-term growth hormone therapy in adulthood results in significant linear growth in siblings with a PROP-1 gene mutation. J Clin Endocrinol Metab. 2004;89(10):4850–6.
91. Brown MR, Parks JS, Adess ME, Rich BH, Rosenthal IM, Voss TC, et al. Central hypothyroidism reveals compound heterozygous mutations in the Pit-1 gene. Horm Res. 1998; 49(2):98–102.
92. Kvistad PH, Løvås K, Boman H, Myking OL. Retarded bone growth in thyroid hormone resistance. A clinical study of a large family with a novel thyroid hormone receptor mutation. Eur J Endocrinol. 2004;150(4):425–30.
93. Moran C, Agostini M, Visser WE, Schoenmakers E, Schoenmakers N, Offiah AC, et al. Resistance to thyroid hormone caused by a mutation in thyroid hormone receptor (TR)α1 and TRα2: clinical, biochemical, and genetic analyses of three related patients. Lancet Diabetes Endocrinol. 2014;2(8):619–26.
94. Smyczyńska J, Stawerska R, Lewiński A, Hilczer M. Do IGF-I concentrations better reflect growth hormone (GH) action in children with short stature than the results of GH stimulating tests? Evidence from the simultaneous assessment of thyroid function. Thyroid Res. 2011;4(1):6.
95. Quevedo MF, Pironis B, Palese T, Counts DR, De Luca F. TSH secretory pattern and thyroid function in children with growth hormone neurosecretory dysfunction. J Pediatr Endocrinol Metab. 2002;15(4):377–80.

96. Portes ES, Oliveira JH, MacCagnan P, Abucham J. Changes in serum thyroid hormones levels and their mechanisms during long-term growth hormone (GH) replacement therapy in GH deficient children. Clin Endocrinol (Oxf). 2000;53(2):183–9.
97. Susperreguy S, Muñoz L, Tkalenko NY, Mascanfroni ID, Alamino VA, Montesinos MM, et al. Growth hormone treatment in children with idiopathic short stature: correlation of growth response with peripheral thyroid hormone action. Clin Endocrinol (Oxf). 2011;74(3):346–53.

# Chapter 5
# Undernutrition, Inflammation and Catabolic Illness, and Growth Hormone Secretion

### Charumathi Baskaran and Madhusmita Misra

> Adapt or perish, now as ever, is nature's inexorable imperative.
>
> H.G. Wells

## Introduction

The adjustment that the human body undergoes in states of fasting and chronic starvation is a fascinating example of nature's indispensable phenomenon of adaptation. In an attempt to preserve basic metabolic functions and to provide essential fuels to the brain, malnourished individuals develop a state of growth hormone (GH) excess, which should facilitate increased lipolysis and availability of gluconeogenic substrates, while hepatic GH resistance results in low insulin-like growth factor-I (IGF-I) levels and conservation of energy otherwise expended for primarily IGF-I-dependent functions (such as statural growth and bone accrual). The neuroendocrine secretion of GH is profoundly sensitive to alterations in nutritional status, with this regulation being species specific. Humans are characterized by GH resistance that is associated with elevated GH and low IGF-I levels. In contrast, rodents exhibit low systemic levels of GH [1] and yet demonstrate GH resistance with decreased IGF-I response to GH injections and infusions [2].

## Normal Growth Hormone Secretion

Growth hormone is secreted in a pulsatile manner with pulse dynamic studies revealing ten pulses lasting for about 104 min over the course of 24 h [3]. The two major regulators of GH secretion are growth hormone-releasing hormone (GHRH), which stimulates GH secretion, and somatostatin (SRIH), which inhibits secretion of GH. Multiple other physiological factors influence the secretion of GH including age, sex, nutritional status, and the state of wakefulness and hunger. As discussed in earlier chapters, by virtue of being a peptide hormone, actions of GH are mediated through receptors and second messengers. GH acts on the liver to induce the production of IGF-I through signaling along the Janus kinase (JAK) signal transduction and activators of transcription (STAT) pathway, which mediates most of GH effects. In the following sections, we will examine alterations in GH secretion and action in conditions of undernutrition.

## Growth Hormone Concentrations in States of Undernutrition

For ease of understanding, we will classify undernutrition as states resulting from (i) decreased availability of substrate (involuntary or self-imposed) and (ii) increased catabolism, as seen in conditions of cachexia and inflammatory conditions.

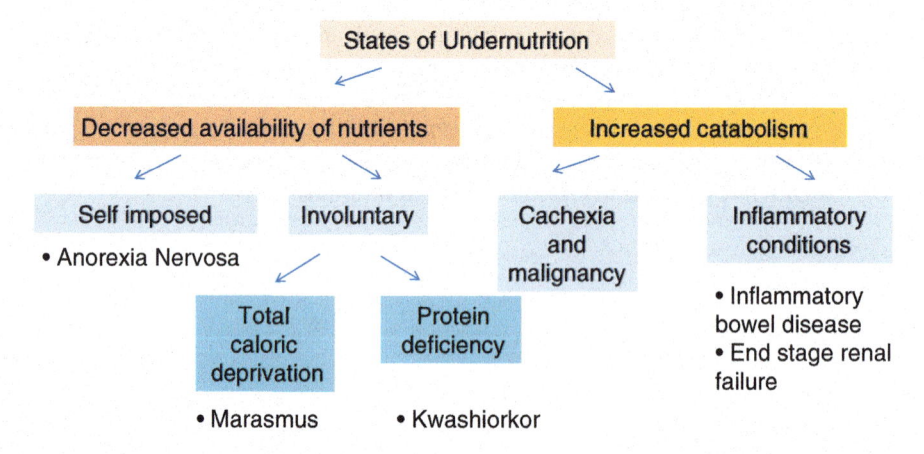

### States of Undernutrition

- Decreased availability of nutrients
  - Self imposed
    - Anorexia Nervosa
  - Involuntary
    - Total caloric deprivation
      - Marasmus
    - Protein deficiency
      - Kwashiorkor
- Increased catabolism
  - Cachexia and malignancy
  - Inflammatory conditions
    - Inflammatory bowel disease
    - End stage renal failure

### *Decreased Availability of Nutrients*

Decreased energy availability can be classified into conditions that result from acute energy limitation as in fasting or from long-term food and nutrient deprivation. Chronic malnutrition consequent to decreased food availability is relatively rare in the modern era, although still evident in developing countries. A chronic reduction in energy availability can further be categorized as complete caloric deprivation as in marasmus or limited to specific nutrients such as proteins as in kwashiorkor.

**Involuntary Reduction in Nutrient Availability**

Both acute and chronic malnutrition result in increased GH levels. In one study in humans, 5 days of fasting led to an increase in GH pulse frequency and maximum pulse amplitude [4] with a decrease in IGF-I levels. Similar to the fasting studies, GH levels have been found to be elevated in patients with marasmus and kwashiorkor [5–8]. Additionally, in some of these studies, because protein supplementation in addition to caloric replenishment, but not caloric replenishment alone, led to restoration of GH levels, severe protein deficiency is believed to be a stimulus for increased GH secretion [6]. These findings lead to the general consensus that GH levels are high in conditions of undernutrition.

Despite high GH levels, children with protein-energy malnutrition have low systemic IGF-I (consistent with a state of GH resistance) that improves with protein supplementation [5]. Furthermore, multiple authors have demonstrated low IGF-I levels in humans following fasting and malnutrition [8, 9]. The concluding evidence for GH resistance came from studies such as that of Shapiro et al., which demonstrated that there was a lack of increase in IGF-I following administration of human/bovine GH in protein-malnourished animals [10].

Of note, in one of the early studies from the 1960s, malnourished infants who failed to demonstrate weight gain despite receiving an appropriate dietary regimen were treated with 2 mg human GH (hGH) extract weekly for 4 weeks. GH therapy led to significant weight gain (15±8 g/day vs. 1.1±0.4 g/day without treatment), possibly from its anabolic effects on the muscle [11]. Indeed, these patients had significant retention of nitrogen, phosphorus, and potassium following GH administration, as indicated by metabolic balance studies, suggesting better utilization of these sources with GH treatment.

Hypoglycemia and stress associated with undernutrition, and predominantly the low IGF-I levels found in these conditions, act as stimuli to increase GH production. The direct lipolytic effect of GH results in increased availability of free fatty acids to the brain, an important metabolic fuel. Additionally, low IGF-I level results in decreased protein synthesis in a compromised state of nutrition. Changes in the GH-IGF-I axis in states of starvation are likely an adaptive response to preserve energy for vital bodily functions at the cost of stunted growth.

Factors Influencing Secretion and Action of GH in Marasmus and Kwashiorkor (Fig. 5.1)

**Hypothalamus: Role of GHRH and SRIH** Animal studies investigating mRNA expression of GHRH and SRIH in chronically food restricted sheep show an increased expression of GHRH in the arcuate nucleus and decreased expression of

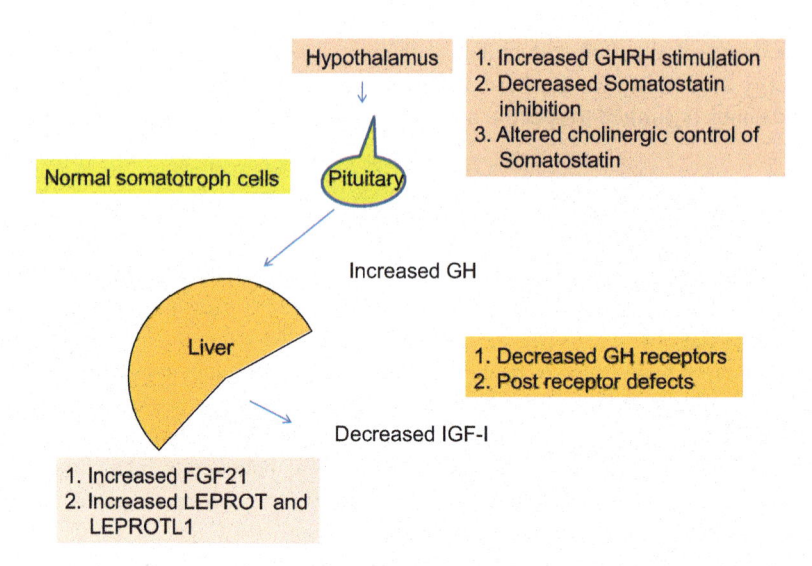

**Fig. 5.1** Mechanism mediating GH resistance in under nutrition

SRIH in the rostral periventricular and ventromedial nuclei of the hypothalamus [12]. Further, some studies have speculated that increased GH secretion by the pituitary somatotrophs may be a consequence of reduced sensitivity of pituitary cells to the inhibitory effect of SRIH [13].

**Pituitary** Studies assessing changes in pituitary morphology and histology in conditions of chronic energy depletion have reported conflicting findings with Paullada [14] reporting no morphological changes in the pituitary, Zubiran and Gomez-Mont reporting degenerative changes in the pituitary, and Tejada and Russfield reporting hypertrophy of trophic cells in autopsies of children with protein-energy malnutrition [15, 16].

Studies evaluating GH secretion in response to provocative stimuli in children with malnutrition have also had variable results. One study suggested that children with marasmus may have impaired GH secretion following arginine stimulation, whereas children with kwashiorkor have a robust response [17]. Subsequent studies confirmed normal GH secretion in both marasmus and kwashiorkor [18, 19].

**Liver: Receptor and post-receptor modifications** A proposed mechanism for low IGF-I production in conditions of chronic energy deficiency despite robust GH secretion is a reduction in GH receptor expression [20]. Young rat pups aged 3, 6, and 8 weeks that were fed a low-protein diet (~5 % of total caloric intake) for a week demonstrated decreased number of hepatic GH receptors associated with low IGF-I levels. However, the lack of an association between decreased hepatic GH receptors and IGF-I levels in older rat pups led the authors to propose a post-receptor defect in the nutrient-deficient state in addition to decreased GH receptor expression. Further evidence of a post-receptor defect comes from a lack of increase in

IGF-I levels in these animals despite normalization of GH receptors with continuous GH infusion [2]. Furthermore, the same authors demonstrated the inability of recombinant IGF-I to produce adequate tail growth in protein-deficient rats suggesting an element of IGF-I resistance in these animals [21].

More recently, multiple other mechanisms have been proposed by researchers to explain this state of GH resistance in malnutrition. FGF21, which belongs to the family of fibroblast growth factors, has gained significant interest in this front with fasting studies showing increased expression of FGF21 in the liver and cartilage [22]. FGF21 has further been shown to mediate GH resistance through its inhibitory action on STAT-5 (which otherwise potentiates GH action) [23] resulting in decreased IGF-I production. In addition, it has been proposed that GH resistance by FGF21 is mediated by increased expression of leptin receptor overlapping transcript (LEPROT) and LEPROT-like 1 (LEPROTL1) [24]. LEPROT and LEPROTL1 are genes that code for small proteins that regulate intracellular protein trafficking. Importantly, overexpression of LEPROT and LEPROTL1 is associated with decreased cell surface GH receptors [25]. When compared with animals fed ad lib, the expression of LEPROT and LEPROTL1 in the liver and cartilage was increased in rats that were food restricted for 4 weeks. Further this increase was not noted in FGF21 knockout animals, indicating that FGF21 might act via the LEPROT and LEPROTL1 to cause GH resistance [24].

Another factor postulated to mediate GH resistance through STAT-5 inhibition is Sirtuin1 (SIRT1). Yamamoto et al. reported that SIRT1 was able to inhibit GH-induced IGF-I production in hepatocytes through its inhibitory effect on STAT-5 [26].

## Self-Imposed Food Restriction: Anorexia Nervosa (AN)

Low body weight is a distinctive feature of this common psychiatric disorder that is characterized by an abnormal body image and an intense fear of gaining weight. This disorder is the most frequent cause of mortality in adolescent girls, and its effects on the GH-IGF-I axis are similar to those observed in marasmus or kwashiorkor. Multiple studies have demonstrated high levels of GH with low levels of IGF-I in patients with AN. Similar to the other states of malnutrition, GH resistance constitutes an important feature of this eating disorder. Advances in techniques to assess secretory hormone dynamics have helped quantify the secretory activity of hormones in this condition. Deconvolution analysis of GH levels in adult women with AN revealed a fourfold increase in the daily pulsatile secretion of GH with a 20-fold increase in basal secretion [27]. In a study conducted by our group, adolescent girls with AN, in addition to having increased pulsatile and basal secretion, also had increased disorderliness of GH secretion associated with low IGF-I levels [28] (Fig. 5.2). Indicators of nutritional status such as body mass index (BMI), leptin, and body fat were inversely correlated with GH in this study, indicating the impact of nutritional status on the neuroendocrine regulation of GH secretion.

**Fig. 5.2** Cluster and deconvolutional analyses in AN patients and controls. (**a**) Cluster analysis in two girls with AN (*two left panels*) and two healthy adolescent girls (*two right panels*). The mean and nadir GH concentrations and the total AUC were greater in girls with AN than in controls. (**b**) Deconvolutional analysis in the two girls with AN and the two healthy controls analyzed by cluster in A. The *upper panels* show GH concentrations over the sampling period; the *lower panels* show the individual secretory bursts. Girls with AN had higher basal GH secretion and a greater number of secretory episodes than healthy adolescents of comparable chronological and bone ages. Republished with permission of the Endocrine Society, from Misra et al., Alterations in growth hormone secretory dynamics in adolescent girls with anorexia nervosa and effects on bone metabolism. J Clin Endocrinol Metab. 2003. 88(12): 5615–23. Permission conveyed through Copyright Clearance Center, Inc.

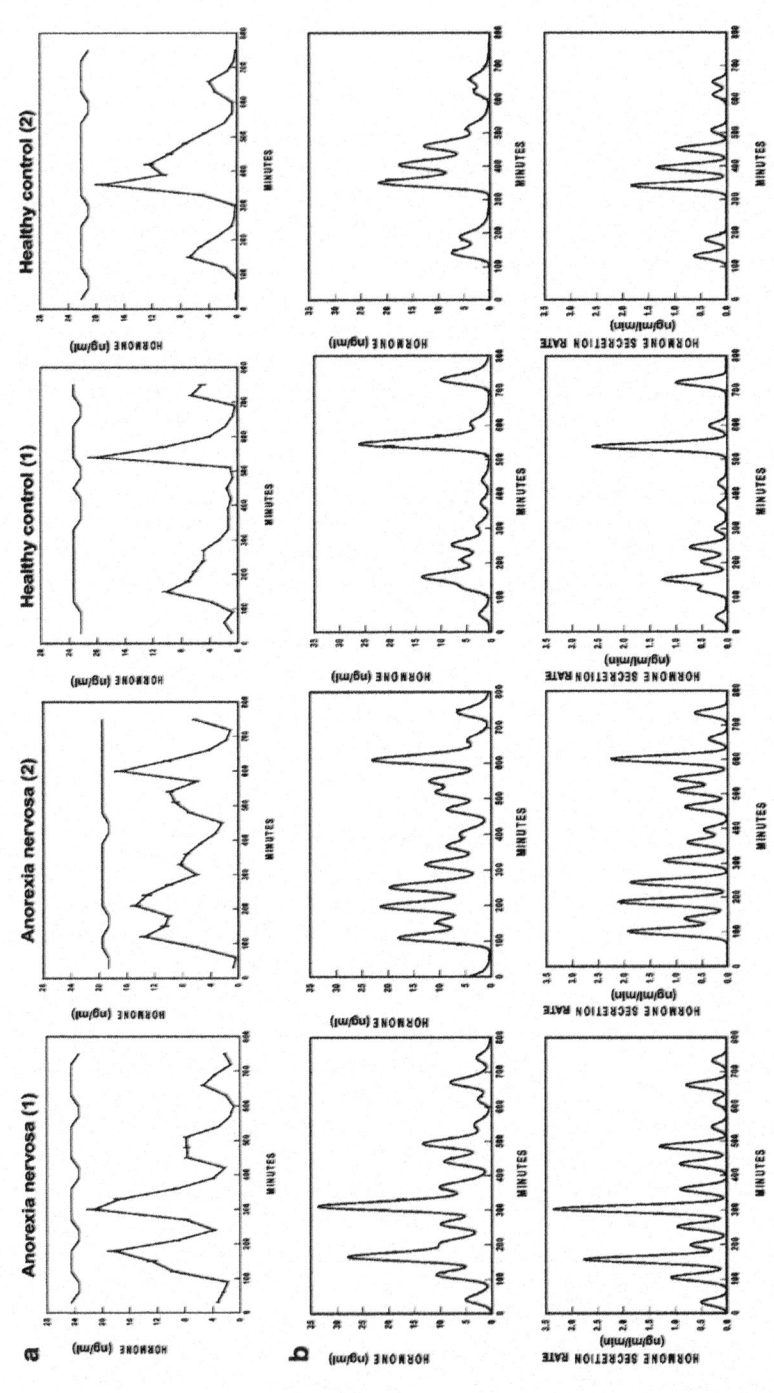

Convincing evidence in support of GH resistance in patients with AN emerged from a randomized placebo-controlled study conducted by our group administering supraphysiological doses of recombinant human growth hormone (rhGH) to women with AN. rhGH at a maximum dose of 1.4 ± 0.12 mg/day was administered to these women for 12 weeks with no resultant increase in IGF-I levels, suggesting no role for high-dose rhGH treatment to overcome GH resistance in AN [29, 30].

Factors Influencing Secretion and Action of GH in Anorexia Nervosa

**Hypothalamus** In addition to GH resistance, there is evidence that GH secretion is dysregulated in AN. However, it is unclear whether increased GH secretion in AN is secondary to decreased negative feedback at the hypothalamus from low IGF-I levels or whether there is a primary hypothalamic defect in GHRH/SRIH secretion. Low-dose rhIGF-I given to AN patients inhibits GHRH-mediated GH release only partially, suggesting a coexistent hypothalamic defect in the regulation of GH secretion [31]. The somatostatinergic control of GH secretion, which is mediated by cholinergic pathways, might also be altered in AN [32, 33]. In one study of eight women with AN and eight age- and sex-matched controls, participants were given one of the following infusions: (a) GHRH, (b) GHRH plus low-dose SRIH, and (c) GHRH plus high-dose SRIH, and GH area under the curve (AUC) was assessed over 120 min following the specific infusion [32]. Compared with controls, women with AN showed an exaggerated GH response to GHRH infusion alone. SRIH infusion in low doses inhibited the GHRH-mediated increase in GH secretion, indicating that the sensitivity of pituitary cells to SRIH is preserved in AN. Nevertheless, this dose was unable to inhibit GHRH-induced GH release in control women indicating alterations in somatostatinergic control of GH secretion.

Similar to these findings, Fassino et al. demonstrated an exaggerated GH response to GHRH in women with AN compared with controls. Additionally, following treatment with cholinergic drugs, GHRH no longer caused this increase in GH levels, suggesting an impaired cholinergic regulation of GH secretion in AN [34].

Another possible mediator of high GH levels in AN is the GH secretagogue, ghrelin. Ghrelin is an orexigenic hormone, and levels of ghrelin are appropriately increased in patients with AN compared with controls [35–37]. Misra et al. reported positive associations of ghrelin with GH secretory parameters, and ghrelin was an independent predictor of GH secretion in AN [36].

**Pituitary** Histopathological examination of pituitary biopsies obtained from patients who died from AN has not revealed specific changes to suggest a primary pituitary abnormality [38].

**Liver** Serum GH-binding protein (GHBP) levels, a good indicator of GH receptor expression, are low in patients in AN suggesting a decrease in GH receptors [39, 40], similar to patients with malnutrition. Further, the binding capacity of GHBP is reduced in AN compared with controls [39]. Studies conducted by our group have demonstrated a positive association of FGF21 with GH-AUC in adolescents with AN even after controlling for body fat and insulin resistance, indicating a possible role of FGF21 in GH resistance in AN, similar to that seen in animal models of malnutrition [29, 30].

Effects of Acquired GH Resistance in AN on End Organs

1. *Body composition and glycemia*: GH has lipolytic effects, and our studies have demonstrated a strong inverse association of GH-AUC with total, and particularly trunk, fat in adolescents with AN, suggesting that reduced body fat in this condition may be consequent to high GH concentrations [35, 37]. This is consistent with the role of GH as a gluconeogenic hormone that, through lipolysis, provides gluconeogenic substrate at times of chronic energy deficiency. Effects of GH on fat are direct end-organ effects not mediated via IGF-I and thus are evident even when IGF-I levels are low. Consistent with this, administration of rhGH in supraphysiological doses to adult women with AN led to a reduction in body fat mass over a 3-month period despite no significant increase in IGF-I levels [29, 30]. In contrast, there was no effect of rhGH on lean mass.

2. *Bone*: In addition to a hepatic resistance to GH in AN as evidenced by low circulating IGF-I levels, AN is characterized by a resistance to GH at the level of the bone, which contributes to impaired bone metabolism. Both GH and IGF-I are bone anabolic hormones, and in normal-weight adolescents, we have shown strong positive associations between GH concentrations and bone turnover markers [28]. However, this association is completely lost in adolescent girls with AN, indicative of GH resistance in the bone [28]. Consistent with these findings, administration of supraphysiological doses of rhGH for 3 months to adult women with AN did not result in a significant increase in levels of bone formation markers compared with placebo [29, 30]. In contrast, administration of rhIGF-I in replacement doses does cause an increase in bone formation markers in both adults and adolescents with AN [41, 42].

## *Disorders Characterized by Increased Catabolism*

### Cachexia

Cachexia is defined as a metabolic syndrome characterized by weight loss of at least 5 % over 12 months (or a BMI < 20 kg/m$^2$) resulting from muscle wasting secondary to chronic disease [43]. Cachexia can be consequent to a number of chronic disease states such as congestive heart failure, chronic kidney disease, and infectious disorders such as HIV or secondary to malignancy. Cachexia is distinct from AN in that it is irreversible with nutritional repletion and thus is not just a consequence of anorexia. Similar to other states of undernutrition, alterations in the GH-IGF-I axis are a major feature of cachexia. Although GH levels may be variable at different stages of the underlying conditions that eventually lead to cachexia, an acquired state of GH resistance is evident once cachexia develops. Cachexic states are thus characterized by elevated GH and low IGF-I levels [44, 45]. However, deconvolution analysis examining secretory dynamics of GH in patients with rheumatoid cachexia with diminished body cell mass did not show any significant differences in GH secretion compared with controls [46]. Because of the anabolic effects of GH and IGF-I, many studies have attempted to use these hormones to improve the underlying nutritional status of cachexic patients with variable results. Administration of rhGH to 21 patients with AIDS induced cachexia resulted in a less significant response in IGF-I levels compared with age-matched controls, suggestive of a partial GH-resistant state [47]. Furthermore, low IGF-I levels are a marker of nutritional status and predict mortality in these subjects. Ghrelin and ghrelin receptor agonists, which are potent GH secretagogues, can improve IGF-I levels in cachexic states [48–50]. Inflammatory cytokines thought to mediate cachexia are also believed to be responsible for GH resistance in this condition.

## Factors Influencing GH Secretion and Action

**Hypothalamus** While there are no studies to our knowledge that address the impact of GHRH and SRIH on GH release in cachexic states, some understanding of the regulation GH secretion in cachexia comes from studies using ghrelin in this condition. Ghrelin is a potent GH secretagogue (GHS) that acts through the GHS type 1 alpha receptor. Ghrelin is believed to be beneficial in these conditions because of its orexigenic and GH-independent anti-inflammatory effects, and studies in cachexia have shown an increase in GH and IGF-I levels following ghrelin administration suggesting a GH-mediated effect as well [49].

**Pituitary** One study from Japan reported that the pituitary gland of patients dying from senile cachexia weighed less than in controls (0.46 g vs. 0.60 g, $p \leq 0.01$), with a significant reduction in somatotrophs [51].

**Liver** Evidence points toward suppressed/decreased transcription of GH receptors in the liver induced by tumor cytokines as a possible mechanism for GH resistance in cachexia. Overexpression of inflammatory cytokines in transgenic mice induces GH resistance with reduced growth. One study reported a tumor necrosis factor (TNF)-mediated reduction in DNA binding of GH receptor gene promoter Sp1/Sp3 transactivators in the mouse liver cells [52]. Further, IL-6 has been implicated in mediating post-receptor defects in GH signaling by upregulating cytokine-inducible inhibitor of signaling (CIS) and suppressor of cytokine-inducible signaling (SOCS)-3 genes, thereby leading to inhibition of STAT-5 phosphorylation [53].

## Inflammatory Conditions

Stunted growth constitutes a major feature of inflammatory conditions in childhood, as seen in conditions such as inflammatory bowel disease (IBD) and juvenile idiopathic arthritis. Varying response to GH stimulation tests have been noted in IBD with Tenore et al. reporting normal GH peak response following insulin and McCaffery et al. showing a blunted GH response to insulin [54, 55]. A more recent retrospective study of children with colitis who presented with growth retardation revealed a spectrum of GH abnormalities ranging from GH deficiency to GH resistance. These children were subjected to insulin tolerance tests, and GH deficiency was diagnosed when the peak GH response was <6 mcg/L. Of the 28 children who underwent testing, 15 had low GH (four children with <3 mcg/L, 11 children with values between 3 and 6 mcg/L and low IGF-I indicating GH deficiency), 11 children had normal GH secretion with low IGF-I indicating GH resistance, and two children had normal to high GH levels and IGF-I-SDS >0 indicating some degree of IGF-I resistance in addition to GH resistance [56]. In rat models that were induced with colitis, 60 % of the subsequent growth retardation was explained by undernutrition and the remaining attributed to the underlying inflammatory process [57]. Thus inflammatory disorders represent a unique situation where GH secretion is impacted not only by the underlying undernutrition but also by the presence of pro-inflammatory cytokines such as TNFα, interleukin (IL)-1 and IL-6.

Deconvolution analysis of GH parameters in premenopausal women with active rheumatoid arthritis has shown nonsignificant elevation of integrated GH levels compared with normal controls, with no difference in secretory dynamics of GH [58] except for a shorter GH half-life in patients with active rheumatoid arthritis. However, in this study IGF-I and IGFBP-3 trended lower than in controls, which along with unaltered 24 h GH secretion suggests GH resistance.

**Cytokines and the GH-IGF-I Axis** Cytokines are pro-inflammatory in nature and are produced by different cell types. They mediate their effect on the GH-IGF-I axis by altering GH action at the level of GH receptors as well as by post-receptor mechanisms (Fig. 5.3).

TNFα inhibits expression of the hepatocyte GH receptor [52]. IL-6, the other major cytokine involved in inflammatory bowel disorders, acts through SOC3 proteins to inhibit the JAK-STAT pathway, thereby resulting in GH resistance [53]. Furthermore, in rat hepatocytes, IL-1 has been shown to decrease the ability of GH to induce acid-labile subunit (ALS) mRNA expression. In effect, this leads to decreased IGF-I levels since ALS is one of the three main components of the circulating 150 Dka complex [59].

Additional evidence for the role played by cytokines in mediating the GH resistance comes from a study where administration of a TNF-alpha receptor blocker to adult patients with inflammatory bowel disease resulted in significant increases in IGF-I and IGFBP-3 levels [60].

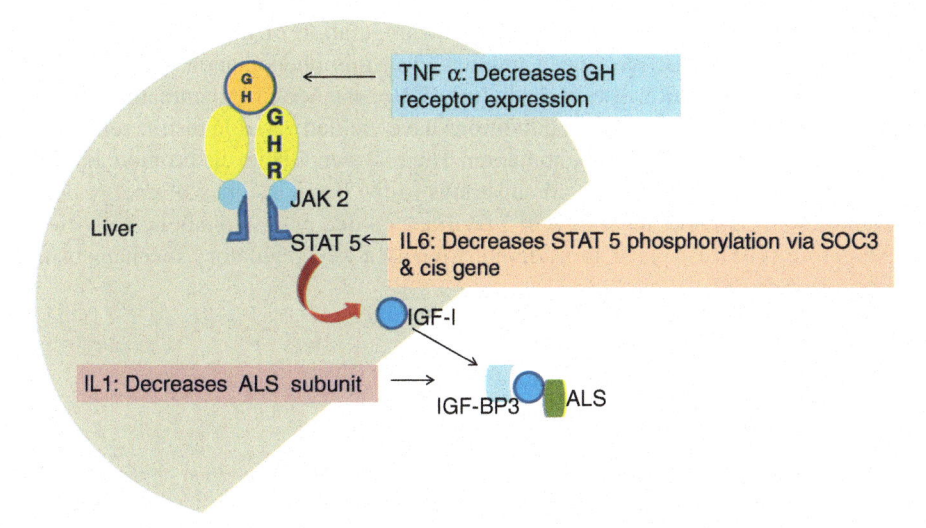

**Fig. 5.3** Influence of cytokines on GH-IGF-I axis

Some rodent studies reveal intriguing details regarding the mucosal protective role played by GH in IBD. Transgenic mice overexpressing GH demonstrated increased survival associated with decreased inflammation and enhanced mucosal repair compared to wild-type controls [61]. However, trials using GH for improvement of inflammatory disease have yielded inconsistent results. In adults with chronically active Crohn's disease, administration of GH (1.5 mg/day for 1 week following a loading dose of 5 mg/day) for four months led to a decrease in Crohn's disease activity index compared to those treated with placebo [62]. In contrast, a pediatric randomized-controlled trial using 0.075 mg/kg/day of GH plus corticosteroid treatment versus corticosteroid alone in 20 patients aged 7–18 years showed no difference in endoscopic disease activity with use of GH. They concluded that despite an increase in height $z$-scores in the GH group, GH therapy did not promote mucosal repair [63].

The confluence of poor nutrition, inflammatory effect of cytokines, and side effects of medications used for these conditions appears to lead to growth failure in inflammatory disorders such as IBD [64]. Similar to the response seen with GH therapy, treatment with cytokine inhibitors has failed to elucidate a unifying response in terms of improvement in growth [64]. At the present, there is limited evidence in favor of endocrine treatments for improving growth in inflammatory conditions.

## Conclusion

Regardless of the underlying mechanism that leads to undernutrition, humans exhibit a state of GH excess with low IGF-I levels in conditions of undernutrition, indicating a state of GH resistance. Alterations at the level of the hypothalamus and the liver, including downregulation of the GH receptor and post-receptor defects, have been implicated in this phenomenon. Additionally, cytokines play a major role in mediating GH resistance in inflammatory states. Attempts at using GH for these conditions have yielded variable results reflecting the adaptive nature of this phenomenon. The elevated GH levels promote lipolysis and availability of fatty acid substrates to the brain at times of energy deficiency, while the low level of IGF-I facilitates a decrease in anabolic activities. Therefore, GH resistance in undernutrition is a key regulatory mechanism to improve survival.

# References

1. Tannenbaum GS, Rorstad O, et al. Effects of prolonged food deprivation on the ultradian growth hormone rhythm and immunoreactive somatostatin tissue levels in the rat. Endocrinology. 1979;104(6):1733–8.
2. Thissen JP, Triest S, et al. Divergent responses of serum insulin-like growth factor-I and liver growth hormone (GH) receptors to exogenous GH in protein-restricted rats. Endocrinology. 1990;126(2):908–13.
3. Toogood AA, Nass RM, et al. Preservation of growth hormone pulsatility despite pituitary pathology, surgery, and irradiation. J Clin Endocrinol Metab. 1997;82(7):2215–21.
4. Ho KY, Veldhuis JD, et al. Fasting enhances growth hormone secretion and amplifies the complex rhythms of growth hormone secretion in man. J Clin Invest. 1988;81(4):968–75.
5. Grant DB, Hambley J, et al. Reduced sulphation factor in undernourished children. Arch Dis Child. 1973;48(8):596–600.
6. Pimstone BL, Barbezat G, et al. Studies on growth hormone secretion in protein-calorie malnutrition. Am J Clin Nutr. 1968;21(5):482–7.
7. Pimstone BL, Wittmann W, et al. Growth hormone and kwashiorkor. Role of protein in growth-hormone homoeostasis. Lancet. 1966;2(7467):779–80.
8. Zamboni G, Dufillot D, et al. Growth hormone-binding proteins and insulin-like growth factor-binding proteins in protein-energy malnutrition, before and after nutritional rehabilitation. Pediatr Res. 1996;39(3):410–4.
9. Hintz RL, Suskind R, et al. Plasma somatomedin and growth hormone values in children with protein-calorie malnutrition. J Pediatr. 1978;92(1):153–6.
10. Shapiro B, Pimstone BL. Sulphation factor (somatomedin activity) in experimental protein malnutrition in the rat. J Endocrinol. 1978;77(2):233–40.
11. Monckeberg F, Donoso G, et al. Human growth hormone in infant malnutrition. Pediatrics. 1963;31:58–64.
12. Henry BA, Rao A, et al. Chronic food-restriction alters the expression of somatostatin and growth hormone-releasing hormone in the ovariectomised ewe. J Endocrinol. 2001;170(1):R1–5.
13. Cordoba-Chacon J, Gahete MD, et al. Somatostatin and its receptors contribute in a tissue-specific manner to the sex-dependent metabolic (fed/fasting) control of growth hormone axis in mice. Am J Physiol Endocrinol Metab. 2011;300(1):E46–54.
14. Paullada JJ. Endocrine changes in malnutrition. I. Clinical aspects. Rev Invest Clin. 1955;7(1):29–54.
15. Tejada C, Russfield AB. A preliminary report on the pathology of the pituitary gland in children with malnutrition. Arch Dis Child. 1957;32(164):343–6.
16. Zubiran S, Gomez-Mont F. Endocrine disturbances in chronic human malnutrition. Vitam Horm. 1953;11:97–132.

17. Beas F, Contreras I, et al. Growth hormone in infant malnutrition: the arginine test in marasmus and kwashiorkor. Br J Nutr. 1971;26(2):169–75.
18. Brun TA, Nezam-Mafi S, et al. Growth hormone response to arginine infusion in malnourished children. Diabete Metab. 1978;4(1):27–33.
19. Youlton R, Riesco J, et al. Serum growth hormone and growth activity in children and adolescents with present or past malnutrition. Am J Clin Nutr. 1972;25(11):1179–83.
20. Maes M, Maiter D, et al. Contributions of growth hormone receptor and postreceptor defects to growth hormone resistance in malnutrition. Trends Endocrinol Metab. 1991;2(3):92–7.
21. Thissen JP, Underwood LE, et al. Failure of insulin-like growth factor-I (IGF-I) infusion to promote growth in protein-restricted rats despite normalization of serum IGF-I concentrations. Endocrinology. 1991;128(2):885–90.
22. Inagaki T, Dutchak P, et al. Endocrine regulation of the fasting response by PPARalpha-mediated induction of fibroblast growth factor 21. Cell Metab. 2007;5(6):415–25.
23. Inagaki T, Lin VY, et al. Inhibition of growth hormone signaling by the fasting-induced hormone FGF21. Cell Metab. 2008;8(1):77–83.
24. Wu S, Grunwald T, et al. Increased expression of fibroblast growth factor 21 (FGF21) during chronic undernutrition causes growth hormone insensitivity in chondrocytes by inducing leptin receptor overlapping transcript (LEPROT) and leptin receptor overlapping transcript-like 1 (LEPROTL1) expression. J Biol Chem. 2013;288(38):27375–83.
25. Touvier T, Conte-Auriol F, et al. LEPROT and LEPROTL1 cooperatively decrease hepatic growth hormone action in mice. J Clin Invest. 2009;119(12):3830–8.
26. Yamamoto M, Iguchi G, et al. SIRT1 regulates adaptive response of the growth hormone – insulin-like growth factor-I axis under fasting conditions in liver. Proc Natl Acad Sci U S A. 2013;110(37):14948–53.
27. Stoving RK, Veldhuis JD, et al. Jointly amplified basal and pulsatile growth hormone (GH) secretion and increased process irregularity in women with anorexia nervosa: indirect evidence for disruption of feedback regulation within the GH-insulin-like growth factor I axis. J Clin Endocrinol Metab. 1999;84(6):2056–63.
28. Misra M, Miller KK, et al. Alterations in growth hormone secretory dynamics in adolescent girls with anorexia nervosa and effects on bone metabolism. J Clin Endocrinol Metab. 2003;88(12):5615–23.
29. Fazeli PK, Lawson EA, et al. Effects of recombinant human growth hormone in anorexia nervosa: a randomized, placebo-controlled study. J Clin Endocrinol Metab. 2010;95(11):4889–97.
30. Fazeli PK, Misra M, et al. Fibroblast growth factor-21 may mediate growth hormone resistance in anorexia nervosa. J Clin Endocrinol Metab. 2010;95(1):369–74.
31. Gianotti L, Pincelli AI, et al. Effects of recombinant human insulin-like growth factor I administration on spontaneous and growth hormone (GH)-releasing hormone-stimulated GH secretion in anorexia nervosa. J Clin Endocrinol Metab. 2000;85(8):2805–9.
32. Gianotti L, Rolla M, et al. Effect of somatostatin infusion on the somatotrope responsiveness to growth hormone-releasing hormone in patients with anorexia nervosa. Biol Psychiatry. 1999;45(3):334–9.
33. Stoving RK, Andersen M, et al. Indirect evidence for decreased hypothalamic somatostatinergic tone in anorexia nervosa. Clin Endocrinol (Oxf). 2002;56(3):391–6.
34. Fassino S, Lanfranco F, et al. Prolonged treatment with glycerophosphocholine, an acetylcholine precursor, does not disclose the potentiating effect of cholinesterase inhibitors on GHRH-induced somatotroph secretion in anorexia nervosa. J Endocrinol Invest. 2003;26(6):503–7.
35. Misra M, Miller KK, et al. Hormonal determinants of regional body composition in adolescent girls with anorexia nervosa and controls. J Clin Endocrinol Metab. 2005;90(5):2580–7.
36. Misra M, Miller KK, et al. Growth hormone and ghrelin responses to an oral glucose load in adolescent girls with anorexia nervosa and controls. J Clin Endocrinol Metab. 2004;89(4):1605–12.
37. Misra M, Miller KK, et al. Secretory dynamics of leptin in adolescent girls with anorexia nervosa and healthy adolescents. Am J Physiol Endocrinol Metab. 2005;289(3):E373–81.

38. Scheithauer BW, Kovacs KT, et al. Anorexia nervosa: an immunohistochemical study of the pituitary gland. Mayo Clin Proc. 1988;63(1):23–8.
39. Hochberg Z, Hertz P, et al. The distal axis of growth hormone (GH) in nutritional disorders: GH-binding protein, insulin-like growth factor-I (IGF-I), and IGF-I receptors in obesity and anorexia nervosa. Metabolism. 1992;41(1):106–12.
40. Murata A, Yasuda T, et al. Growth hormone-binding protein in patients with anorexia nervosa determined in two assay systems. Horm Metab Res. 1992;24(6):297–9.
41. Grinspoon S, Thomas L, et al. Effects of recombinant human IGF-I and oral contraceptive administration on bone density in anorexia nervosa. J Clin Endocrinol Metab. 2002;87(6):2883–91.
42. Misra M, McGrane J, et al. Effects of rhIGF-I administration on surrogate markers of bone turnover in adolescents with anorexia nervosa. Bone. 2009;45(3):493–8.
43. Evans WJ, Morley JE, et al. Cachexia: a new definition. Clin Nutr. 2008;27(6):793–9.
44. Cicoira M, Kalra PR, et al. Growth hormone resistance in chronic heart failure and its therapeutic implications. J Card Fail. 2003;9(3):219–26.
45. Ross R, Miell J, et al. Critically ill patients have high basal growth hormone levels with attenuated oscillatory activity associated with low levels of insulin-like growth factor-I. Clin Endocrinol (Oxf). 1991;35(1):47–54.
46. Rall LC, Walsmith JM, et al. Cachexia in rheumatoid arthritis is not explained by decreased growth hormone secretion. Arthritis Rheum. 2002;46(10):2574–7.
47. Lieberman SA, Butterfield GE, et al. Anabolic effects of recombinant insulin-like growth factor-I in cachectic patients with the acquired immunodeficiency syndrome. J Clin Endocrinol Metab. 1994;78(2):404–10.
48. Akamizu T, Kangawa K. Ghrelin for cachexia. J Cachexia Sarcopenia Muscle. 2010;1(2):169–76.
49. Pietra C, Takeda Y, et al. Anamorelin HCl (ONO-7643), a novel ghrelin receptor agonist, for the treatment of cancer anorexia-cachexia syndrome: preclinical profile. J Cachexia Sarcopenia Muscle. 2014;5(4):329–37.
50. Zhang H, Garcia JM. Anamorelin hydrochloride for the treatment of cancer-anorexia-cachexia in NSCLC. Expert Opin Pharmacother. 2015;16(8):1245–53.
51. Takanashi R, Sugawara O, et al. Decreased growth hormone secreting cells of the hypophysis in senile cachexia. Rinsho Byori. 2001;49(1):61–5.
52. Denson LA, Menon RK, et al. TNF-alpha downregulates murine hepatic growth hormone receptor expression by inhibiting Sp1 and Sp3 binding. J Clin Invest. 2001;107(11):1451–8.
53. Denson LA, Held MA, et al. Interleukin-6 inhibits hepatic growth hormone signaling via upregulation of Cis and Socs-3. Am J Physiol Gastrointest Liver Physiol. 2003;284(4):G646–54.
54. McCaffery TD, Nasr K, et al. Severe growth retardation in children with inflammatory bowel disease. Pediatrics. 1970;45(3):386–93.
55. Tenore A, Berman WF, et al. Basal and stimulated serum growth hormone concentrations in inflammatory bowel disease. J Clin Endocrinol Metab. 1977;44(4):622–8.
56. Wong SC, Smyth A, et al. The growth hormone insulin-like growth factor 1 axis in children and adolescents with inflammatory bowel disease and growth retardation. Clin Endocrinol (Oxf). 2010;73(2):220–8.
57. Ballinger A. Fundamental mechanisms of growth failure in inflammatory bowel disease. Horm Res. 2002;58 Suppl 1:7–10.
58. Blackman MR, Muniyappa R, et al. Diurnal secretion of growth hormone, cortisol, and dehydroepiandrosterone in pre- and perimenopausal women with active rheumatoid arthritis: a pilot case-control study. Arthritis Res Ther. 2007;9(4):R73.
59. Boisclair YR, Wang J, et al. Role of the suppressor of cytokine signaling-3 in mediating the inhibitory effects of interleukin-1beta on the growth hormone-dependent transcription of the acid-labile subunit gene in liver cells. J Biol Chem. 2000;275(6):3841–7.
60. Vespasiani Gentilucci U, Caviglia R, et al. Infliximab reverses growth hormone resistance associated with inflammatory bowel disease. Aliment Pharmacol Ther. 2005;21(9):1063–71.

61. Williams KL, Fuller CR, et al. Enhanced survival and mucosal repair after dextran sodium sulfate-induced colitis in transgenic mice that overexpress growth hormone. Gastroenterology. 2001;120(4):925–37.
62. Slonim AE, Bulone L, et al. A preliminary study of growth hormone therapy for Crohn's disease. N Engl J Med. 2000;342(22):1633–7.
63. Denson LA, Kim MO, et al. A randomized controlled trial of growth hormone in active pediatric Crohn disease. J Pediatr Gastroenterol Nutr. 2010;51(2):130–9.
64. Altowati MA, Russell RK, et al. Endocrine therapy for growth retardation in paediatric inflammatory bowel disease. Paediatr Drugs. 2014;16(1):29–42.

# Chapter 6
# Obesity and Growth Hormone Secretion

Takara L. Stanley

## Introduction

An association between obesity and reduced growth hormone (GH) secretion has been recognized for several decades. In children and adults, both spontaneous [1–5] and stimulated [6–8] GH secretion decreases with increasing body mass index (BMI). In response to provocative testing, approximately 25–30 % of otherwise normal obese adults will meet criteria for frank GH deficiency (GHD) [9, 10]. This chapter will discuss obesity-related alterations in the GH-insulin-like growth factor-I (IGF-I) axis along with the physiological effects and clinical implications of these changes.

## Abdominal Adiposity and GH Secretion

In detailed studies of body composition and GH secretion, central adiposity emerges as a stronger determinant of GH secretion than overall adiposity or BMI, suggesting an interrelationship between abdominal fat in particular and GH secretion [11]. In adults, Makimura et al. demonstrated that the decline observed in peak stimulated GH with increasing BMI could be explained by measures of central adiposity. Figure 6.1 shows peak GH responses for 75 men who underwent GH-releasing hormone (GHRH)-arginine stimulation testing by weight status and waist circumference. In modeling including both BMI and waist circumference, waist circumference showed a significant independent association with peak stimulated GH, whereas BMI was not significantly associated with peak GH after

---

T.L. Stanley (✉)
Pediatric Endocrine Unit, Massachusetts General Hospital for Children
and Harvard Medical School, Boston, MA, USA
e-mail: tstanley@partners.org

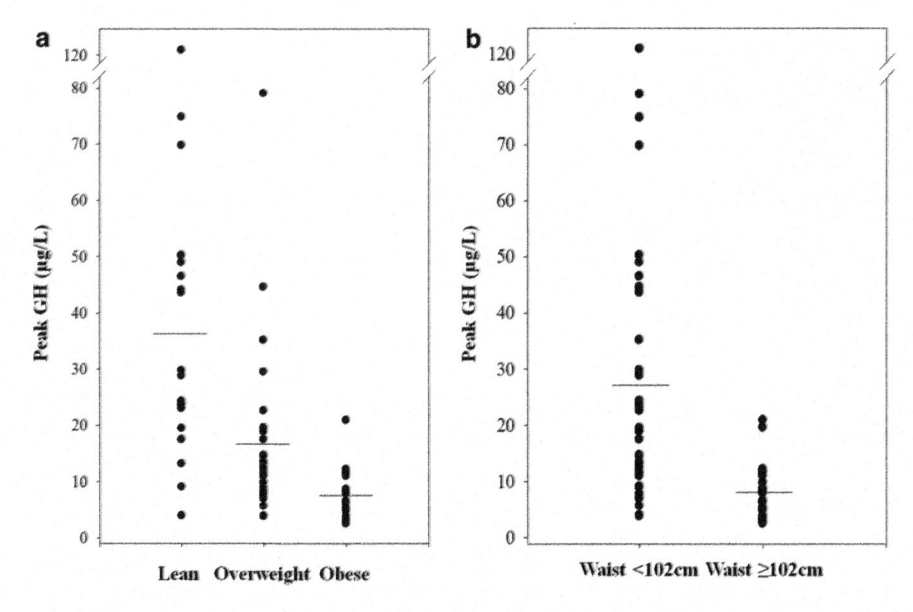

**Fig. 6.1** Scatter plot of peak stimulated GH levels following GHRH-arginine stimulation testing according to (**a**) weight category (lean [BMI <25 kg/m$^2$, $N$=23], overweight [BMI ≥ 25 kg/m$^2$ and <30 kg/m$^2$, $N$=28], and obese [BMI ≥ 30 kg/m$^2$, $N$=24]) and (**b**) waist circumference (<102 cm [$N$=47] or ≥102 cm [$N$=28]) [12]. Republished with permission of The Endocrine Society, from Makimura et al., The effects of central adiposity on growth hormone (GH) response to GH-releasing hormone-arginine stimulation testing in men. *J Clin Endocrinol Metab.* 2008. 93(11): 4254–60. Permission conveyed through Copyright Clearance Center, Inc.

adjusting for waist circumference. Similarly, in modeling including both BMI and visceral fat as measured by computed tomography (CT), visceral fat was significantly associated with peak GH, whereas BMI no longer predicted peak GH after adjusting for visceral fat [12]. A similar independent association between abdominal fat and peak GH, adjusted for BMI, has also been shown in other populations, including women and adolescent girls [8, 13]. The finding that abdominal fat, rather than overall adiposity, is most strongly associated with reductions in GH likely reflects the mechanisms of GH reduction in obesity. As discussed below, decreased GH likely results, at least in part, from hyperinsulinism and increased free fatty acids (FFA), both of which are more strongly associated with abdominal adiposity than with general adiposity.

## Mechanisms of Altered Growth Hormone Secretion in Obesity

In both children and adults, obesity-related reductions in GH secretion is reversed after significant weight loss [14, 15]. Thus, although stimulated peak GH levels in obese individuals overlap with levels in patients who have true pituitary GHD, the relative GHD of obesity is considered to be functional. Obesity is characterized by decreased GH pulse amplitude, with substantially less GH released per secretory burst [4, 16–18], as well as increased GH clearance [4, 17–20]. The reasons for increased GH clearance remain unclear but appear to include increased renal fractional excretion [19].

Multiple mechanisms have been proposed to explain obesity-related reductions in GH secretion, including suppression of GH secretion by insulin and/or FFA, increased somatostatin tone, and reductions in ghrelin. Short-term nutritional status is an important mediator of GH secretion. Short-term caloric reduction significantly increases GH in obese individuals [21], whereas short-term overfeeding reduces GH secretion in normal-weight controls [22]. In both experimental conditions, changes in GH secretion occur prior to any measurable changes in body composition, suggesting the importance of metabolic regulators such as insulin or FFA. In healthy, normal-weight men who consumed approximately 4000 kcal daily, significant reductions in GH was seen after 3 days of overfeeding, in conjunction with a significant increase in circulating insulin levels [22]. The suppressive effect of insulin on GH secretion is strongly supported by in vitro studies, in which insulin added to pituitary cell culture dose-dependently decreases mRNA expression of GH as well as GHRH-receptor and GH secretagogue receptor (ghrelin receptor) [23, 24]. Free fatty acids also suppress GH secretion, and obesity-related elevation in FFA may be another mechanism whereby GH is reduced in obesity [25]. In support of this hypothesis, administration of the anti-lipolytic agent acipimox to obese individuals partially restores GH responsiveness to provocative stimuli [26]. The precise mechanisms by which FFA suppress GH remains unclear. FFA may directly inhibit GH secretion and/or increase somatostatin, which mediates the effect. Obesity is thought to be associated with increased somatostatin tone [27, 28], and this is yet another proposed mechanism for decreased GH in obesity.

Finally, reductions in ghrelin may also cause decreased GH in obesity. In a recent study of GH and ghrelin in obese women, ghrelin secretion was the only significant independent predictor of reduced GH secretion in modeling including body composition and insulin measures [29]. It is likely that many or all of these factors act together to reduce GH secretion in obesity. In addition, as discussed below, it is possible that changes in free IGF-I due to obesity-related alterations in IGF-binding proteins may affect GH levels through negative feedback at the level of the pituitary.

## Obesity-Related Changes in IGF-I and IGF-Binding Proteins

Whereas the inverse association between adiposity and GH secretion is highly reproducible, the relationship between obesity and circulating levels of IGF-I and IGF-binding proteins is less clear. Multiple studies have investigated the levels of IGF-I and binding proteins in obese vs. lean individuals, with varying results (see Table 6.1).

With regard to total IGF-I, levels are generally reported to be unchanged or modestly decreased with increasing BMI. Studies in children have generally shown no

**Table 6.1** Effect of obesity on levels of IGF-I and IGF-binding proteins

| First author, year | N | IGF-I | Free IGF-I | IGFBP-1 | IGFBP-2 | IGFBP-3 |
|---|---|---|---|---|---|---|
| *Children and adolescents* | | | | | | |
| Argente, 1997 [30] | 65 obese | ↔ | ↑ | ↓ | ↓ | ↑ |
| | 37 controls | | | | | |
| Attia, 1998 [31] | 19 obese | ↓ | ↔/↑ | ↓ | ↔ | ↓ |
| | 20 controls | | | | | |
| Ballerini, 2004 [32] | 22 obese | ↔ | NR | NR | ↓ | ↔ |
| | 17 controls | | | | | |
| Park, 1999 [33] | 36 obese | ↔ | ↔ | ↔ | NR | ↑ |
| | 39 controls | | | | | |
| Radetti, 1998 [34] | 21 obese | ↔ | NR | ↓ | ↓ | ↑ |
| | 32 controls | | | | | |
| Saitoh, 1998 [35] | 20 obese | ↔ | NR | ↓ | NR | ↔ |
| | 20 controls | | | | | |
| Wabitsch, 1996 [36] | 73 obese | ↑ | NR | ↑ | ↑ | ↑ |
| | 100 controls | | | | | |
| *Adults* | | | | | | |
| Frystyk, 1999 [37] | 24 obese | ↔ | ↑ | ↓ | ↓ | ↑ |
| | 26 lean | | | | | |
| Frystyk, 2009 [38] | 34 F | ↓ | ↔ (bioactive) | ↓ | NR | ↔ |
| Gomez, 2004 [39] | 24 obese M | ↔ | ↔ | NR | NR | ↔ |
| | 110 lean M | | | | | |
| | 36 obese F | ↓ | ↓ | NR | NR | ↔ |
| | 98 lean F | | | | | |
| Nam, 1997 [40] | 45 obese | ↔ | ↑ | ↓ | ↓ | ↔ |
| | 45 controls | | | | | |

NR indicates data not reported

*IGF-I* insulin-like growth factor-I, *IGFBP* insulin-like growth factor-binding protein

difference in total IGF-I levels between obese and normal-weight groups, but these studies have relatively limited sample size and may have limited statistical power (see Table 6.1). In adults, studies suggest that total IGF-I is unchanged or modestly decreased [41]. The discrepancy between studies is likely due, at least in part, to significant variation in the assays used, differential selection of control groups, and relatively limited sample sizes. In addition, gender, hormonal status, and nutritional status are also likely to mediate changes in IGF-I in the context of low GH secretion. Utz et al. have shown that, in obese women, free androgen levels are increased and appear to contribute to preservation of IGF-I levels in spite of decreased GH secretion [42]. In a study of 620 pre- and postmenopausal women, Lukanova et al. showed no change in IGF-I with increasing BMI in premenopausal women but demonstrated that, in postmenopausal women, IGF-I levels were highest in those women with BMI between 24 and 25 kg/m$^2$ and decreased at lower or higher BMIs [43]. Further study is needed to better clarify the roles of gonadal steroids, body composition, and nutritional status as determinants of IGF-I in obesity. Additionally, GH sensitivity appears to be increased in obesity and requires further characterization in this population [44, 45]. Nonetheless, available data demonstrate that, although IGF-I levels may be modestly decreased in obese individuals, they are not reduced to the degree expected by the magnitude of reduction in GH.

A second critical question is the status of "free" or bioavailable IGF-I in obesity. Discussion of this question must first acknowledge two significant challenges in the assessment of free IGF-I. First, free IGF-I assays are technically difficult, and, given that free IGF-I represents only about 1 % of total IGF-I in the circulation, factors such as temperature that may change the equilibrium between bound and unbound hormone may significantly bias the results [46]. Second, IGF-binding proteins (IGFBP) may modulate IGF-I action at the receptor level, such that free IGF-I measurements may not perfectly reflect IGF-I bioactivity [38, 46]. Hepatic IGFBP-1 expression is suppressed by insulin, and IGFBP-1 is generally shown to be decreased in obesity [30, 34, 37, 40]. Most studies also indicate decreased IGFBP-2 in obesity [30, 34, 37, 40], although the mechanisms underlying this reduction are less clear. IGFBP-3 is variably reported as unchanged, increased, or decreased in obesity, with most reports indicating no significant change (see Table 6.1). The net effect of obesity-related alterations in GH secretion and IGFBPs on free IGF-I levels is controversial. Multiple studies have suggested that free IGF-I levels are increased in obesity [30, 40]. Indeed, one hypothesis proposed to explain reduced GH in obesity is that obesity-related reductions in IGFBP-1 and IGFBP-2 lead to increased free IGF-I levels, which, in turn, inhibit GH secretion. Other studies show unchanged free IGF-I, however, and a more recent investigation using an IGF-I receptor activation assay [47] showed no difference in bioactive IGF-I according to BMI [38].

Although further study is required to clarify obesity-related changes in IGF-I and IGFBPs, existing data allow for important preliminary conclusions. First, IGFBPs 1 and 2 appear to be decreased in obesity, whereas IGFBP-3 is probably not substantially altered. Second, total IGF-I levels may be normal or modestly decreased but clearly are not reduced to the degree expected by reductions in GH, likely reflecting increased GH sensitivity in obesity. Finally, free or bioactive IGF-I levels are likely to be unchanged or somewhat increased in obesity. The relative preservation of total and free IGF-I in obesity is clinically important, as it suggests that obesity-related reductions in GH is likely to be relevant only for those physiological actions of GH that are independent of IGF-I.

## Physiological Effects of Altered GH Secretion in Obesity

As above, those effects of GH that are largely mediated by IGF-I appear to be relatively unaffected in obesity. For example, obese children are often taller than their peers during childhood and reach normal adult height. Additionally, there is no evidence that bone mineral density is compromised in obese individuals due to GHD. In contrast, GH has IGF-I independent effects on lipid metabolism, body composition, and inflammatory and fibrinolytic pathways, and it is in these areas that obesity-related reductions in GH may be physiologically relevant.

Patients with untreated pituitary GHD have increased abdominal fat, dyslipidemia, and increased measures of systemic inflammation and cardiovascular risk [48–53]. That many obese patients share this phenotype has led to the hypothesis that the relative GHD in obesity may contribute to dyslipidemia, systemic inflammation, and increased measures of cardiovascular risk. Although many studies support correlations between reduced GH and cardiometabolic risk measures, fewer reports are available demonstrating independent associations between GH and these measures after controlling for abdominal obesity. In obese women, Utz et al. demonstrate that reduced GH is associated with lower high-density lipoprotein cholesterol (HDL), higher c-reactive protein (CRP), and higher tumor necrosis factor receptor 2 (TNFR2), after adjusting for BMI and truncal adiposity [10]. Peak GH is also significantly associated with intrahepatic and intramyocellular lipid in obese women, independent of age and visceral adiposity [54]. In a cohort including both men and women, we have demonstrated that reduced GH is independently associated with increased carotid intima-media thickness (cIMT), after adjusting for visceral fat and other markers of cardiovascular risk [55]. Decreased GH also predicts atherogenic reductions in LDL and HDL particle size, independent of BMI and other cardiovascular risk factors [56]. In obese adolescent girls compared to healthy controls, Russell et al. also report strong associations between reduced GH and multiple serum markers of inflammation, including CRP, TNFR2, and IL-6 [57]. Many of these associations persisted when controlling for cortisol and adiponectin, but modeling did not include measures of visceral fat.

It is important to note that the relationship between decreased GH and increased visceral fat may be bidirectional. Plausible mechanisms such as hyperinsulinism and increased FFA levels exist to explain how visceral adiposity decreases GH secretion. It is also possible, however, that reductions in GH exacerbates the accumulation of visceral adiposity. GH increases lipolysis via hormone-sensitive lipase (HSL), an effect which may be most relevant to the highly lipolytic visceral depot, such that reductions in GH facilitates visceral fat accumulation. Thus a self-reinforcing cycle may exist whereby obesity-related reductions in GH further exacerbates visceral fat accumulation, and both reduced GH and visceral obesity contribute to dyslipidemia and increased cardiovascular risk (Fig. 6.2).

The effects of GH on body composition, lipids, and markers of cardiovascular risk are elucidated by trials of GH or GHRH in obese individuals. Studies of GH in obesity performed through 2007, summarized in a meta-analysis by Mekala and Tritos [59], have generally demonstrated that treatment with GH reduces visceral fat and modestly increases lean mass, without overall changes in body weight [59]. Modest reductions in LDL is also seen, as are increases in glucose and insulin levels [59]. As a counter-regulatory hormone, GH increases glucose, particularly in the first several weeks of treatment. Of note, however, longer term treatment often shows less significant or even neutral effects on glucose homeostasis, likely because beneficial reductions in visceral fat and increases in lean mass offset the direct actions of GH on glucose homeostasis. For example, in a randomized trial of 30

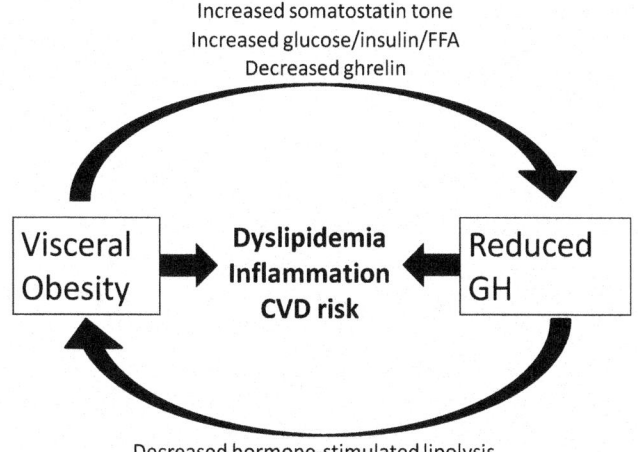

Increased somatostatin tone
Increased glucose/insulin/FFA
Decreased ghrelin

Visceral Obesity → Dyslipidemia Inflammation CVD risk ← Reduced GH

Decreased hormone-stimulated lipolysis

**Fig. 6.2** Potential mutually reinforcing relationship between visceral adiposity and reduced GH secretion, both of which may contribute independently to increased metabolic and cardiovascular risk [58]. Republished with permission of The Growth Hormone Research Society and The International Society for IGF Research, from Stanley and Grinspoon, Effects of growth hormone-releasing hormone on visceral fat, metabolic, and cardiovascular indices in human studies. *Growth Horm IGF Res.* 2015. 25(2):59–65. Permission conveyed through Copyright Clearance Center, Inc.

abdominally obese men receiving GH or placebo, glucose disposal rate worsened after 6 weeks in the GH group as compared to placebo, whereas, after 9 months of treatment, the glucose disposal rate was actually improved compared to placebo [60]. A similar effect was seen in a study of 40 postmenopausal women, in whom glucose disposal rate as assessed by euglycemic hyperinsulinemic clamp improved compared to placebo after 12 months of GH treatment, in association with reductions in liver fat [61].

Whereas many of the studies included in the meta-analysis used supraphysiologic dosing of GH, studies have been performed more recently using physiologic dosing to achieve IGF-I levels at the population mean (i.e., IGF-I standard deviation scores (SDS) of approximately 0) in both obese men and obese premenopausal women. In obese men, physiologic GH administration decreased visceral adipose tissue, intrahepatic lipid, CRP, and apolipoprotein B when compared to placebo [62]. In premenopausal obese women, physiologic GH reduced CRP and total abdominal adiposity compared to placebo, but it did not significantly reduce visceral adiposity [63]. Elevated glucose was observed in a minority of subjects [63]. Also of note, improvements in body composition and metabolic and inflammatory parameters reverted to baseline within 6 months after discontinuation of GH [64]. Makimura et al. have recently reported results of a strategy to increase endogenous GH through the use of GHRH in obese men and women. Over 1 year, treatment with GHRH reduced visceral adiposity, triglycerides, CRP, and (cIMT) in comparison to placebo [65]. No effects on glucose parameters were seen, but further, larger studies are needed to better define the effects of this strategy and the duration of effects following treatment discontinuation. It is critical to note that insufficient evidence exists to recommend either GH or GHRH for obesity, and use in obese individuals is purely investigational.

# Clinical Implications of Reduced GH in Obesity

## Interpretation GH-IGF-I Axis Testing

Perhaps one of the most important clinical implications of the reduction in growth hormone secretion with increasing body weight lies in the interpretation of provocative GH testing. In children, multiple studies have demonstrated that children with short stature and relatively high BMI are more likely to be classified as having GHD on the basis of provocative testing. In 116 children with short stature and no known pituitary pathology who underwent GH provocative testing, we demonstrated that BMI was a significant independent determinant of peak GH, even within the range of normal body weight. Figure 6.3, which shows the percentage of patients testing GH deficient by BMI category for multiple diagnostic thresholds for GHD, demonstrates that the percentage of children meeting diagnostic criteria for GHD significantly increases as BMI-SDS rises [66]. In a larger cohort of children with short

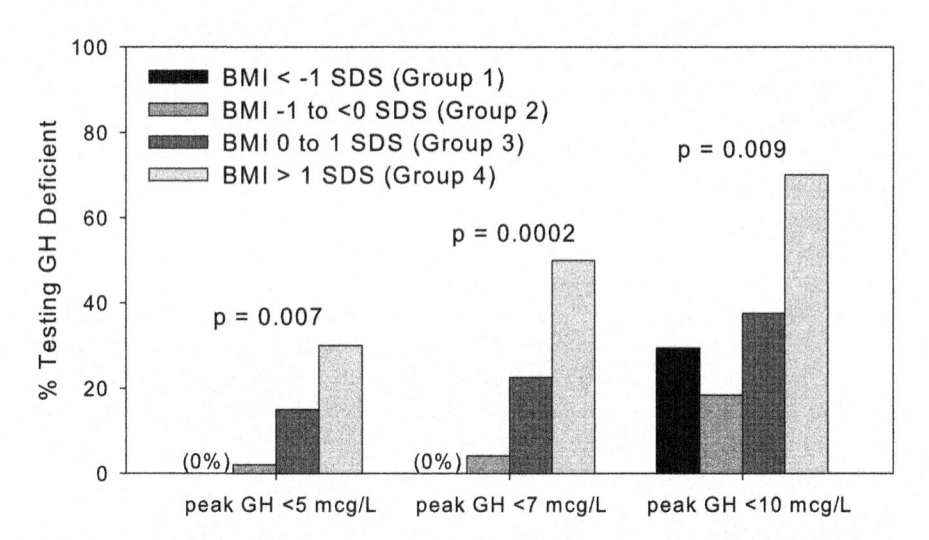

**Fig. 6.3** Percentage of patients testing GH deficient by BMI category for three different peak GH cutoffs: <5, <7, and <10 µg/L. *P*-value is shown for each cutoff [66]. Republished with permission of the Endocrine Society, from Stanley et al., Effect of body mass index on peak growth hormone response to provocative testing in children with short stature. *J Clin Endocrinol Metab.* 2009. 94(12):4875–81. Permission conveyed through Copyright Clearance Center, Inc.

stature who underwent provocative testing with clonidine, Loche et al. showed similar results, with BMI-SDS explaining 21.4 % of the variability in peak GH and with the percentage of children who "failed" GH provocative testing increasing with increasing BMI-SDS [67]. These data suggest that children with relatively high BMI, even within the normal range, may be at risk of overdiagnosis of GHD based on GH provocative testing.

In adults, body weight also affects optimal diagnostic thresholds for GHD. Corneli et al. demonstrated that the optimal threshold for defining GHD following GHRH-arginine stimulation in obese individuals (4.2 µg/L) is less than half that in lean individuals (11.2 µg/L) [68]. More recently, Dichtel et al. showed that the common diagnostic threshold for GHD of 3 µg/L for the glucagon stimulation test classifies 45% of normal controls with BMI ≥25 kg/m$^2$ as having GHD [69]. In this analysis, a peak GH value of 0.94 µg/L for the glucagon stimulation test provided the best combination of sensitivity (90 %) and specificity (94 %) in overweight and obese individuals [69]. Further study is needed to define optimal thresholds for various provocative agents, and currently there are no standard BMI-based thresholds for provocative agents used in pediatrics or for glucagon in adults. These analyses clearly suggest the potential for overdiagnosis of GHD in individuals with higher BMI, and clinicians should consider BMI when interpreting the results of provocative GH testing.

## *Metabolic Effects of GH in Other Indications*

The investigation of relative GHD in obesity highlights potential body composition and metabolic benefits of GH used in other settings. GH is used in individuals with pituitary GHD, Prader–Willi Syndrome (PWS), Turner Syndrome, and small for gestational age (SGA), all of whom may have abnormalities in body composition or metabolic parameters. Many of the effects of GH that are seen in obese individuals are also relevant in these populations (Table 6.2). In children and adults with pituitary GHD, physiologic replacement with GH generally reduces fat mass, particularly visceral fat, increases lean mass, reduces low-density lipoprotein cholesterol (LDL), increases HDL, decreases systemic inflammatory markers, and, in adults, reduces cIMT [71–80]. Awareness of these effects is particularly important in the adolescent transition period, when many adolescents with GHD have their GH replacement stopped for several months or longer. Recent studies have shown that prolonged cessation of GH therapy in adolescents with true GHD decreases lean mass accrual, increases fat mass, and increases LDL [48, 94–96]. Timely retesting and, when indicated, reinitiation of GH treatment in adolescents with GHD may prevent adverse changes in body composition and metabolic profile associated with reduced GH levels.

Whereas long-term cardiovascular effects of GH have not been characterized in other syndromes, including PWS and Turner syndrome, effects on body composition and lipids are well described. In PWS, GH significantly improves lean mass and muscle strength while decreasing fat mass [81, 82, 97]. Effects on lipid

**Table 6.2** Reported effects of GH for various indications on body composition and metabolic parameters

|  | Fat mass | Lean mass | LDL | HDL | Insulin resistance[a] | Inflammatory markers[b] |
|---|---|---|---|---|---|---|
| Obesity [59–63, 70] | ↓ | ↑ | ↓/↔ | ↔ | ↑/↔ | ↓ |
| GHD [71–80] | ↓ | ↑ | ↓/↔ | ↑/↔ | ↑/↔ | ↓ |
| PWS [81–86] | ↓ | ↑ | ↓/↔ | ↑/↔ | ↑/↔ | ↔ |
| Turner [87–89] | ↓ | ↑ | ↓ | ↑ | ↑/↔ | [c] |
| SGA [74, 90–93] | ↓ | ↑ | ↓ | ↔ | ↑/↔ | ↔ |

[a]Insulin resistance was measured variously in different studies as fasting or 2 h glucose, fasting or 2 h insulin, or homeostasis model assessment-estimated insulin resistance (HOMA-IR)
[b]Systemic inflammatory markers such as c-reactive protein, components of the tumor necrosis factor alpha family, and others
[c]Indicates no published data available
*GHD* GH deficiency, *PWS* Prader–Willi syndrome, *SGA* small for gestational age, *LDL* low-density lipoprotein cholesterol, *HDL* high-density lipoprotein cholesterol, *cIMT* carotid intima-media thickness

parameters vary among reports and may be modest or neutral [83, 84]. Similarly, in Turner syndrome, GH reduces fat mass and increases lean mass [87, 88], with one study also showing beneficial effects of increased HDL and reduced LDL [89]. Small for gestational age children are often characterized by lower lean mass and increased fat mass, particularly in the visceral depot [90, 98], whereas GH treatment ameliorates these changes [90, 91]. In addition, GH reduces LDL and triglycerides, with no effect demonstrated on HDL [91]. Of note, as in obesity, GH can be antagonistic to insulin sensitivity in all of these conditions, particularly in the short term (see Table 6.2). Over long-term treatment, however, beneficial changes in body composition, particularly reductions in visceral fat, may counterbalance direct effects of GH on glucose. Thus, while increased insulin levels may persist, clinically relevant abnormalities in glucose are less common [82, 89, 92].

In conditions with altered body composition and possible metabolic dysregulation, clinical consideration of GH use should include the possible benefits of GH on body composition and lipids, as well as the potential effects on glucose homeostasis. Whereas treatment with GH, GHRH, or other GH secretagogues remains entirely investigational in adults with general obesity, further study is needed to determine if some of the benefits of GH with respect to reducing systemic inflammation and improving cardiovascular risk markers are also applicable to other populations such as those mentioned above.

## Conclusion

Adiposity, particularly in the visceral depot, is associated with significant reductions in GH that may, in turn, exacerbate cardiometabolic risk independent of adiposity. Although treatment of obese individuals with GH has shown potential metabolic benefits, it may also be associated with worsening of insulin resistance. These findings raise the question of whether reduced GH in states of obesity is adaptive or maladaptive. At least in some respects, decreased GH is likely to be beneficial in obesity. For example, reductions in GH may ameliorate worsening of glucose homeostasis with progressive weight gain. Alternatively, as discussed above, reductions in GH decreases lipolysis, which may exacerbate fat accumulation, particularly in the visceral compartment. Additionally, evidence suggests that relative reductions in GH is independently associated with unfavorable changes in lipids and systemic inflammatory markers, such that they may potentially worsen the adverse cardiovascular profile of obesity. Additional investigation will be required to determine the degree to which obesity-related alterations in GH are beneficial or disadvantageous. Until further information is available, there is insufficient information to suggest that the relative GHD of obesity is a pathologic condition that requires treatment. Nonetheless, an understanding of altered GH secretion in obesity is critical in the interpretation of tests of the GH-IGF-I axis, and a heightened awareness of the metabolic effects of GH may inform its use in other indications associated with dysmetabolism or abnormal body composition.

# References

1. Albertsson-Wikland K, et al. Analysis of 24-hour growth hormone profiles in healthy boys and girls of normal stature: relation to puberty. J Clin Endocrinol Metab. 1994;78(5):1195–201.
2. Martha Jr PM, et al. Endogenous growth hormone secretion and clearance rates in normal boys, as determined by deconvolution analysis: relationship to age, pubertal status, and body mass. J Clin Endocrinol Metab. 1992;74(2):336–44.
3. Rose SR, et al. Spontaneous growth hormone secretion increases during puberty in normal girls and boys. J Clin Endocrinol Metab. 1991;73(2):428–35.
4. Iranmanesh A, Lizarralde G, Veldhuis JD. Age and relative adiposity are specific negative determinants of the frequency and amplitude of growth hormone (GH) secretory bursts and the half-life of endogenous GH in healthy men. J Clin Endocrinol Metab. 1991;73:1081–8.
5. Riedel M, et al. Pulsatile growth hormone secretion in normal-weight and obese men: differential metabolic regulation during energy restriction. Metabolism. 1995;44(5):605–10.
6. Ghigo E, et al. Arginine potentiates but does not restore the blunted growth hormone response to growth hormone-releasing hormone in obesity. Metabolism. 1992;41(5):560–3.
7. Kopelman PG, et al. Impaired growth hormone response to growth hormone releasing factor and insulin-hypoglycaemia in obesity. Clin Endocrinol (Oxf). 1985;23(1):87–94.
8. Misra M, et al. Lower growth hormone and higher cortisol are associated with greater visceral adiposity, intramyocellular lipids, and insulin resistance in overweight girls. Am J Physiol Endocrinol Metab. 2008;295(2):E385–92.
9. Di Somma C, et al. Prevalence of the metabolic syndrome in moderately-severely obese subjects with and without growth hormone deficiency. J Endocrinol Invest. 2010;33(3):171–7.
10. Utz AL, et al. Growth hormone deficiency by growth hormone releasing hormone-arginine testing criteria predicts increased cardiovascular risk markers in normal young overweight and obese women. J Clin Endocrinol Metab. 2008;93(7):2507–14.
11. Vahl N, et al. Abdominal adiposity rather than age and sex predicts mass and regularity of GH secretion in healthy adults. Am J Physiol. 1997;272(6 Pt 1):E1108–16.
12. Makimura H, et al. The effects of central adiposity on growth hormone (GH) response to GH-releasing hormone-arginine stimulation testing in men. J Clin Endocrinol Metab. 2008;93(11):4254–60.
13. Carmichael JD, et al. GH peak response to GHRH-arginine: relationship to insulin resistance and other cardiovascular risk factors in a population of adults aged 50–90. Clin Endocrinol (Oxf). 2006;65(2):169–77.

14. Rasmussen MH, et al. Massive weight loss restores 24-hour growth hormone release profiles and serum insulin-like growth factor-I levels in obese subjects. J Clin Endocrinol Metab. 1995;80(4):1407–15.
15. Rasmussen MH, Juul A, Hilsted J. Effect of weight loss on free insulin-like growth factor-I in obese women with hyposomatotropism. Obesity (Silver Spring). 2007;15(4):879–86.
16. Stanley TL, et al. Effects of a growth hormone-releasing hormone analog on endogenous GH pulsatility and insulin sensitivity in healthy men. J Clin Endocrinol Metab. 2011;96(1):150–8.
17. Veldhuis JD, et al. Dual defects in pulsatile growth hormone secretion and clearance subserve the hyposomatotropism of obesity in man. J Clin Endocrinol Metab. 1991;72(1):51–9.
18. Veldhuis JD, et al. Differential impact of age, sex steroid hormones, and obesity on basal versus pulsatile growth hormone secretion in men as assessed in an ultrasensitive chemiluminescence assay. J Clin Endocrinol Metab. 1995;80(11):3209–22.
19. Buijs MM, et al. Renal contribution to increased clearance of exogenous growth hormone in obese hypertensive patients. J Clin Endocrinol Metab. 2005;90(2):795–9.
20. Langendonk JG, et al. Influence of obesity and body fat distribution on growth hormone kinetics in humans. Am J Physiol. 1999;277(5 Pt 1):E824–9.
21. Kasa-Vubu JZ, et al. Incomplete modified fast in obese early pubertal girls leads to an increase in 24-hour growth hormone concentration and a lessening of the circadian pattern in leptin. J Clin Endocrinol Metab. 2002;87(4):1885–93.
22. Cornford AS, Barkan AL, Horowitz JF. Rapid suppression of growth hormone concentration by overeating: potential mediation by hyperinsulinemia. J Clin Endocrinol Metab. 2011;96(3):824–30.
23. Luque RM, Kineman RD. Impact of obesity on the growth hormone axis: evidence for a direct inhibitory effect of hyperinsulinemia on pituitary function. Endocrinology. 2006;147(6):2754–63.
24. Luque RM, et al. Examination of the direct effects of metabolic factors on somatotrope function in a non-human primate model *Papio anubis*. J Mol Endocrinol. 2006;37(1):25–38.
25. Casanueva FF, et al. Free fatty acids block growth hormone (GH) releasing hormone-stimulated GH secretion in man directly at the pituitary. J Clin Endocrinol Metab. 1987;65(4):634–42.
26. Cordido F, et al. Impaired growth hormone secretion in obese subjects is partially reversed by acipimox-mediated plasma free fatty acid depression. J Clin Endocrinol Metab. 1996;81(3):914–8.
27. Zhou X, et al. Cafeteria diet-induced obese rats have an increased somatostatin protein content and gene expression in the periventricular nucleus. J Endocrinol Invest. 1997;20(5):264–9.
28. Maccario M, et al. In obesity the somatotrope response to either growth hormone-releasing hormone or arginine is inhibited by somatostatin or pirenzepine but not by glucose. J Clin Endocrinol Metab. 1995;80(12):3774–8.
29. Pena-Bello L, et al. Effect of oral glucose administration on rebound growth hormone release in normal and obese women: the role of adiposity, insulin sensitivity and ghrelin. PLoS One. 2015;10(3), e0121087.
30. Argente J, et al. Multiple endocrine abnormalities of the growth hormone and insulin-like growth factor axis in prepubertal children with exogenous obesity: effect of short- and long-term weight reduction. J Clin Endocrinol Metab. 1997;82(7):2076–83.
31. Attia N, et al. The metabolic syndrome and insulin-like growth factor I regulation in adolescent obesity. J Clin Endocrinol Metab. 1998;83(5):1467–71.
32. Ballerini MG, et al. Differential impact of simple childhood obesity on the components of the growth hormone-insulin-like growth factor (IGF)-IGF binding proteins axis. J Pediatr Endocrinol Metab. 2004;17(5):749–57.
33. Park MJ, et al. Serum levels of insulin-like growth factor (IGF)-I, free IGF-I, IGF binding protein (IGFBP)-1, IGFBP-3 and insulin in obese children. J Pediatr Endocrinol Metab. 1999;12(2):139–44.
34. Radetti G, et al. Growth hormone bioactivity, insulin-like growth factors (IGFs), and IGF binding proteins in obese children. Metabolism. 1998;47(12):1490–3.
35. Saitoh H, et al. Serum concentrations of insulin, insulin-like growth factor(IGF)-I, IGF binding protein (IGFBP)-1 and -3 and growth hormone binding protein in obese children: fasting IGFBP-1 is suppressed in normoinsulinaemic obese children. Clin Endocrinol (Oxf). 1998;48(4):487–92.

36. Wabitsch M, et al. Insulin-like growth factors and their binding proteins before and after weight loss and their associations with hormonal and metabolic parameters in obese adolescent girls. Int J Obes Relat Metab Disord. 1996;20(12):1073–80.
37. Frystyk J, et al. Circulating levels of free insulin-like growth factors in obese subjects: the impact of type 2 diabetes. Diabetes Metab Res Rev. 1999;15(5):314–22.
38. Frystyk J, et al. Bioactive insulin-like growth factor-I in obesity. J Clin Endocrinol Metab. 2009;94(8):3093–7.
39. Gomez JM, et al. The IGF-I system component concentrations that decrease with ageing are lower in obesity in relationship to body mass index and body fat. Growth Horm IGF Res. 2004;14(2):91–6.
40. Nam SY, et al. Effect of obesity on total and free insulin-like growth factor (IGF)-1, and their relationship to IGF-binding protein (BP)-1, IGFBP-2, IGFBP-3, insulin, and growth hormone. Int J Obes Relat Metab Disord. 1997;21(5):355–9.
41. Maccario M, et al. Relationships between IGF-I and age, gender, body mass, fat distribution, metabolic and hormonal variables in obese patients. Int J Obes Relat Metab Disord. 1999;23(6):612–8.
42. Utz AL, et al. Androgens may mediate a relative preservation of IGF-I levels in overweight and obese women despite reduced growth hormone secretion. J Clin Endocrinol Metab. 2008;93(10):4033–40.
43. Lukanova A, et al. Body mass index, circulating levels of sex-steroid hormones, IGF-I and IGF-binding protein-3: a cross-sectional study in healthy women. Eur J Endocrinol. 2004;150(2):161–71.
44. Gleeson HK, Lissett CA, Shalet SM. Insulin-like growth factor-I response to a single bolus of growth hormone is increased in obesity. J Clin Endocrinol Metab. 2005;90(2):1061–7.
45. Yuen KC, et al. Individual igf-I responsiveness to a fixed regimen of low-dose growth hormone replacement is increased with less variability in obese compared to non-obese adults with severe growth hormone deficiency. Horm Res. 2006;65(1):6–13.
46. Frystyk J. Free insulin-like growth factors – measurements and relationships to growth hormone secretion and glucose homeostasis. Growth Horm IGF Res. 2004;14(5):337–75.
47. Chen JW, et al. A highly sensitive and specific assay for determination of IGF-I bioactivity in human serum. Am J Physiol Endocrinol Metab. 2003;284(6):E1149–55.
48. Colao A, et al. The cardiovascular risk of adult GH deficiency (GHD) improved after GH replacement and worsened in untreated GHD: a 12-month prospective study. J Clin Endocrinol Metab. 2002;87(3):1088–93.
49. Colao A, et al. Improved cardiovascular risk factors and cardiac performance after 12 months of growth hormone (GH) replacement in young adult patients with GH deficiency. J Clin Endocrinol Metab. 2001;86(5):1874–81.
50. Colao A, et al. Short-term effects of growth hormone (GH) treatment or deprivation on cardiovascular risk parameters and intima-media thickness at carotid arteries in patients with severe GH deficiency. J Clin Endocrinol Metab. 2005;90(4):2056–62.
51. Devin JK, et al. Markedly impaired fibrinolytic balance contributes to cardiovascular risk in adults with growth hormone deficiency. J Clin Endocrinol Metab. 2007;92(9):3633–9.
52. Lanes R, et al. Cardiac mass and function, carotid artery intima-media thickness, and lipoprotein levels in growth hormone-deficient adolescents. J Clin Endocrinol Metab. 2001;86(3):1061–5.
53. Lanes R, et al. Growth hormone deficiency, low levels of adiponectin, and unfavorable plasma lipid and lipoproteins. J Pediatr. 2006;149(3):324–9.
54. Bredella MA, et al. Peak growth hormone-releasing hormone-arginine-stimulated growth hormone is inversely associated with intramyocellular and intrahepatic lipid content in premenopausal women with obesity. J Clin Endocrinol Metab. 2009;94(10):3995–4002.
55. Makimura H, et al. Reduced growth hormone secretion is associated with increased carotid intima-media thickness in obesity. J Clin Endocrinol Metab. 2009;94(12):5131–8.
56. Makimura H, et al. Reduced growth hormone secretion in obesity is associated with smaller LDL and HDL particle size. Clin Endocrinol (Oxf). 2012;76(2):220–7.

57. Russell M, et al. Relative growth hormone deficiency and cortisol excess are associated with increased cardiovascular risk markers in obese adolescent girls. J Clin Endocrinol Metab. 2009;94(8):2864–71.
58. Stanley TL, Grinspoon SK. Effects of growth hormone-releasing hormone on visceral fat, metabolic, and cardiovascular indices in human studies. Growth Horm IGF Res. 2015;25(2):59–65.
59. Mekala KC, Tritos NA. Effects of recombinant human growth hormone therapy in obesity in adults: a meta analysis. J Clin Endocrinol Metab. 2009;94(1):130–7.
60. Johannsson G, et al. Growth hormone treatment of abdominally obese men reduces abdominal fat mass, improves glucose and lipoprotein metabolism, and reduces diastolic blood pressure. J Clin Endocrinol Metab. 1997;82(3):727–34.
61. Franco C, et al. Growth hormone treatment reduces abdominal visceral fat in postmenopausal women with abdominal obesity: a 12-month placebo-controlled trial. J Clin Endocrinol Metab. 2005;90:1466–74.
62. Bredella MA, et al. Effects of GH on body composition and cardiovascular risk markers in young men with abdominal obesity. J Clin Endocrinol Metab. 2013;98(9):3864–72.
63. Bredella MA, et al. Effects of GH in women with abdominal adiposity: a 6-month randomized, double-blind, placebo-controlled trial. Eur J Endocrinol. 2012;166(4):601–11.
64. Lin E, et al. Effects of growth hormone withdrawal in obese premenopausal women. Clin Endocrinol (Oxf). 2013;78(6):914–9.
65. Makimura H, et al. Metabolic effects of a growth hormone-releasing factor in obese subjects with reduced growth hormone secretion: a randomized controlled trial. J Clin Endocrinol Metab. 2012;97(12):4769–79.
66. Stanley TL, et al. Effect of body mass index on peak growth hormone response to provocative testing in children with short stature. J Clin Endocrinol Metab. 2009;94(12):4875–81.
67. Loche S, et al. Effect of body mass index on the growth hormone response to clonidine stimulation testing in children with short stature. Clin Endocrinol (Oxf). 2011;74(6):726–31.
68. Corneli G, et al. The cut-off limits of the GH response to GH-releasing hormone-arginine test related to body mass index. Eur J Endocrinol. 2005;153(2):257–64.
69. Dichtel LE, et al. Overweight/obese adults with pituitary disorders require lower peak growth hormone cutoff values on glucagon stimulation testing to avoid overdiagnosis of growth hormone deficiency. J Clin Endocrinol Metab. 2014;99(12):4712–9.
70. Franco C, et al. Growth hormone reduces inflammation in postmenopausal women with abdominal obesity: a 12-month, randomized, placebo-controlled trial. J Clin Endocrinol Metab. 2007;92(7):2644–7.
71. Colao A, et al. Growth hormone treatment on atherosclerosis: results of a 5-year open, prospective, controlled study in male patients with severe growth hormone deficiency. J Clin Endocrinol Metab. 2008;93(9):3416–24.
72. Boot AM, et al. Changes in bone mineral density, body composition, and lipid metabolism during growth hormone (GH) treatment in children with GH deficiency. J Clin Endocrinol Metab. 1997;82(8):2423–8.
73. Roemmich JN, et al. Alterations in body composition and fat distribution in growth hormone-deficient prepubertal children during growth hormone therapy. Metabolism. 2001;50(5):537–47.
74. Schweizer R, et al. Similar effects of long-term exogenous growth hormone (GH) on bone and muscle parameters: a pQCT study of GH-deficient and small-for-gestational-age (SGA) children. Bone. 2007;41(5):875–81.
75. van der Sluis IM, et al. Long-term effects of growth hormone therapy on bone mineral density, body composition, and serum lipid levels in growth hormone deficient children: a 6-year follow-up study. Horm Res. 2002;58(5):207–14.
76. Attanasio AF, et al. Human growth hormone replacement in adult hypopituitary patients: long-term effects on body composition and lipid status--3-year results from the HypoCCS Database. J Clin Endocrinol Metab. 2002;87(4):1600–6.
77. Ciresi A, et al. Metabolic parameters and adipokine profile during GH replacement therapy in children with GH deficiency. Eur J Endocrinol. 2007;156(3):353–60.
78. Soares DV, et al. Carotid artery intima-media thickness and lipid profile in adults with growth hormone deficiency after long-term growth hormone replacement. Metabolism. 2005;54(3):321–9.

79. Deepak D, et al. The influence of growth hormone replacement on peripheral inflammatory and cardiovascular risk markers in adults with severe growth hormone deficiency. Growth Horm IGF Res. 2010;20(3):220–5.
80. Hoffman AR, et al. Growth hormone (GH) replacement therapy in adult-onset gh deficiency: effects on body composition in men and women in a double-blind, randomized, placebo-controlled trial. J Clin Endocrinol Metab. 2004;89(5):2048–56.
81. Lafortuna CL, et al. Skeletal muscle characteristics and motor performance after 2-year growth hormone treatment in adults with Prader–Willi syndrome. J Clin Endocrinol Metab. 2014;99(5):1816–24.
82. Bakker NE, et al. Eight years of growth hormone treatment in children with Prader–Willi syndrome: maintaining the positive effects. J Clin Endocrinol Metab. 2013;98(10):4013–22.
83. de Lind van Wijngaarden RF, et al. Cardiovascular and metabolic risk profile and acylation-stimulating protein levels in children with Prader–Willi syndrome and effects of growth hormone treatment. J Clin Endocrinol Metab. 2010;95(4):1758–66.
84. l'Allemand D, et al. Cardiovascular risk factors improve during 3 years of growth hormone therapy in Prader–Willi syndrome. Eur J Pediatr. 2000;159(11):835–42.
85. Jorgensen AP, et al. Glucose homeostasis in adults with Prader–Willi syndrome during treatment with growth hormone: results from a 12-month prospective study. Growth Horm IGF Res. 2014;24(1):16–21.
86. Hoybye C. Inflammatory markers in adults with Prader–Willi syndrome before and during 12 months growth hormone treatment. Horm Res. 2006;66(1):27–32.
87. Gravholt CH, et al. Short-term growth hormone treatment in girls with Turner syndrome decreases fat mass and insulin sensitivity: a randomized, double-blind, placebo-controlled, crossover study. Pediatrics. 2002;110(5):889–96.
88. Ari M, et al. The effects of growth hormone treatment on bone mineral density and body composition in girls with turner syndrome. J Clin Endocrinol Metab. 2006;91(11):4302–5.
89. van Teunenbroek A, et al. Carbohydrate and lipid metabolism during various growth hormone dosing regimens in girls with Turner syndrome. Dutch Working Group on Growth Hormone. Metabolism. 1999;48(1):7–14.
90. Boonstra VH, et al. Food intake of children with short stature born small for gestational age before and during a randomized GH trial. Horm Res. 2006;65(1):23–30.
91. Sas T, Mulder P, Hokken-Koelega A. Body composition, blood pressure, and lipid metabolism before and during long-term growth hormone (GH) treatment in children with short stature born small for gestational age either with or without GH deficiency. J Clin Endocrinol Metab. 2000;85(10):3786–92.
92. Sas T, et al. Carbohydrate metabolism during long-term growth hormone treatment in children with short stature born small for gestational age. Clin Endocrinol (Oxf). 2001;54(2):243–51.
93. Willemsen RH, et al. Long-term GH treatment is not associated with disadvantageous changes of inflammatory markers and adipocytokines in children born small for gestational age. Clin Endocrinol (Oxf). 2008;68(2):198–205.
94. Johannsson G, Albertsson-Wikland K, Bengtsson BA. Discontinuation of growth hormone (GH) treatment: metabolic effects in GH-deficient and GH-sufficient adolescent patients compared with control subjects. Swedish Study Group for Growth Hormone Treatment in Children. J Clin Endocrinol Metab. 1999;84(12):4516–24.
95. Carroll PV, et al. Comparison of continuation or cessation of growth hormone (GH) therapy on body composition and metabolic status in adolescents with severe GH deficiency at completion of linear growth. J Clin Endocrinol Metab. 2004;89(8):3890–5.
96. Koltowska-Haggstrom M, et al. Discontinuation of growth hormone (GH) treatment during the transition phase is an important factor determining the phenotype of young adults with nonidiopathic childhood-onset GH deficiency. J Clin Endocrinol Metab. 2010;95(6):2646–54.
97. de Lind van Wijngaarden RF, et al. Efficacy and safety of long-term continuous growth hormone treatment in children with Prader–Willi syndrome. J Clin Endocrinol Metab. 2009;94(11):4205–15.
98. Ibanez L, et al. Visceral adiposity without overweight in children born small for gestational age. J Clin Endocrinol Metab. 2008;93(6):2079–83.

# Chapter 7
# Metabolic Benefits of Growth Hormone Therapy

**Roberto Lanes**

## Introduction

Cardiovascular morbidity and mortality have been found to be increased in adult subjects with growth hormone (GH) deficiency (GHD). Long-term follow-up of a large cohort of patients with adult-onset (AO) GHD suggests that GH therapy may contribute to a reduced risk of nonfatal stroke, particularly in women, and in a decline in nonfatal cardiac events in GHD men [1, 2].

A cluster of cardiovascular risk factors such as increased visceral adiposity, abnormalities in lipoprotein metabolism, premature atherosclerosis, impaired fibrinolytic activity, peripheral insulin resistance, abnormal cardiac structure and function, and endothelial dysfunction have been reported in adult hypopituitary patients with untreated GHD [3, 4]. Several of these risk factors have now been confirmed in double-blind, randomized, placebo-controlled trials [5, 6]. Metabolic abnormalities have been evaluated only in a small number of GHD children and adolescents. In this chapter, we will review these abnormalities and their underlying mechanisms, and we will discuss the beneficial effect of GH treatment in GHD subjects.

## Body Composition

Obesity, and in particular abdominal adiposity, appears to be a major risk factor for cardiovascular disease, possibly through their association with atherosclerosis and arterial stiffness. Several studies have reported abnormalities in body composition

---

R. Lanes (✉)
Pediatric Endocrine Unit, Hospital de Clinicas Caracas, Caracas, Venezuela
e-mail: lanesroberto@gmail.com

in GHD adults, adolescents, and children, with a reduction in lean body mass and an increase in fat mass, particularly with abdominal/visceral obesity; GH therapy reduces the volume of the adipose tissue and increases the amount of muscle. Two double-blind, randomized, placebo-controlled trials in GH-treated men and women confirmed significant decreases in total body and trunk fat and increases in lean body mass over baseline [5, 6]. Body fat was increased in young adults with childhood-onset GHD (CO), while lean mass and muscle strength were decreased in this group, when compared to subjects with AO GHD [7]. During GH treatment, the increase in lean mass was more marked in CO patients, so that after 5 years of therapy, there was no difference between the CO and the AO group in any variable reflecting body composition.

During treatment, Kuromaru et al. [8] reported a decrease in the mean obesity index value of 6.1 % in boys and of 9.7 % in GHD girls, while the waist-hip ratio did not change appreciably in either sex. Body fat decreased significantly in both boys and girls during the first 6 months of therapy, remained constant in boys, and increased in girls after 2 years, while lean body mass increased significantly in both sexes throughout the treatment period. Capalbo et al. recently [9] found that GHD children at study entry had a higher waist-to-height ratio than healthy controls; GH therapy was associated with a significant reduction in this parameter. After discontinuing GH treatment once adult height was attained and during a 2-year observation period, Johannsson and collaborators [10] detected a decrease in lean body mass and an increase in body fat and in the amount of truncal fat in GHD adolescents. Carrol et al. [11] reported that maintaining GH once adult height was attained resulted in ongoing accrual of lean body mass over the next year, whereas skeletal muscle mass remained static once GH was discontinued. These studies suggest that discontinuation of GH therapy in adolescents with GHD at adult height could lead to long-term adverse physical and metabolic consequences.

Not only does muscle mass increase in GHD patients on GH treatment, but an increase in muscle strength and improved exercise performance have been noted in these patients. Svensson et al. [12] demonstrated how GH replacement therapy in subjects with AO GHD normalized isometric and isokinetic knee flexor and extensor strength, while handgrip strength increased. Ter Maaten et al. [13] demonstrated an increase in the maximal workload and in oxygen consumption in GHD adults after long-term GH therapy.

## Fasting and Postprandial Lipids

Elevated cholesterol and triglyceride levels have been reported in untreated GHD subjects. Elevated fasting cholesterol and triglyceride levels were reported by our group (Table 7.1) in two cohorts of untreated GHD adolescents [14, 15], and similar results were reported by Johansson et al. [10] who noted an increase in total and low-density lipoprotein (LDL) cholesterol after discontinuation of GH treatment in GHD adolescents who had reached adult height. Recent blinded, randomized,

**Table 7.1** Total, LDL and HDL cholesterol, triglycerides, lipoprotein(a), fibrinogen, PAI-1, homocysteine, folate, and vitamin B12 in untreated and treated GHD adolescents and healthy controls

|  | Untreated GHD (n=10) | Treated GHD (n=15) | Non-GHD controls (n=15) | P< |
|---|---|---|---|---|
| Total cholesterol (mg/dL) | 178.8±46.7 | 187.3±38.3 | 167.5±28.7 | 0.05* |
| HDL cholesterol (mg/dL) | 53.1±3.3 | 53.3±13.3 | 46.6±8.5 | NS |
| LDL cholesterol (mg/dL) | 112.1±43.8 | 112.2±29.5 | 110.9±27.3 | NS |
| Triglycerides (mg/dL) | 105.5±51.2 | 86.9±29.6 | 69.0±35.6 | 0.05** |
| Lipoprotein(a) (mg/dL) | 26.0±29.3 | 32.5±35.5 | 28.9±31.3 | NS |
| Fibrinogen (mg/dL) | 169.4±30 | 194.2±59.4 | 149.2±23.3 | 0.01+ |
| PAI-1 (ng/mL) | 35.5±13.6 | 46.2±11.9 | 38.3±16.3 | NS |
| Homocysteine (μmol/L) | 10.5±2.7 | 7.4+1.3 | 7.3+2.8 | 0.04** |
| Folate (mg/dL) | 2.3±0.7 | 4.3±1.7 | 5.3±3.9 | 0.04** |
| Vitamin B12 (mg/dL) | 396.2±164.0 | 609.3±251.8 | 430.0±166.0 | 0.02* |

Modified from Lanes et al. Hormone Res. 2003;60:291–295
* On GH vs controls
** Off GH vs on GH and controls
+On and off GH vs controls

placebo-controlled trials have confirmed a significant decrease in total cholesterol and in LDL cholesterol levels following GH treatment in GHD adults when compared with those of placebo-treated subjects [16, 17].

Abnormalities in serum lipids in GHD patients may be due to an increase in the secretion rate and a reduction in the clearance rate of very low-density lipoproteins (VLDL). Increased VLDL-apo B secretion is probably related to abdominal obesity in GHD patients, as abdominal obesity when combined with insulin resistance increases VLDL-apo B secretion from the liver. Short-term GH treatment has been shown to increase the VLDL-apo B clearance rate.

Considerable evidence suggesting a positive correlation between the postprandial triglyceride response to an oral lipid load and atherosclerosis of the carotid and coronary arteries has been reported in adults. Elevated plasma levels of triglycerides and triglyceride-rich lipoprotein particles (TRP), consisting of VLDL containing apo B-100 of hepatic origin and chylomicrons containing apo B48 of intestinal origin, have been found to be associated with increased carotid artery intima-media thickness (IMT) and cardiovascular mortality. In adult GHD subjects, Al-Shoumer et al. [18] and Twickler et al. [19] reported increased fasting and postprandial levels of triglycerides and TRP, suggesting that these changes may contribute to their increased vascular morbidity and mortality. Our group reported a significant increase in postprandial triglycerides following an oral lipid load in untreated GHD adolescents, when compared to that of both treated GHD subjects and to that of healthy controls (Fig. 7.1) [15]. The accumulation of postprandial TRP in GHD may be explained by a decrease in their removal from the circulation via hepatic lipoprotein receptors, as the expression of several hepatic surface receptors such as LDL and LDL receptor-related protein receptors has been found to be lower in GHD states than in healthy subjects.

Growth hormone therapy would seem to improve both the fasting and the postprandial atherogenic lipoprotein profile in AO GHD, as demonstrated by a decrease

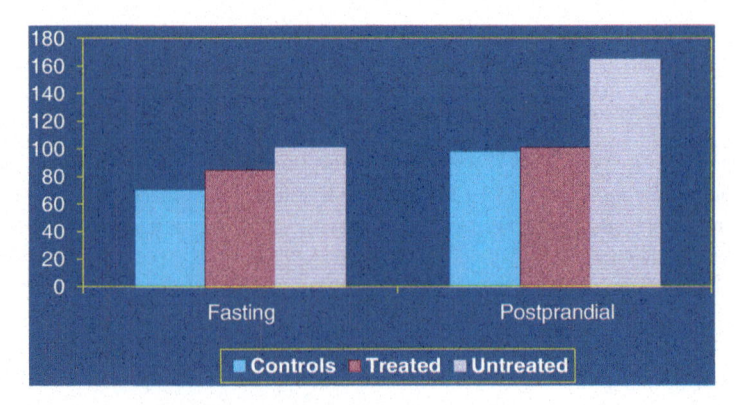

**Fig. 7.1** Fasting and postprandial triglycerides in GHD adolescents and healthy controls (Modified from Lanes et al. Hormone Res. 2003;60:291–295)

of fasting lipids and of postprandial lipoprotein remnants following GH administration [20]. This beneficial effect of GH was also noted by us, as both fasting and postprandial triglyceride levels of treated GHD teenagers were found to be significantly lower than those of untreated ones [15]. In two recent studies, De Marco et al. [21] and Capalbo et al. [9] reported significantly higher levels of asymmetric dimethylarginine (ADMA), triglycerides, total cholesterol, and LDL cholesterol at baseline in GHD children when compared to healthy controls. After 12 months of GH treatment, ADMA, total cholesterol, and LDL cholesterol significantly decreased, reaching values comparable to those in controls. This beneficial effect of GH treatment has been shown to result from an increased expression of hepatic surface receptors.

Lipoprotein(a) is an independently atherogenic lipoprotein that can be thrombogenic and may be used as a plasmatic marker for individuals at risk for cardiovascular events. While we [14] found both treated and untreated GHD adolescents to have elevated lipoprotein(a) levels when compared to healthy controls, Capalbo et al. [9] found no difference in lipoprotein(a) levels between untreated CO GHD adults and healthy controls.

## Coagulation Factors

Fibrinogen, tissue plasminogen activator inhibitor-1 (PAI-1), and factor VII concentrations have been reported to be elevated in GHD adults, suggesting a defective fibrinolytic system. Colao et al. [17] demonstrated that both treated and untreated GHD adults had elevated fibrinogen levels when compared to healthy subjects. In a cohort of young adult GHD patients diagnosed either at childhood or at adulthood, 12 months of GH replacement significantly reduced fibrinogen, but without reaching normal levels. Our results in adolescents were similar to those of Colao et al., as both our treated and untreated GHD subjects had elevated fasting fibrinogen levels (Table 7.1) [15];

and in a recent study by Capalbo et al. [9] in 71 GHD children, fibrinogen concentrations were elevated prior to treatment when compared to controls, with a significant reduction of this parameter following 2 years of GH treatment. While elevated PAI-1 concentrations were detected in untreated GHD adults [22] and children [23], levels of PAI-1 were not increased in either our treated or untreated GHD adolescents [15]. Fibrinogen has been shown to be an independent risk factor for stroke and myocardial infarction [24], while PAI-1 activity has been associated with an increased risk for recurrent myocardial infarction [25]. Additionally, abdominal adiposity has been found to be associated with increased concentrations of fibrinogen and PAI-1 activity, so the increase of these parameters in subjects with GHD may be linked to their increased waist-hip ratio; and elevated triglycerides might contribute to the elevated PAI-1 activity. This prothrombotic state, with reduced fibrinolytic activity, may therefore contribute to an increased risk for atherothrombotic events in GHD patients.

## Homocysteine

Elevated homocysteine plasma levels are believed to be independent risk factors for cardiovascular events. Experimental and clinical evidence indicate that homocysteine is prothrombotic, and therefore, high concentrations are associated with vascular endothelial injury and dysfunction. Evans et al. [26], in a preliminary report in a small number of subjects, reported a doubling of plasma homocysteine levels in GHD adults when compared to matched controls. Sesmilo et al. [27] found the median homocysteine level at baseline in GHD adults to be almost identical to the reported 90th percentile of a comparable subset from a large cross-sectional US study of non-GHD adults; when treated with GH, a significant decrease in homocysteine was noted. However, Abdu et al. [28] did not detect an elevation in plasma homocysteine in GHD adults when compared to controls. Folate intake is inversely correlated with fasting homocysteine, and folate supplements, with or without vitamins B6 and B12, have been reported to reduce homocysteine levels. In their group of AO GHD patients, Sesmilo et al. [27] found homocysteine at baseline to be negatively correlated with plasma levels of folate. These results are in agreement with our finding of increased homocysteine concentrations and decreased folate and vitamin B12 levels in young untreated GHD adolescents, when compared to both treated GHD subjects and to healthy controls (Table 7.1) [15] and to the findings of Capalbo et al. [9] of elevated homocysteine concentrations in GHD children prior to treatment, with a significant reduction of these levels following 2 years of GH therapy.

## Endothelial Dysfunction

Endothelial dysfunction in GHD patients may be a direct consequence of the low levels of GH and insulin-like growth factor-I (IGF-I) seen in these patients. GH and IGF-I stimulate the production and the release of nitric oxide in the endothelium and induce vasodilation. IGF-I is a potent stimulator of the phosphatidylinositol 3-kinase/protein kinase B/endothelial NO synthase pathway. In healthy middle-age volunteers, GH treatment induced markers of increased NO bioavailability and enhanced circulating endothelial progenitor cell numbers, and this effect was mediated via an increase in IGF-I plasma levels; blocking of the IGF-I receptor in vivo abolished the GH-mediated effect on markers of increased NO bioavailability [29]. However, recent data suggest that GH may also regulate vascular reactivity through a direct action on the GH receptor in the vascular endothelium to increase endothelial nitric oxide synthase phosphorylation and activity [30]. This conclusion is based on data that indicate that GH exerts an acute vasodilatory effect independent of both systemic and local IGF-I production, that human aortic endothelial cells express abundant amount of GH receptors and that GH causes a time-dependent increase in the phosphorylation and activity of endothelial nitric oxide synthase.

Endothelial dysfunction may also occur due to an indirect action in the atherogenic process induced by alterations in lipoprotein metabolism and the accumulation of lipoproteic remnants. In the postprandial phase, these remnants are predominantly and highly atherogenic stimulating an increased formation of macrophages and the induction of vascular inflammation. An increase in plasma triglyceride levels during daily regular meals and of postprandial lipoprotein remnant concentrations has been reported in GHD adults. Twickler et al. [19, 20] recently demonstrated that plasma levels of proinflammatory cytokines such as interleukin (IL)-6 and tumor necrosis factor-alpha (TNF-α) are increased during the postprandial period in GH-deficient adults and are related to the presence of elevated levels of lipoprotein remnants, suggesting that lipoprotein remnants may induce an inflammatory response in endothelial cells and macrophages. GH replacement therapy has been shown to reduce the levels of lipoprotein remnants and of serum levels of both C-reactive protein (CRP) and IL-6 and to decrease the IMT of GHD adults.

In addition, Leonsson et al. [31] have demonstrated that untreated GHD adults have increased levels of CRP and IL-6 and that IL-6 concentrations are independently associated with the degree of common carotid artery IMT. In GHD adolescents, we have reported elevated serum levels of CRP, TNF-α, and fibrinogen when compared to healthy controls [32], so that a pronounced inflammatory response seems to exist as early as in adolescence in GHD subjects. GH replacement has been shown to reduce the increased monocytic production and the serum levels of proinflammatory cytokines in GHD adults, suggesting that GH may play a role in the regulation of the vascular wall inflammation.

While endothelial cells were long considered inactive, acting only as a semipermanent barrier between blood and tissue, there are now increasing data that support the role of the vascular endothelium in the maintenance of homeostasis and vascular tone. When activated, the vascular endothelium changes the balance between mechanisms that control vasoconstriction and thrombosis and those favoring vasodilation and fibrinolysis. In response to their activation, endothelial cells are known to express a number of molecules, including adhesion molecules such as E-selectin, intercellular adhesion molecule-1 (ICAM-1), and vascular cell adhesion protein-1 (VCAM-1), which play a role in the modulation of leukocyte recruitment and platelet adhesion during thrombosis and inflammation. Upregulation of endothelial adhesion molecules plays a key role in the earliest phases of atherogenesis by allowing leukocyte and monocyte adhesion to the endothelial cell surface and their migration to the subendothelial space, where they facilitate the atherogenic process. Activated platelets also participate in this process by modulating chemotactic and adhesive properties of endothelial cells. Elevation of several biochemical markers of endothelial cell activation, such as VCAM-1 and P-selectin, have been reported by our group in GHD adolescents [33], with flow-mediated endothelium-dependent vasodilation following hyperemia correlating with P-selectin in these patients. An association between biochemical and biophysical markers of endothelial dysfunction has also been detected in adults with hypopituitarism and severe GH deficiency [34], suggesting a role for GHD, as early as in adolescence, in the development of the atherogenic process.

## Adiponectin

While adipose tissue was considered until recently to be an organ for fat storage and mobilization, recent evidence suggests that it is a highly active endocrine organ. Adiponectin, an adipocytokine that is exclusively and abundantly expressed in adipose tissue, has been proposed to contribute to the development of insulin resistance and type 2 diabetes, coronary artery disease, and endothelial dysfunction in adults. Adiponectin seems to be secreted principally by visceral adipose tissue, so that the size of the visceral fat depot is an important correlate of adiponectin levels. In obese adolescents, several studies have demonstrated that adiponectin is positively correlated to HDL cholesterol and negatively associated with triglycerides and insulin resistance. In addition, a recent report provided the first evidence of early atherosclerotic lesions associated with hypoadiponectinemia in obese juveniles [35]. Subjects of all ages with GHD display many features of the metabolic syndrome including increased abdominal fat with more visceral adiposity than normal healthy controls for a given body mass index (BMI), elevated levels of LDL cholesterol and triglycerides, and endothelial dysfunction. Several reports have suggested that these abnormalities can be reversed by GH therapy. The effect of GH replacement on adiponectin levels in adult GHD patients has been evaluated by several recent studies and has led to conflicting results [36, 37]. We have found adiponectin concentrations to be decreased in untreated GHD adolescents when compared to both treated GHD subjects and to healthy controls (Table 7.2); adiponectin correlated positively with HDL cholesterol concentrations in both treated and untreated patients and negatively with BMI, waist-hip ratio, fasting total and LDL cholesterol, triglycerides, apo B, and insulin levels in our untreated GHD adolescents [38]. In a recent study, Capalbo et al. [9] found 2 years of GH therapy to be associated with a significant increase in adiponectin levels in GHD children.

Increased circulating adiponectin levels have been shown to inhibit both the expression of hepatic gluconeogenic enzymes and the rate of endogenous glucose production, with an improvement in insulin sensitivity. However, the mechanism explaining the

**Table 7.2** Fasting adiponectin, insulin, lipids, and lipoproteins in treated and untreated GHD adolescents and healthy controls

|  | Treated GHD ($n=12$) | Untreated GHD ($n=12$) | Non-GHD controls ($n=12$) | $p<$ |
|---|---|---|---|---|
| Adiponectin (µg/mL) | 16.5±7.4 | 12.7±6.1 | 16.2±5.1 | 0.008* |
| Insulin (µLU/mL) | 7.9±5.2 | 5.3±2.7 | 3.8±2.1 | 0.05^ |
| Total cholesterol (mg/dL) | 154.9±38.6 | 190.4±51.6 | 155.1±26.6 | 0.03* |
| LDL cholesterol (mg/dL) | 95.9±28.9 | 123.9±52.3 | 100.8±39.1 | 0.01* |
| HDL cholesterol (mg/dL) | 47.8±26.9 | 43.8±10.1 | 45.0±9.9 | NS |
| Triglycerides (mg/dL) | 74.6±29.8 | 88.3±37.2 | 76.2±40.3 | 0.001* |
| Apolipoprotein A-1 (mg/dL) | 84.5±41.1 | 109.6±40.5 | 97.2±45.6 | NS |
| Apolipoprotein B (mg/dL) | 40.3±15.4 | 59.6±21.3 | 44.8±22.9 | 0.009* |

Modified Lanes et al. J Pediatr. 2006;149:324–329
*untreated GHD vs treated GHD and controls
^treated GHD vs controls

link between adiponectin and triglycerides is not clear. In a recent study in obese adolescents, Weiss et al. [39] suggested that adiponectin might affect the production of VLDL particles from the liver, thereby regulating serum triglycerides, so that one could speculate that in untreated GHD, low adiponectin may contribute to the increased secretion of VLDL-apo B-100 and triglycerides.

## Cardiac Mass and Function

The impairment in cardiac performance in young GHD adults is manifested by a reduction in left ventricular mass, an inadequate ejection fraction, and in abnormalities of left ventricular diastolic filling [40]. GH administration has been shown to increase left ventricular mass and function in these patients [41]. In an initial study in untreated GHD adolescents, we were unable to find any abnormalities in cardiac mass, as the interventricular septal thickness, the left ventricular posterior wall thickness, and the left ventricular mass after correction for body surface area were all similar to that of healthy controls. Cardiac function of untreated GHD adolescents was also not different from that of healthy controls, as our adolescents had normal left ventricular ejection fraction at rest, as well as normal pulmonary venous flow velocities. Cardiac mass or function was also not different in treated vs. untreated GHD patients [14].

While Colao et al. [42] and Salerno et al. [43] found no change in the heart rate, systolic and diastolic blood pressure, and in the left ventricular ejection fraction of GHD adolescents upon discontinuing GH for 6 months, GH withdrawal slightly decreased cardiac size and impaired the diastolic filling of GHD adolescents. This is in agreement with the echocardiographic findings of two other studies in children with severe classical GHD by Shulman and ourselves [44, 45], which demonstrated that cardiac growth may be impeded by severe childhood GHD (Table 7.3); moreover, an increase in left ventricular mass normalized for changes in body size was

Table 7.3 Cardiac dimensions and volumes in GHD patients with and without GH replacement compared to healthy controls

|  | Off GH (n=12) | On GH (n=10) | Controls (n=14) | P< |
|---|---|---|---|---|
| Interventricular septal thickness (mm) | 6.9±1.1 | 6.9±0.6 | 7.0±1.1 | NS |
| LV posterior wall thickness (mm) | 6.5±1.1 | 6.6±1.3 | 6.9±1.3 | NS |
| Left ventricular mass (g/m$^2$) | 42.2±2.4 | 43.5±6.3 | 49.9±9.0 | 0.05* |
| Ventricular ejection fraction (%) | 64.9±5.4 | 68.6±3.0 | 65.0±5.0 | NS |

Modified from Lanes et al. J Clin Endocrinol Metab. 2005;90:3978–3982
* untreated and treated GHD vs controls

noted by Shulman following GH therapy [44]. Recently, Nygren et al. [46] reported that left ventricular mass indexed to body surface area increased significantly during 2 years of GH treatment in a large population of GHD children, irrespective of randomized dose. This change was already apparent at 3 months of treatment, when standard deviation scores (SDS) of wall thickness and diameter were increased; at 24 months, left ventricular diameter SDS remained increased, whereas myocardial thickness SDS returned to baseline values. Similar findings were also recently reported by Esen et al. [47]. These two studies demonstrated that GH therapy causes an increase in myocardial mass without changing the geometry or function of the myocardium. Therefore, the increase in myocardial mass appears to be concentric, thus causing remodeling instead of hypertrophy.

## Intima-Media Thickness and Vascular Reactivity

Increased IMT, with more atheromatous plaques in the carotid and the femoral arteries when compared to controls matched for age, sex, and body weight, was recently detected in GHD adults [48]. This increased IMT, which represents the earliest morphological change in the arterial wall in the process of atherogenesis, has been detected in the absence of clear-cut abnormalities of classic vascular risk factors.

Growth hormone treatment has been recently shown to reverse early atherosclerotic changes, with a decrease in carotid artery IMT and an improvement of flow-mediated dilation of the brachial artery in GHD adults [48]. With long-term GH substitution, this improvement in arterial performance is maintained [49]. While no significant difference in the carotid artery IMT of untreated GHD adolescents and that of healthy controls or treated GHD subjects was noted by Colao et al. [42] and ourselves [14, 45], a clear tendency toward an increase in IMT was detected in our untreated GHD adolescents (Table 7.4) [45] and in the patients of Colao et al. after discontinuing GH for 6 months. The flow-mediated endothelium-dependent increase in the diameter of the brachial artery during hyperemia was found by us to be lower in untreated GHD adolescents than in GHD-treated subjects or healthy controls,

**Table 7.4** Carotid artery intima-media thickness and brachial artery diameter and blood flow in GHD patients on and off GH replacement compared to healthy controls

|  | Off GH ($n=12$) | On GH ($n=10$) | Controls ($n=14$) | $P<$ |
|---|---|---|---|---|
| Carotid artery intima-media thickness (mm) | 0.9±0.2 | 0.7±0.1 | 0.8±0.2 | NS |
| Increase in brachial artery diameter (%) | 15.4±1.1 | 23.7±1.3 | 29.8±2.1 | 0.02* |
| Increase in brachial artery blood flow (%) | 179±69 | 253.2±43 | 144.4±70.7 | 0.001^ |

Modified from Lanes et al. J Clin Endocrinol Metab. 2005;90:3978–3982
*untreated GHD vs treated GHD and controls
^treated GHD vs untreated GHD and controls

while the blood flow increase of the brachial artery after hyperemia was greater in treated than in untreated adolescents (Table 7.4) [45].

However, not all studies have demonstrated a positive effect of GH therapy on these parameters. While GH treatment had a reversible beneficial effect on body composition, on the metabolic profile, and on cardiac morphology in a large Brazilian kindred with lifelong severe and isolated GHD due to a homozygous mutation in the GHRH receptor gene, it resulted in a progressive increase in the IMT and in the number of atherosclerotic carotid plaques [50], casting doubts on the positive effects of GH replacement therapy on these parameters.

## Insulin Resistance

Growth hormone has antagonistic effects to that of insulin, and a decrease in insulin sensitivity has been reported in acromegaly, in puberty, or during GH replacement therapy. Children with GHD have a larger tendency to present with hypoglycemia both fasting and induced, possibly due to an alteration in the regulation of counter-regulatory hormones and an increase in insulin sensitivity. This susceptibility to hypoglycemia tends to diminish with age, and adults with GHD present with insulin resistance even before GH administration; this could be due to changes in body composition, metabolic responses to GH, or to the interaction with sex hormones.

In children with GHD, Husbands and collaborators [51] measured the glucose disappearance rate following a modified insulin tolerance test and demonstrated that these patients were more sensitive to insulin than children with normal GH secretion. This effect decreased with advancing age and puberty, possibly due to the development of central obesity and the secretion of sex steroids. Recently [23], children with GHD were found to have lower levels of glucose, insulin, and HOMA-IR index when compared to those of healthy controls. After 6 months of treatment, glucose levels increased, though not significantly, while insulin levels and HOMA-IR index rose to normal levels. A positive correlation between changes in insulin status/HOMA-IR index and levels of aPAI-1, fibrinogen, vWF, CRP, and IL-6 was detected. However, in a group of GHD adolescents, Carroll et al. [11] demonstrated that after cessation of GH treatment, insulin sensitivity increased at both 6 and 12 months; these increases were noted despite a trend toward increased fat mass and no gain in lean body mass over the same time period. In adults with hypopituitarism, insulin resistance has been reported even without replacement therapy. The administration of GH further decreases insulin sensitivity, but after this initial deterioration, an improvement of insulin sensitivity with a return to basal levels was noted.

Growth hormone replacement therapy increases lipolysis with an increment in the concentrations of free fatty acids, which could diminish the uptake of glucose into skeletal muscle. Studies using acipimox, a free fatty acid blocker, have confirmed the inverse relation that exists between circulating free fatty acid concentrations and insulin sensitivity in adults with GHD. Bramnert et al. [52] recently demonstrated how the administration of GH increases lipid oxidation with an increase of the circulating levels of free fatty acids and a deterioration of insulin sensitivity. The effect of GH in the long term is, however, beneficial with a reduction in body fat mass and an improvement in insulin sensitivity. Individualization of GH therapy, with an initial administration of smaller GH doses and a gradual increase in dose based on the clinical response and on IGF-I titration, could probably minimize the changes in insulin sensitivity noted in adults during the first few months of GH treatment.

## Conclusions

GHD subjects may present with an abnormal body composition, with elevated fasting cholesterol and triglycerides levels, and with increased postprandial triglyceride concentrations. In addition, concentrations of peripheral inflammatory and fibrinolytic markers have been found to be increased in GHD. Increased carotid artery IMT and vascular rigidity, as well as abnormalities in cardiac mass and function, have also been noted in GHD. Many of these abnormalities seem to be already detectable early on in life, so that children and adolescents with severe GHD need to be followed carefully as they enter into adulthood. GH treatment has a beneficial impact on body fat distribution, lipid abnormalities, and on flow-mediated dilation (a biophysical marker of endothelial function) and may lead to a reduction of the risk of cardiac events in adult GHD subjects.

## References

1. Holmer H, Svensson J, Rylander L, Johannsson G, Rosen T, Bengtsson BA, Thoren M, Hoybye C, Degerblad M, Bramnert M, Hagg E, Engstrom BE, Ekman B, Norrving B, Hagmar L and Erfurth EM. 2007 Nonfatal stroke, cardiac disease, and diabetes mellitus in hypopituitary patients on hormone replacement including growth hormone. J Clin Endocrinol Metab 92: 3560–3567.

2. Hagmar L, Erfurth EM. Nonfatal stroke, cardiac disease, and diabetes mellitus in hypopituitary patients on hormone replacement including growth hormone. J Clin Endocrinol Metab. 2007;92:3560–7.
3. Bengtsson BA, Christiansen JS, Cuneo RC, Sacca L. Cardiovascular effects of GH. J Endocrinol. 1997;152:1–3.
4. Rosen T, Eden S, Larson G, Wilhelmsen L, Bengtsson BA. Cardiovascular risk factors in adult patients with growth hormone deficiency. Acta Endocrinol (Copenh). 1997;129:195–200.
5. Hoffman AR, Kuntze JE, Baptista J, Baum HBA, Baumann GP, Biller BM, Clark RV, Cook D, Inzucchi SE, Kleinberg D, Klibanski A, Phillips LS, Ridgway EC, Robbins RJ, Schechte J, Sharma M, Thorner MO, Vance ML. Growth hormone (GH) replacement therapy in adult-onset GH deficiency: effects on body composition in men and women in a double-blind, randomized, placebo-controlled trial. J Clin Endocrinol Metab. 2004;89:2048–56.
6. Maison P, Griffin S, Nicoue-Beglah M, Haddad N, Balkau B, Chanson P. Impact of growth hormone (GH) treatment on cardiovascular risk factors in GH-deficient adults: a meta-analysis of blinded, randomized, placebo-controlled trials. J Clin Endocrinol Metab. 2004;89:2192–9.
7. Koranyi J, Gothesrstrom G, Sunnerhagen KS, Bengtsson BA, Johansson G. Baseline characteristics and the effects of five years of GH replacement therapy in adults with GH deficiency of childhood or adulthood onset: a comparative, prospective study. J Clin Endocrinol Metab. 2001;86:4693–9.
8. Kuromaru R, Kohno H, Ueyama N, Hassan HMS, Hara T. Long-term prospective study of body composition and lipid profiles during and after growth hormone (GH) treatment in children with GH deficiency: gender-specific metabolic effects. J Clin Endocrinol Metab. 1998;83:3890–6.
9. Capalbo D, Mattace Raso G, Di Mase R, Barbieri F, Mell R, Bruzzesse D, Salerno M. Cluster of cardiometabolic risk factors in children with GH deficiency: a prospective, case–control study. Clin Endocrinol. 2013;80:856–62.
10. Johannsson G, Albertsson-Wikland K. Discontinuation of growth hormone (GH) treatment: metabolic effects in GH-deficient and GH-sufficient adolescent patients compared with control subjects. J Clin Endocrinol Metab. 1999;84:4516–24.
11. Carroll PV, Drake WM, Maher KT, Metcalfe MK, Shaw NJ, Dunger DB, Cheetham TD, Camacho-Hubner C, Savage MO, Monson JP. Comparison of continuation or cessation of growth hormone (GH) therapy on body composition and metabolic status in adolescents with severe GH deficiency at completion of linear growth. J Clin Endocrinol Metab. 2004;89:3890–5.
12. Svensson J, Sunnerhagen KS, Johannsson G. Five years of growth hormone replacement therapy in adults: age- and gender-related changes in isometric and isokinetic muscle strength. J Clin Endocrinol Metab. 2003;88:2061–9.
13. Ter Maaten JC, De Boer H, Kamp O, Stuurman L, Van Der Veen EA. Long term effects of growth hormone (GH) replacement in men with childhood-onset GH deficiency. J Clin Endocrinol Metab. 1999;84:2373–80.
14. Lanes R, Gunczler P, Lopez E, Esaa S, Villaroel O, Revel-Chion R. Cardiac mass and function, carotid artery intima-media thickness and lipoprotein levels in growth hormone deficient adolescents. J Clin Endocrinol Metab. 2001;88:1061–5.
15. Lanes R, Paoli M, Carrillo E, Villaroel O, Palacios A. The Cardiovascular risk of young growth hormone deficient adolescents; differences in growth hormone treated and untreated subjects. Horm Res. 2003;60:291–5.
16. Murray RD, Wieringat GE, Lissett CA, Darzy KH, Smethurst LE, Shalet SM. Low dose replacement improves the adverse lipid profile associated with the adult GH deficiency syndrome. Clin Endocrinol. 2002;56:525–32.
17. Colao A, Di Somma C, Cuocolo A, Spinelli L, Tedesco N, Pivonello R, Bonaduce D, Salvatore M, Lombardi G. Improved cardiovascular risk factors and cardiac performance after 12 months of growth hormone (GH) replacement in young adult patients with GH deficiency. J Clin Endocrinol Metab. 2001;86:1874–81.

18. Al-Shoumer KAS, Cox KH, Hughes CL, Richmond Y, Johnston DG. Fasting and postprandial lipid abnormalities in hypopituitary women receiving conventional replacement therapy. J Clin Endocrinol Metab. 1997;82:2653–9.
19. Twickler TB, Wilmink HW, Schreuder NJ, Casto Cabezas M, van Dam PS, Koppeschaar D, Erkelens DW, Dallinga-Thie GM. Growth hormone (GH) treatment decreases postprandial remnant-like particle cholesterol concentration and improves endothelial function in adult-onset GH deficiency. J Clin Endocrinol Metab. 2000;85:4683–9.
20. Twickler TB, Dallinga-Thie GM, Visseren FLJ, de Vries WE, Erkelens DW, Koppershaar HPF. Induction of postprandial inflammatory response in adult onset growth hormone deficiency is related to plasma remnant-like particle cholesterol concentration. J Clin Endocrinol Metab. 2003;88:1228–32.
21. De Marco S, Marcovecchio ML, Caniglia D, De Leonibus C, Chiarelli F, Mohn A. Circulating asymmetric dimethylarginine and lipid profile in pre-pubertal children with growth hormone deficiency: effect of 12-month growth hormone replacement therapy. Growth Hormon IGF Res. 2014;24(5):216–20.
22. Johansson JO, Landin K, Tengborn L, Rosen T, Bengsson BA. High fibrinogen and plasminogen activator inhibitor activity in growth hormone deficient adults. Arterosclerosis Thrombosis. 1999;76:422–8.
23. Cañete R, Valle M, Martos R, Sanchez Carion A, Cañete MD, van Donkelaar EL. Short-term effects of GH treatment on coagulation, fibrinolysis, inflammation biomarkers, and insulin resistance status in prepubertal children with GH deficiency. EurJ Endocrinol. 2012;167(2):255–60.
24. Wilhemsen L, Svardsudd K, Korsan-Bengtsen K, Larsson B, Weiin L, Tibblin G. Fibrinogen as a risk factor for stroke and myocardial infarction. N Engl J Med. 1984;311:501–5.
25. Hamsten A, deFaire U, Walldius G, Dahlen G, Szamosi A, Landou C, Blomback M, Wiman B. Plasminogen activator inhibitor in plasma: risk factor for recurrent myocardial infarction. Lancet. 1987;2:3–9.
26. Evans LM, Davies JS, Anderson RA, Jackson SK, Smith JC, Morgan CLL, McDowell I, Rees AY, Scanlon MF. Elevated plasma homocysteine levels are associated with enhanced oxidative stress and endothelial dysfunction in adult hypopituitary patients with growth hormone deficiency. J Endocrinol. 1999;160(Suppl):22.
27. Sesmilo G, Biller BM, Llevado J, Hayden D, Hanson G, Rifai N, Klibanski A. Effects of growth hormone (GH) administration on homocysteine levels in men with GH deficiency: a randomized controlled trial. J Clin Endocrinol Metab. 2001;86:1518–24.
28. Abdu TA, Elhadd TA, Akber M, Hartland A, Neary R, Clayton N. Plasma homocysteine is not a major risk factor for vascular disease in growth hormone deficient adults. Clin Endocrinol. 2001;55:635–8.
29. Thum T, Fleissner F, Klink I, Tsikas D, Jakob M, Bauersachs J, Stichtenoth DO. Growth hormone treatment improves markers of systemic nitric oxide bioavailability via insulin-like growth factor 1. J Clin Endocrinol Metab. 2007;92:4172–9.
30. Li G, del Rincon JP, Jahn LA, Wu Y, Gaylinn B, Thorner MO, Liu Z. Growth hormone exerts acute vascular effects independent of systemic or muscle insulin-like growth factor 1. J Clin Endocrinol Metab. 2008;93:1379–85.
31. Leonsson M, Hulthe J, Johannsson G, Wiklund O, Wikstrandt J, Bengtsson BA, Oscarsson J. Increased interleukin-6 levels in pituitary-deficient patients are independently related to their carotid intima-media thickness. Clin Endocrinol. 2003;59:242–50.
32. Lanes R, Paoli M, Carrillo E, Villaroel O, Palacios A. Peripheral inflammatory and fibrinolytic markers in adolescents with growth hormone deficiency. Relation to postprandial dyslipidemia. J Pediatr. 2004;145:657–61.
33. Lanes R, Marcano H, Villaroel O, Moriilo E, Gunczler P, Paoli M, Perez M, Maulino N, Palacios A. Circulating levels of highly sensitive C-reactive protein and soluble markers of vascular cell activation in growth hormone deficiency. Horm Res. 2008;70:230–5.
34. Elhadd TA, Abdu TA, Oxtoby J, Kennedy G, McLaren M, Neary R, Belch JJF, Clayton RN. Biochemical and biophysical markers of endothelial dysfunction in adults with hypopituitarism and severe GH deficiency. J Clin Endocrinol Metab. 2001;86:4223–32.

35. Pilz S, Horejsi R, Moller R, Almer G, Scharnagl H, Stojakovic T, Dimitrova R, Weihrauch G, Borkenstein M, Maerz W, Schauenstein K, Mangge H. Early atherosclerosis in obese juveniles is associated with low serum levels of adiponectin. J Clin Endocrinol Metab. 2005;90:4792–6.
36. Eden Engstrom B, Burman P, Holdstock C, Karlsson F. Effects of growth hormone (GH) on ghrelin, leptin and adiponectin in GH-deficient patients. J Clin Endocrinol Metab. 2003;88:5193–8.
37. Hana V, Silha J, Justova V, Lacinova Z, Stepan J, Murphy I. The effects of GH replacement in adult GH-deficient patients: changes in body composition without concomitant changes in adipokines and insulin resistance. Clin Endocrinol (Oxf). 2004;60:442–50.
38. Lanes R, Soros A, Gunczler P, Paoli M, Carrillo E, Villaroel O, Palacios A. Growth hormone deficiency in adolescence is associated with low serum levels of adiponectin and with an unfavorable serum lipid and lipoprotein profile. J Pediatr. 2006;149:324–9.
39. Weiss R, Otvos JD, Flyvbjerg A, Miserez AR, Frystyk J, Sinnreich R, Kark JD. Adiponectin and lipoprotein particle size. Diabetes Care. 2009;32:1317–9.
40. Longobardi S, Cuocolo A, Merola B, et al. Left ventricular function in young adults with childhood and adulthood onset growth hormone deficiency. Clin Endocrinol. 1998;48:137–43.
41. Vacaldi R, Gaddi O, Zini M, et al. Cardiac performance and mass in adults with hypopituitarism: Effects of one year of growth hormone treatment. J Clin Endocrinol Metab 1995;86:659–666.
42. Colao A, Di Somma C, Salerno MC, Spinelli L, Orio F, Lombardi G. The cardiovascular risk of GH-deficient adolescents. J Clin Endocrinol Metab. 2002;87:3650–5.
43. Salerno M, Esposito V, Spinelli L, Di Somma C, Farina V, Muzzica S, Tanfurri de Horatio L, Lombardi G, Coalo A. Left ventricular mass and function in children with GH deficiency before and during 12 months GH replacement therapy. Clin Endocrinol. 2004;60:630–6.
44. Shulman DI, Root AW, Diamond FB, Bercu BB, Martinez R, Boucek RJ. Effects of one year of recombinant human growth hormone (GH) therapy on cardiac mass and function in children with classical GH deficiency. J Clin Endocrinol Metab. 2003;88:4095–199.
45. Lanes R, Soros A, Flores K, Gunczler P, Carrillo E, Bandel J. Endothelial function, carotid artery intima-media thickness, epicardial adipose tissue and left ventricular mass and function in growth hormone deficient adolescents. J Clin Endocrinol Metab. 2005;90:3978–82.
46. Nygren A, Telen D, Jonzon A, Björkherm G, Lindell S, Albertsson-Wikland K, Kristom B. Rapid Cardiovascular Effects of Growth Hormone treatment in short prepubertal children. Impact of treatment duration. Clin Endocrinol. 2012;77(6):877–84.
47. Esen I, Cetin L, Demirel F, Ekici F. The effect of recombinant human growth hormone therapy on left-ventricular chamber size and function in children with growth hormone deficiency. Pediatr Cardiol. 2013;34(8):1854–9.
48. Borson-Chazot F, Serusclat A, Kalfallah Y, Ducottet X, Sassolas G, Bernard S, Labrousse F, Pastene J, Sassolas A, Roux Y, Berthezene F. Decrease in carotid intima-media thickness after one year growth hormone (GH) treatment in adults with GH deficiency. J Clin Endocrinol Metab. 1999;84:1329–33.
49. Smith JC, Evans LM, Wilkinson I, Goodfellow J, Cockcroft JR, Scanlon MF, Davies JS. Effects of GH replacement on endothelial function and large-artery stiffness in GH-deficient adults; a randomized, double-blind, placebo-controlled study. Clin Endocrinol. 2002;5:493–501.
50. Oliveira JLM, Aguiar-Oliveira MH, D'Oliveira A, Pereira RMC, Oliveira CRP, Farias CT, Barreto-Filho JA, Anjos-Andrade FD, Marques-Santos C, Nascimento-Junior AC, Alves EO, Oliveira FT, Campos VC, Ximenes R, Blackford A, Parmigiani G, Salvator R. Congenital growth hormone (GH) deficiency and atherosclerosis: effects of GH replacement in GH-naïve adults. J Clin Endocrinol Metab. 2007;92:4664–70.
51. Husbands S, Ong KKL, Gilbert J, Wass JAH, Dunger DB. Increased insulin sensitivity in young, growth hormone deficient children. Clin Endocrinol. 2001;55:87–92.
52. Bramnert M, Segerlantz M, Luarila E, Daugaard JR, Manhe P, Groop L. Growth hormone replacement therapy induces insulin resistance by activating the glucose-fatty acid cycle. J Clin Endocrinol Metab. 2003;88:1455–63.

# Part II
# Diagnosis of Human Growth Hormone Deficiency

# Chapter 8
# Laboratory Diagnosis of Growth Hormone Deficiency in Children

**Constantin Polychronakos**

This chapter is an expansion of proposed guidelines based on a systematic review of the literature by a committee of pediatric endocrinologists of the Pediatric Endocrine Society [1]. Opinions expressed are those of the author, who considers them completely compatible with the spirit of the systematic review. Growth hormone (GH) is arguably the only hormone for the clinical testing of which (and its interpretation) an entire textbook chapter needs to be written. Questions of purity and stability of standard, affinities, and specificities of different antibodies and other technical sources of variability are certainly issues with the clinical testing of every peptide hormone. What makes GH testing unique is that interpretation of its results needs to address the pulsatile nature of its secretion, as a consequence of which healthy individuals spend most of their day at levels indistinguishable from those of profound deficiency, and the important consequences of making, or failing to make, the diagnosis of deficiency on the basis of a single threshold. This diagnosis involves long treatment of children with daily injections of a very expensive biological preparation and is usually made based on a single point in time and without provisions to revisit until the treatment (for growth purposes) is completed. This chapter will review the diagnostic application of GH testing for the specific purpose of treating a child to permit or enhance growth. It will concentrate less on the technical aspects of the clinical chemistry and more on the interpretation of the results. Standard practices will be critically reviewed in the light of the evidence base—or lack thereof. Diagnosis for indications other than growth promotion will not be addressed.

---

C. Polychronakos (✉)
Departments of Paediatrics and Human Genetics,
Child Health and Human Development, The McGill University Health Centre,
1001 Decarie Blvd, Block E, Rm M03211, Montreal, QC, Canada, H4A3J1
e-mail: constantin.polychronakos@mcgill.ca

## Analytical Aspects of GH Testing

A number of factors can affect the quality of GH assays and result in lack of reproducibility across different methodologies and laboratories. Circulating GH is not homogeneous, consisting of monomers, dimers, and posttranslationally modified forms, and can exist free or bound to GH-binding protein (GHBP, the soluble extracellular part of the GH receptor) [2]. The standards against which the sample is measured could also have some aspects of the same variability. Different antibodies, recognizing only one epitope each, or different epitopes with different affinities, are an obvious source of discrepancies [3]. Moreover, differences in detecting antibody-bound vs. free analyte can differ across methodologies and instrumentations.

Much of what we know about GH diagnosis and treatment has been established using polyclonal radioimmunoassays and purified pituitary standards. Currently used immunometric assays with monoclonal antibodies and recombinant standards have higher specificity, but the use of different standards and antibodies with specificities for different GH isoforms has resulted in non-negligible discrepancies between assays.

Using three reference assays (two using the same standard, 88/624), Hauffa et al. reexamined 699 peak samples from GH provocative testing [4]. The mean difference among assays varied from 5.4 to 10.3 mU/L. Assignment to GH-deficient (GHD) vs. GH-sufficient groups varied substantially among different assays in a subset of 132 subjects who had standardized insulin and arginine testing, resulting in misclassification of up to 29 % of cases. In another study, samples from 47 provocative tests were assayed with four different methods [5]; discrepancies were found with significant effects on diagnostic outcome. One immunometric assay classified 36 % of tests as indicating GHD compared to 14.9 % for the standard radioimmunoassay. A more systematic, multi-laboratory effort at standardization of assays in Finland between 1998 and 2003 showed considerable improvement in concordance, but, even in the last year of the effort, discrepancies persisted [6]. Another harmonization effort in Germany found a 27 % misclassification rate prior to adjusting results by a conversion factor, but good concordance afterward [7]. In Japan, a systematic effort at harmonization using a uniform biosynthetic standard resulted in lowering of the cutoff of a peak GH value from 10 to 6 µg/L due largely to the immunometric methods measuring much lower than the original radioimmunoassay [8]. These examples highlight the importance of considering measurement method when using the literature of the past few decades to obtain the evidence base for rational decision-making regarding GH treatment.

In more recent years, standardization or, at least, harmonization has been recognized as required to meaningfully evaluate and compare results [3]. If different methods give the same result for the same serum pools, the assay can be considered standardized. If not, harmonization is achieved by documenting sample-independent differences and deriving correction factors to obtain the same numbers for the same sample by the use of commutable serum pools [9]. An important first step is the adoption of recombinant primary reference material, the most current and widely used of which is 98/574 [3]. It represents the 22 kD isoform and has high purity, proven biological activity, and stability [10]. However, none of these characteristics necessarily guarantees its commutability (similar results with different antibodies and detection methods). Clinicians and third-party payers should only accept results from clinical laboratories that use methodologies whose manufacturers employ this standard and actively participate in standardization and harmonization efforts.

## Clinical Interpretation of Biochemical GH Results

Purely analytical problems can be solved, but, beyond these, interpretation of GH results for the purpose of making a diagnosis and initiating treatment is far from straightforward. GH is secreted in irregularly timed pulsatile peaks, with long troughs in between, during which healthy individuals are indistinguishable from patients with profound deficiency [11]. This precludes diagnostic inference from a single sample and has given rise to the development of stimulation tests (also referred to as "provocative tests") that evaluate peak response to the administration of one of several substances known to induce GH release during a trough. Insulin, arginine, clonidine, glucagon, and L-dopa are the most commonly used such substances [12], accepted in current clinical and reimbursement practice as interchangeable despite very limited knowledge of their exact mechanism of action and how it is affected by the various causes of GHD. Many of these stimuli may bypass one or more of the multiple inputs into the hypothalamus that determine the release of GH-releasing hormone and/or somatostatin [13].

### *Consistency Across Different Stimulating Agents*

This is the first GH testing aspect that requires a critical appraisal. Using the same analytical assay to measure peak GH concentrations of 68 normally growing children, Zadik et al. found good agreement between insulin- and arginine-stimulated GH peaks (14.2 ± 6.3 vs. 13.1 ± 6.1 µg/L), but clonidine, another widely used stimulus, gave much higher levels (21.0 ± 10.7 µg/L) [14]. These results were corroborated in a large, registry-based study of 3233 cases in the French registry [15], in which correlation coefficients (r) between peaks in two GH tests on the same patient ranged from 0.35 to 0.6, meaning that the $r^2$ (expressing the fraction of variance explained by the fact that the two tests were performed on the same subject) ranged from 12 to 36 %. These results also suggested imperfect reproducibility of the same test in the same patient, with the highest correlation, that being for insulin/insulin, having a coefficient of only 0.72 ($r^2 = 52$ %).

## Peak Response and the Diagnosis of GHD

In terms of existing clinical guidelines, as well as in regulatory approvals and third-party reimbursement policies, a single threshold of peak response, below which the diagnosis of GHD can be made, is typically established regardless of the stimulus used [16]. These thresholds vary substantially in different jurisdictions, from 6 µg/L in Japan to 7–10 µg/L in North America and Europe (Australia, interestingly, has completely done away with provocative testing as a criterion for treatment [17]). The evidence base for establishing such thresholds will be reviewed below. To the extent that it exists, it indicates that most of these thresholds are well within the range of peak responses seen in healthy, normally growing children. These inflated thresholds result in poor specificity and compromised ability to predict response along the spectrum that ranges from the difference between "pituitary dwarfism" (complete GHD) and resultant adult normal stature (seen in complete GHD [18, 19]) to a gain in the order of 5–6 cm in adult stature, seen in children treated despite normal GH testing [20–24].

The main problem is the absence of a prospective gold standard for the diagnosis of GH deficiency. "Classical" GHD, as described by Lawson Wilkins, involves the complete or near-complete inability to secrete GH, resulting in zero or near-zero growth velocity and adult height (AH) many standard deviations below the mean [18]. Classical GHD usually starts at a young age, and early treatment restores normal growth, with catch-up to a percentile compatible with midparental height, including the upper percentiles of adult stature. In these cases, the effect of the treatment is dramatic. "Pituitary dwarfs" have disappeared in affluent countries since the availability of GH treatment. In the majority of these cases, classical GHD is associated with hypothalamic-pituitary abnormalities on imaging [25, 26], multiple pituitary hormone deficiencies, or a history of insult to the area such as tumor, surgery, or cranial irradiation. In observational studies of these children, provocative tests show low levels very distinct from the normal range such that test precision, reproducibility, agent used for stimulation, and assay performance may not be crucial barriers to precise diagnosis. These tests were never validated as a basis for intervention with a formal randomized control trial (RCT) to AH, but observational studies tend to show that very low peak response correlates with dramatic response to treatment [27]. In the pre-recombinant era, the scarce supply of GH purified from human cadavers permitted the treatment of only the most seriously affected cases with near-zero GH response to stimuli, which made the absence of standardized testing or prospective RTC evidence of the spectacular benefit from GH treatment less of a problem.

With the availability of recombinant GH in the mid-1980s, the opportunity arose to treat children with less complete GHD, and the threshold for declaring GHD was arbitrarily raised. This increase was compounded by the adoption of testing methods using purer standards and two-antibody immunometric assays that dramatically increased specificity of testing compared to the old methods, resulting in smaller actual numbers [8]. These changes drastically increased sensitivity at the expense of specificity to an extent that has never been properly determined for either metric.

The sensitivity and specificity of a diagnostic test is formally determined by the receiver-operator characteristic (ROC) curve, which plots sensitivity against (1—specificity) for any given threshold value, in order to choose one that maximizes the more desirable of the two (sensitivity in this case) without unacceptably compromising the other (specificity) [28]. Construction of this curve requires a gold standard that unequivocally distinguishes "normal" from "abnormal." The "hard" end-points (zero height velocity, presence of other anterior or posterior pituitary deficiencies, brain-imaging abnormalities, history of cranial irradiation) cannot be used because they would exclude "idiopathic" isolated GHD, as well as the hypothesized cases of partial GHD that the relaxed thresholds were meant to include.

In the absence of such gold standard, it might have made sense to use a more utilitarian definition of a "positive" test as one that meets a threshold beyond which treating the condition diagnosed will do more good than harm. Proper use of this criterion would require quantification of the assumed psychological and social harm from shortness, its reversal by treatment, and the possible psychological harm from stigmatizing shortness by prescribing years of daily injections that, in many cases, will end up making the individual only a few centimeters less short. From a broader perspective, one might add a cost-benefit analysis of how much health and quality of life can be purchased by using the considerable cost of years of GH treatment to enhance some other aspect of health or well-being. We will not review here the scant literature on such outcomes [29–31], other than to say that no study has correlated them to a peak-response threshold used to justify treatment. Not even the crude end-point of effect of treatment on AH gain for any given peak GH response has been assessed with a formal RCT. We know that treatment of short children with peak responses >10 µg/L (idiopathic short stature (ISS)) results in an AH gain of 5–6 cm [20–24], but no AH data exist to show that this outcome is any better for children in the "gray zone" of peak response of 5–10 µg/L.

## Normative Data

A reference range for a quantitative test is commonly used to determine diagnostic threshold in the absence of direct outcome-based evidence. This would involve obtaining peak-response values in children who definitely do not have GHD, i.e., healthy children of normal stature and growing at a normal velocity, and then establishing the threshold at the lower end of the distribution of these values, typically -2SD. Given the voluminous literature on GH testing, the paucity of such studies is surprising, but the results are telling.

In 68 children of normal stature and growing at normal growth velocity, Zadik et al. measured GH by radioimmunoassay and found peak responses (mean ± SD) to arginine and insulin, commonly used GH stimulants, at 13.1 ± 6.1 and 14.2 ± 6.3 µg/L, respectively, indicating that mean-1SD for healthy children is already well below the 10 µg/L cutoff [14]. In the same data, 5th percentile values were <5 µg/L. Using a lower-measuring, more specific immunometric method (HGH-CPK,

Sorin, Italy), Ghigo et al. examined peak responses to a wide variety of stimulants in 472 children and adolescents, of whom 295 were within the normal range for height and the rest were short, but all otherwise healthy and growing at a normal height velocity [15]. Results were no different in the two groups and were pooled. *Mean* peak-response values for commonly used stimulants ranged from 9.7 µg/L for clonidine to 11.7 µg/L for arginine with mean-1SD for all provocative tests around 7 µg/L.

Therefore, the normative data, such as they are, provide little support for the most widely used peak-response thresholds for diagnosing GHD. The requirement for two tests below the threshold, combined with the poor correlation between two tests performed on the same individual [15], somewhat mitigates this serious loss of specificity, but, even then, it is clear that the 10 µg/L threshold misclassifies large numbers of non-GHD children.

## *Outcome-Based Estimation of a Diagnostic Threshold*

Any attempt at setting an outcome-based threshold in the absence of evidence from controlled studies on AH, the meaningful outcome, would have to be limited to a good proxy from post-marketing surveys. One such outcome could be first-year response to GH, a quite reliable predictor in children treated to AH [32]. Data from KIGS (a Europe-based *Pfizer* post-marketing database) were mathematically modeled from 593 GH-treated prepubertal children diagnosed as having GHD on the basis of a GH response <10 µg/L [33]. Adding peak GH response to a model of auxological parameters increased the percentage of variance explained from 45 to 60 %, making it a statistically significant, but rather modest predictor. However, when individual values for the improvement in first-year height velocity prediction attributable to the GH peak are plotted, it becomes clear that the prediction comes from peak levels <5 µg/L; at this level, the GH peak increases the prediction by as much as 4 cm of growth in the first year. Similar results were shown in 236 prepubertal children enrolled in the National Cooperative Growth Study (NCGS, *Genentech*) in the USA [34]. In both studies, first-year increase in height SDS (Δ-Ht SDS) was indistinguishable between children with peak GH responses 5–10 or >10 µg/L. Δ-Ht SDS >1.5 SD was seen only with GH peaks <5 µg/L. The specificity of the 10 µg/L cutoff was estimated at only 25 % and driven exclusively by the lower values. In 1192 children enrolled in the International Cooperative Growth Study (ICGS) in Japan [18] (also industry sponsored), a much better Δ-Ht SDS was seen in children with GH peaks <5 µg/L in two tests, compared to those with at least one test with a peak >5 µg/L. Adult height analyses from the post-marketing studies would not be meaningful because of a strong bias to continue treatment (and/or data submission) only in good early responders. However, it is clear that first-year response, a good predictor of AH [32], is no different between children peaking at 5–10 or >10 µg/L.

## Alternatives to Provocative Testing

Given the limitations of provocative testing, the idea of testing spontaneous secretion as a profile with serial sampling [35] or as an integrated level by continuous withdrawal [36] is attractive. It seems plausible that a child unable to normally secrete GH could still respond to the unphysiological pharmacology of provocative testing.

This hypothesis was tested by Spiliotis et al. [35]. Seven short children with abnormally low growth velocity, who had provocative responses >10 µg/L but low spontaneous secretion, were treated with GH. Short-term acceleration of growth was observed, but not compared to that seen in treated GH-sufficient children to demonstrate superiority and AH data were not presented. In addition, a major weakness of this study was that four of the seven patients were of pubertal age with severe bone-age delay. Onset of puberty during treatment was not evaluated and could account for much or all of this acceleration. A similar first-year growth acceleration was reported in two other studies of children diagnosed by the same criteria [37, 38]. Both of these studies suffered from the same limitations.

We could find a report of the effects on AH in only one retrospective study [25] that showed AH gain of 1.03 SDS following GH treatment in children who met the criteria for neurosecretory dysfunction, compared to untreated short stature cases with normal spontaneous secretion. This gain is virtually identical to that obtained in treated ISS [20–24], making the prognostic contribution of the spontaneous GH study very questionable.

Normative data for spontaneous GH secretion were established by a study that showed that 4/10 normal-height, normally growing children and 8/35 with constitutional delay, but normal growth velocity, had overnight secretory patterns compatible with the diagnosis of neurosecretory GHD [39, 40]. Another attempt at establishing normative data for spontaneous secretion by frequent GH sampling showed a troubling inconsistency when normal children were studied on two separate occasions under identical conditions [41].

## Patient-Specific Factors Affecting Interpretation of Biochemical GH Testing

### *Obesity*

Studies show that GH response to provocative testing depends on body mass index (BMI) and that GH response to stimulation is considerably lower in obese children [42–44]. In a prospective study of 65 normally growing obese children, spontaneous GH secretion was less than half of reference, and it normalized after weight loss [44]. *Prima facie*, these results would mandate halving the threshold for diagnosing GHD in the presence of obesity. However, the information that would be required to individualize this adjustment based on the patient's individual BMI is not available (see Chap. 6 for more details).

## Pubertal Delay

In children with constitutional delay of growth and puberty and normal AH prognosis, the normal decline in prepubertal growth velocity with age (normally interrupted by the pubertal growth spurt) is prolonged and may lead to frankly abnormal growth velocity [45]. This is accompanied by a reduction in the GH response to provocative stimuli that normalizes after the onset of puberty [46]. Thus, in prepubertal children of pubertal age, GH testing may lead to a false diagnosis of GHD. Fortunately, strong evidence reassures that this problem can be solved if testing is preceded by brief treatment with sex steroids. Administration of 1–2 mg of β-estradiol to 44 children with ISS raised the lower 95 % confidence interval of GH peak response to a sequential arginine-clonidine test from a clearly abnormal 3.7 to 8.3 µg/L. This very substantial gain in specificity was not accompanied by a loss of sensitivity, as response was unaltered in 15 children with GHD [47]. Similar results were found in a cross-sectional study of 84 normal, untreated children, where the percentage of those who would have been classified as GHD by the stricter cutoff of 7 µg/L declined from 61 % at Tanner stage I to zero at stages IV and V [48]. No gynecomastia in boys or other side effects have been reported with the recommended doses of sex steroid priming. However, for boys, an alternative would be an injection of 100 mg of a depot testosterone preparation. No systematic controlled evidence exists to favor any of the proposed protocols over another, but they all seem to be effective. Failing to use them in children of normal pubertal age (i.e., >10 years old in girls and >12 in boys) will result in false-positive results and unnecessary treatment.

## Systemic Health Problems

In a child growing at subnormal velocity, it is usually easy to exclude other health problems or congenital malformations as, by the time a morbidity is severe enough to impair growth, it will almost invariably have systemic or organ-specific symptomatology that will direct to the correct diagnosis. There is not much point in testing for GHD if there is an alternative explanation for poor growth, until the growth problem persists after it has been medically controlled. This also applies to other hormone deficiencies, specifically hypothyroidism, as thyroid hormone is necessary for GH secretion [49]. Serum thyroid-stimulating hormone (TSH) and free thyroxine should be measured and GH testing carried out only if both are normal. In low-TSH hypothyroidism, GH testing should proceed immediately after normalization of T4 with treatment, while if TSH is high, GH testing will only be needed in the unlikely event of growth failure persisting after treating the hypothyroidism.

## Decision-Making in the Face of Uncertainty

In view of what has been discussed, it is clear that the use of biochemical testing to make the diagnosis of GHD is nowhere near as well documented in evidence base as one might be led to believe from the confidence expressed in professional body guidelines [16, 50] and reimbursement policies in different jurisdictions and by different third-party payers. In what follows, I will attempt to make suggestions about how the clinician can use this analysis to rationally use (or avoid using) biochemical GH testing.

First, only children with clearly abnormal height velocity should be tested. To follow the third percentile curve, a velocity in the 25th centile is required [51]. A diagnosis of GHD cannot be made on a child growing at this rate or better, regardless of GH peak response (this may appear too obvious to state but in some of the literature reviewed, GHD was diagnosed in children with normal growth velocity). In children with delayed puberty, velocity should, of course, be assessed on the basis of bone age rather than chronological age.

Faced with an otherwise asymptomatic child growing at subnormal velocity, the first concern of the pediatric endocrinologist should be not to miss the life-threatening and treatable possibility of a tumor in the hypothalamic-pituitary region. The uncertainties of GH testing matter surprisingly little in this context. In provocative testing, these cases will invariably peak well below the gray zone of uncertainty and will most of the time have at least one additional pituitary deficiency, and MRI imaging will quickly confirm the diagnosis. Unpublished data from our own clinic will be reassuring in this respect. Although the public system in the province of Québec accepts 8 μg/L as the reimbursement threshold, our clinic has always used 5 μg/L (by immunometric methods) as the cutoff for further investigation or GH treatment. Over the decades, we are not aware of a single case of a tumor that was missed because of having tested higher than 5 μg/L by the time they are documented to grow at a velocity <25th centile (Guyda et al. unpublished observations).

Having ruled out a tumor, provocative GH testing is still useful to diagnose classical GH deficiency of the "idiopathic" isolated kind, where GH treatment can make a difference of several SDs of AH, i.e. the difference between what was formerly called "dwarfism" and normal height (90th percentile if this is what one has inherited from one's parents). To be generous, I suggest 5 μg/L as the cutoff for this diagnosis even though normative data show that a non-negligible proportion of normal, normally growing children will test below that. Most of these children with profound but isolated GHD will have MR imaging abnormalities, usually the classical triad indicating disrupted hypothalamic-pituitary communication [25]. In the presence of these imaging findings and at least one additional pituitary deficiency, confirmation with provocative testing is unnecessary if growth velocity remains abnormal after correction of the other pituitary deficiencies.

What to do for the child growing at a subnormal velocity who tests between 5 and 10 μg/L? If accepted by the third-party payer, GH treatment is an option, with a very important difference however. Where the difference lies is in what justification for the treatment and promise of results can be given to the child and family. With peak responses clearly <5, an extremely short stature without and satisfactory normalization with treatment is an honest most likely scenario. Beyond this level, the evidence reviewed in this chapter makes it dishonest to promise that response to GH treatment can be expected to be better than that seen in short children with idiopathic short stature who test >10 μg/L, i.e., 5–6 cm of AH gain. One should also consider the psychological harm of presenting shortness as something so bad that requires years of daily injections so one can be 5 cm less short.

Given the limitations discussed, an alternative is the long-established Australian policy of completely doing away with GH testing and treating strictly on auxological criteria (growth velocity <25th centile). It has been pointed out that this policy did not result in an unjustified and unmanageable surge in GH prescriptions [17]. In fact, adjusted for population, GH use in Australia under this regime has been only 68.7 % of that in the USA [17]. This might suggest that auxological criteria are not respected by US practitioners, who rely too heavily on biochemical GH testing with inflated diagnostic thresholds.

## Conclusion

A critical review of the evidence base points to serious flaws in what is generally accepted as the standard-of-care way in which GH testing results are interpreted and used to make treatment decisions. This creates the ethical imperative that physicians proposing GH treatment of short children, whose response to provocative testing is in the gray zone of values that may be also seen in healthy, normally-growing children, moderate the promise of the expected effect. In these cases, the effect may be much closer to that for ISS rather than the spectacular effects seen in complete GHD.

## References

1. Guidelines for growth hormone and insulin-like growth factor-I treatment in children and adolescents: the growth hormone deficiency, idiopathic short stature, primary insulin-like growth factor-I deficiency spectrum. In peer review
2. Baumann G. Growth hormone heterogeneity: genes, isohormones, variants, and binding proteins. Endocr Rev. 1991;12:424–49.
3. Clemmons DR, On behalf of the conference participants. Consensus statement on the standardization and evaluation of growth hormone and insulin-like growth factor assays. Clin Chem. 2011;57(4):555–9.
4. Hauffa BP, Lehmann N, Bettendorf M, Mehls O, Dorr HG, Partsch CJ, Schwarz HP, Stahnke N, Steinkamp H, Said E, Sander S, Ranke MB. Central reassessment of GH concentrations measured at local treatment centers in children with impaired growth. Eur J Endocrinol. 2004;150(3):291–7.
5. Rakover Y, Lavi I, Masalah R, Issam T, Weiner E, Ben-Shlomo I. Comparison between four immunoassays for growth hormone (GH) measurement as guides to clinical decisions following GH provocative tests. J Pediatr Endocrinol Metab. 2000;13(6):637–43.

6. Morsky P, Tiikkainen U, Ruokonen A, Markkanen H. Problematic determination of serum growth hormone: experience from external quality assurance surveys 1998–2003. Scand J Clin Lab Invest. 2005;65(5):377–86.
 7. Muller A, Scholz M, Blankenstein O, Binder G, Pfaffle R, Korner A, Kiess W, Heider A, Bidlingmaier M, Thiery J, Kratzsch J. Harmonization of growth hormone measurements with different immunoassays by data adjustment. Clin Chem Lab Med. 2011;49(7):1135–42.
 8. Tanaka T, Tachibana K, Shimatsu A, Katsumata N, Tsushima T, Hizuka N, Fujieda K, Yokoya S, Irie M. A nationwide attempt to standardize growth hormone assays. Horm Res. 2005;64 Suppl 2:6–11.
 9. Ross HA, Lentjes EW, Menheere PM, Sweep CG, Endocrinology Section and project group "Calibration 2000" of the SKML (Dutch Foundation for Quality Assessment in Clinical Laboratories). Harmonization of growth hormone measurement results: the empirical approach. Clin Chim Acta. 2014;432:72–6.
10. Bristow AF, Jespersen AM. The Second International Standard for somatropin (recombinant DNA-derived human growth hormone): preparation and calibration in an international collaborative study. Biologicals. 2001;29:97–106.
11. Buckler JM. Spontaneous variations in serum growth hormone levels. Acta Endocrinol (Copenh). 1970;65(2):342–51.
12. Stanley T. Diagnosis of growth hormone deficiency in childhood. Curr Opin Endocrinol Diabetes Obes. 2012;19(1):47–52. doi:10.1097/MED.0b013e32834ec952. Review.
13. Murray PG, Higham CE, Clayton PE. 60 Years of neuroendocrinology: the hypothalamo-GH axis: the past 60 years. J Endocrinol. 2015;226(2):T123–40. doi:10.1530/JOE-15-0120.
14. Zadik Z, Chalew SA, Kowarski A. Assessment of growth hormone secretion in normal stature children using 24-hour integrated concentration of GH and pharmacological stimulation. J Clin Endocrinol Metab. 1990;71(4):932–6.
15. Carel JC, Tresca JP, Letrait M, Chaussain JL, Lebouc Y, Job JC, Coste J. Growth hormone testing for the diagnosis of growth hormone deficiency in childhood: a population register-based study. J Clin Endocrinol Metab. 1997;82(7):2117–21.
16. Wilson TA, Rose SR, Cohen P, Rogol AD, Backeljauw P, Brown R, Hardin DS, Kemp SF, Lawson M, Radovick S, Rosenthal SM, Silverman L, Speiser P, Lawson Wilkins Pediatric Endocrinology Society Drug and Therapeutics Committee. Update of guidelines for the use of growth hormone in children: the Lawson Wilkins Pediatric Endocrinology Society Drug and Therapeutics Committee. J Pediatr. 2003;143(4):415–21.
17. Werther GA. Growth hormone measurements versus auxology in treatment decisions: the Australian experience. J Pediatr. 1996;128(5 Pt 2):S47–51.
18. Martin M, Wilkins L. Pituitary dwarfism: diagnosis and treatment. J Clin Endocrinol Metab. 1958;18(7):679–93.
19. Dean HJ, Friesen HG, The Members of the Therapeutic Trial of Growth Hormone Committee. Long-term growth of children with growth hormone deficiency and hypoglycemia. J Pediatr. 1989;115:598–600.
20. Leschek EW, Rose SR, Yanovski JA, Troendle JF, Quigley CA, Chipman JJ, Crowe BJ, Ross JL, Cassorla FG, Blum WF, Cutler Jr GB, Baron J. Effect of growth hormone treatment on adult height in peripubertal children with idiopathic short stature: a randomized, double-blind, placebo-controlled trial. J Clin Endocrinol Metab. 2004;89(7):3140–8.
21. Albertsson-Wikland K, Aronson AS, Gustafsson J, Hagenas L, Ivarsson SA, Jonsson B, Kristrom B, Marcus C, Nilsson KO, Ritzen EM, Tuvemo T, Westphal O, Aman J. Dose-dependent effect of growth hormone on final height in children with short stature without growth hormone deficiency. J Clin Endocrinol Metab. 2008;93(11):4342–50.
22. Deodati A, Cianfarani S. Impact of growth hormone therapy on adult height of children with idiopathic short stature: systematic review. BMJ. 2011;342:c7157.
23. Deodati A, Peschiaroli E, Cianfarani S. Review of growth hormone randomized controlled trials in children with idiopathic short stature. Horm Res Paediatr. 2011;76 Suppl 3:40–2. doi:10.1159/000330157.

24. Finkelstein BS, Imperiale TF, Speroff T, Marrero U, Radcliffe DJ, Cuttler L. Effect of growth hormone therapy on height in children with idiopathic short stature: a meta-analysis. Arch Pediatr Adolesc Med. 2002;156(3):230–40.
25. Coutant R, Rouleau S, Despert F, Magontier N, Loisel D, Limal JM. Growth and adult height in GH-treated children with nonacquired GH deficiency and idiopathic short stature: the influence of pituitary magnetic resonance imaging findings. J Clin Endocrinol Metab. 2001;86(10):4649–54.
26. Deal C, Hasselmann C, Pfaffle RW, Zimmermann AG, Quigley CA, Child CJ, Shavrikova EP, Cutler Jr GB, Blum WF. Associations between pituitary imaging abnormalities and clinical and biochemical phenotypes in children with congenital growth hormone deficiency: data from an international observational study. Horm Res Paediatr. 2013;79(5):283–92.
27. Guyda H, Friesen H, Bailey JD, Leboeuf G, Beck JC. Medical Research Council of Canada therapeutic trial of human growth hormone: first 5 years of therapy. Can Med Assoc J. 1975;112(11):1301–9.
28. Fawcett T. An introduction to ROC analysis. Pattern Recogn Lett. 2006;27:861–74.
29. Gardner M, Sandberg DE. Growth hormone treatment for short stature: a review of psychosocial assumptions and empirical evidence. Pediatr Endocrinol Rev. 2011;9(2):579–88. quiz 589.
30. Lee JM, Appugliese D, Coleman SM, Kaciroti N, Corwyn RF, Bradley RH, Sandberg DE, Lumeng JC. Short stature in a population-based cohort: social, emotional, and behavioral functioning. Pediatrics. 2009;124(3):903–10. doi:10.1542/peds.2008-0085.
31. Dean HJ, McTaggart TL, Fish DG, Friesen HG. Evaluation of educational, vocational and marital status of growth hormone deficient adults treated with growth hormone during childhood. Am J Dis Child. 1985;139:1105–10.
32. de Ridder MA, Stijnen T, Hokken-Koelega AC. Prediction of adult height in growth-hormone-treated children with growth hormone deficiency. J Clin Endocrinol Metab. 2007;92(3):925–31.
33. Ranke MB, Lindberg A, Chatelain P, Wilton P, Cutfield W, Albertsson-Wikland K, Price DA. Derivation and validation of a mathematical model for predicting the response to exogenous recombinant human growth hormone (GH) in prepubertal children with idiopathic GH deficiency. J Clin Endocrinol Metab. 1999;84(4):1174–83.
34. Bright GM, Julius JR, Lima J, Blethen SL. Growth hormone stimulation test results as predictors of recombinant human growth hormone treatment outcomes: preliminary analysis of the national cooperative growth study database. Pediatrics. 1999;104(4):1028–31.
35. Spiliotis BE, August GP, Hung W, Sonis W, Mendelson W, Bercu BB. Growth hormone neurosecretory dysfunction. A treatable cause of short stature. JAMA. 1984;251(17):2223–30.
36. Kowarski A, Thompson RG, Migeon CJ, Blizzard RM. Determination of integrated plasma concentrations and true secretion rates of human growth hormone. J Clin Endocrinol Metab. 1971;32(3):356–60.
37. Hernandez M, Nieto JA, Sobradillo B, Pombo M, Ferrandez A, Rejas J. Multicenter clinical trial to evaluate the therapeutic use of recombinant growth hormone from mammalian cells in the treatment of growth hormone neurosecretory dysfunction. Horm Res. 1991;35(1):13–8.
38. Rochiccioli P, Dechaux E, Tauber MT, Pienkowski C, Tiberge M. Growth hormone treatment in patients with neurosecretory dysfunction. Horm Res. 1990;33 Suppl 4:97–101.
39. Radetti G, Buzi F, Cassar W, Paganini C, Stacul E, Maghnie M. Growth hormone secretory pattern and response to treatment in children with short stature followed to adult height. Clin Endocrinol (Oxf). 2003;59(1):27–33.
40. Lanes R. Diagnostic limitations of spontaneous growth hormone measurements in normally growing prepubertal children. Am J Dis Child. 1989;143(11):1284–6.
41. Blizzard RM, Johanson A. Disorders of growth. In: Kappy MS, Blizzard RM, Migeon CJ, editors. Wilkins – the diagnosis and treatment of endocrine disorders in childhood and adolescence. 4th ed. Springfiled: Charles C. Thomas; 1994. p. 383–455.
42. Stanley TL, Levitsky LL, Grinspoon SK, Misra M. Effect of body mass index on peak growth hormone response to provocative testing in children with short stature. J Clin Endocrinol Metab. 2009;94(12):4875–81. doi:10.1210/jc.2009-1369.

43. Loche S, Guzzetti C, Pilia S, Ibba A, Civolani P, Porcu M, Minerba L, Casini MR. Effect of body mass index on the growth hormone response to clonidine stimulation testing in children with short stature. Clin Endocrinol (Oxf). 2011;74(6):726–31. doi:10.1111/j.1365-2265.2011.03988.x.
44. Argente J, Caballo N, Barrios V, Pozo J, Munoz MT, Chowen JA, Hernandez M. Multiple endocrine abnormalities of the growth hormone and insulin-like growth factor axis in prepubertal children with exogenous obesity: effect of short- and long-term weight reduction. J Clin Endocrinol Metab. 1997;82(7):2076–83.
45. Butenandt O, Kunze D. Growth velocity in constitutional delay of growth and development. J Pediatr Endocrinol Metab. 2010;23(1–2):19–25.
46. Saggese G, Cesaretti G, Giannessi N, Bracaloni C, Cinquanta L, Cioni C. Stimulated growth hormone (GH) secretion in children with delays in pubertal development before and after the onset of puberty: relationship with peripheral plasma GH-releasing hormone and somatostatin levels. J Clin Endocrinol Metab. 1992;74(2):272–8.
47. Martinez AS, Domene HM, Ropelato MG, Jasper HG, Pennisi PA, Escobar ME, Heinrich JJ. Estrogen priming effect on growth hormone (GH) provocative test: a useful tool for the diagnosis of GH deficiency. J Clin Endocrinol Metab. 2000;85(11):4168–72.
48. Marin G, Domené HM, Barnes KM, Blackwell BJ, Cassorla FG, Cutler Jr GB. The effects of estrogen priming and puberty on the growth hormone response to standardized treadmill exercise and arginine-insulin in normal girls and boys. J Clin Endocrinol Metab. 1994;79(2):537–41.
49. Giustina A, Wehrenberg WB. Influence of thyroid hormones on the regulation of growth hormone secretion. Eur J Endocrinol. 1995;133(6):646–53.
50. GH Research Society. Consensus guidelines for the diagnosis and treatment of growth hormone (GH) deficiency in childhood and adolescence: summary statement of the GH Research Society. J Clin Endocrinol Metab. 2000;85:3990–3.
51. Tanner JM, Whitehouse RH. Clinical longitudinal standards for height, weight, height velocity, weight velocity, and stages of puberty. Arch Dis Child. 1976;51:170.

# Chapter 9
# Laboratory Diagnosis of Growth Hormone Deficiency in Adults

Kevin C.J. Yuen

## Introduction

Physiological growth hormone (GH) secretion is pulsatile and accounts for more than 85 % of the total daily GH secretion [1]. Due to its circadian and pulsatile nature of secretion, serum GH levels can vary between peaks and troughs. In addition, GH secretion is influenced by many factors such as gender, pubertal status, nutrition, sleep patterns, physical activity, body composition, stress, gonadal steroids, and prevailing insulin levels [2]. Peripheral GH actions are primarily mediated through insulin-like growth factor-I (IGF-I) synthesized in the liver. IGF-I is a 70 amino acid protein that has a longer half-life in the circulation than GH and is considered to provide an integrated measure of GH secretion.

Growth hormone deficiency (GHD) in adults is a well-recognized clinical syndrome that affects many organs and systems, and is characterized by alterations in body composition, decreased aerobic exercise capacity, impaired quality of life, and adverse changes of carbohydrate metabolism and cardiovascular function. Without the salient sign of impaired linear growth seen in children, the symptoms and signs of GHD in adults are nonspecific; hence laboratory testing to assess GH secretion is essential for diagnosis. However, as serum IGF-I levels decline with normal aging, and tend to be low in obesity and in some common medical conditions such as liver disease, poorly controlled diabetes, and fibromyalgia, serum IGF-I levels can

---

*Author disclosure summary*: KCJY has received research grants from Pfizer, Novo Nordisk, Eli Lilly, Versartis, Prolor, OPKO, and Teva and has served on the advisory boards for Pfizer and Novo Nordisk.

K.C.J. Yuen (✉)
Swedish Pituitary Center, Swedish Neuroscience Institute,
550 17th Avenue, Suite 400, Seattle, WA 98122, USA
e-mail: kevin.yuen@swedish.org

often overlap in normal subjects and in adults with GHD. Furthermore, because states of GH sufficiency and deficiency lie on a continuum, the diagnosis of adult GHD cannot be established by a single random measurement of serum GH or IGF-I level, but is dependent on the demonstration of a subnormal rise in peak serum GH level in response to one or more dynamic laboratory GH stimulation tests. The concept underlying the use of GH stimulation test(s) is to assess the peak level of GH response to a stimulatory agent in normal subjects as compared to adults with GHD, with the final objective of being able to clearly discriminate between the two groups. Various GH stimulatory agents, either used alone or in combination, have been proposed in the past, and although the data of many of these tests have been reported in the literature, very few of these tests have been extensively and vigorously validated.

## Diagnosis of Adult GHD: Current Perspectives

Currently, there is no ideal stimulation test; hence the decision to embark on a stimulation test to assess the GH status of an individual must factor in the validity of the chosen test, its appropriate cut-point limits, and the availability of local resources and expertise. In addition, GH immunoassay results may vary between different assay methods. Reasons for the variability in GH assay results include the heterogeneity of the analyte, the availability of different preparations for calibration, and the interference from matrix components such as GH-binding protein [3]. Furthermore, the reporting of results in mass units or international units together with the application of variable conversion factors may lead to confusion. The current international reference standard advocated by the Growth Research Society (GRS) for GH assays is International Reference Preparation 88/624 (1 mg = 3.0 U) and for IGF-I assays is International Reference Preparation 87/518, but the society acknowledges that further comparative studies are needed to achieve standardization of GH and IGF-I assays [4]. The GRS also calls for assay manufacturers to publish the validation of their assays, which should include specification of the GH isoforms detected (20 kDa GH, 22 kDa GH, and other isoforms) and the presence or absence of any effects due to GH-binding protein, and mandates that GH and IGF-I results should be expressed in mass, not international units [4].

Current published guidelines recommend the evaluation of adult GHD to be based on clinical findings and medical history (e.g., patients with hypothalamic-pituitary disease, those who have received cranial irradiation or tumor treatment, and those with a history of traumatic brain injury or subarachnoid hemorrhage), using the appropriate laboratory GH stimulation test(s) for biochemical confirmation [4–6]. In certain subgroups of patients, the timing for testing for adult GHD is critical. For example, childhood-onset GHD may persist into adulthood and requires retesting at least 4 weeks after stopping GH replacement to confirm the diagnosis. The diagnostic cutoff having the optimal sensitivity and specificity in this transition period appears to be higher than in adults but has not been well established. In those with a history of traumatic brain injury, GHD should be tested at 3 and 12 months after the injury since there is a possibility that GH secretion may recover over time. By contrast, in patients with three or more pituitary hormone deficiencies and low serum IGF-I levels below the reference range in the appropriate clinical context, the diagnosis of adult GHD can be made without requiring GH stimulation testing. Testing should also be performed under stable conditions with adequate replacement of other pituitary hormone deficits in patients with hypopituitarism.

The insulin tolerance test (ITT) is currently accepted as the gold standard test for evaluation of GHD and is endorsed by several consensus guidelines [4–6]. However, this test is labor intensive and unpleasant for some patients, has potential risks, and is contraindicated in the elderly and in patients with seizure disorders and coronary artery disease. Thus, there remains a genuine unmet medical need for an alternative test to the ITT that is safe, accurate, convenient, and reproducible. Following the publication of several validation studies [7–10] and recommendations from current consensus guidelines [4–6], the GH-releasing hormone (GHRH) plus arginine (GHRH-arginine) test was accepted as the alternative GH stimulation test to the ITT. However, when EMD Serono Inc. discontinued production of Geref® (a GHRH analogue) in the United States in 2008 [11], the Endocrine Society [6] and the American Association of Clinical Endocrinologists [5] endorsed the glucagon stimulation test (GST) as the alternative test when the ITT is contraindicated.

## Stimulatory Tests Used in Diagnosing Adult GHD

### *Insulin Tolerance Test (Table 9.1)*

Following the seminal work in 1969 by Plumpton and Besser [12], the ITT has become a valuable tool in the investigation of pituitary function. This test remains widely considered as the gold standard test for the assessment of GHD in adults because insulin-induced hypoglycemia is a powerful stimulator of endogenous GH secretion. Another advantage of this test is that it can also simultaneously assess the hypothalamic-pituitary-adrenal (HPA) axis for adrenal insufficiency. The reliability of the ITT as a GH stimulation test with a GH cut point of 5 ng/mL was demonstrated by results indicating 96 % sensitivity and 92 % specificity when evaluated by a receiver-operator characteristic curve analysis [8]. The caveat for this test is that results of the ITT are gender dependent and patients with obesity and/or glucose intolerance demonstrate falsely blunted GH responses, resulting in a false-positive diagnosis of adult GHD [13]. In addition, there have also been some concerns raised by some investigators about its reproducibility and specificity [14, 15].

**Table 9.1** Recommended protocol for performing the ITT

| | |
|---|---|
| *Contraindications*: | |
| | History of epileptic seizures, coronary artery disease, cerebrovascular disease, pregnancy, or age >55 years |
| *Precautions*: | |
| | Patients commonly develop neuroglycopenic symptoms during the test and should be encouraged to report these symptoms (administration of IV antiemetics can be considered) |
| | Late hypoglycemia may occur (patients should be advised to eat small and frequent meals after completion of the test) |
| *Procedure*: | |
| | Ensure patient is fasted from midnight for 8–10 h from solids and liquids (except water) |
| | Withhold all morning medications (if the HPA axis is simultaneously assessed; glucocorticoids should be withheld ≥12 h before testing) |
| | Weigh patient |
| | Place IV cannula in both forearms[a] |
| | Administer IV human regular insulin (standard dose, 0.05–0.1 units/kg for nondiabetic subjects with a BMI <30 kg/m$^2$, and high dose, 0.15–0.3 units/kg for subjects with a BMI ≥30 kg/m$^2$ and subjects with insulin resistance)[b] |
| *Sampling and measurements*: | |
| *Baseline* | |
| | Blood is drawn for glucose measurement with a glucometer |
| | Blood drawn for baseline glucose, GH, and IGF-I (cortisol and ACTH, if HPA axis is assessed simultaneously) levels will be sent to the laboratory for further analysis |
| *During the test* | |
| | Blood samples are drawn from the IV line every 5–10 min for measurement of glucose levels using a glucometer |
| | Signs and symptoms of neuroglycopenia are recorded |
| | When blood glucose levels from the glucometer approaches 45 mg/dL (2.5 mmol/L), blood samples are sent to the laboratory for measurements of blood glucose levels |
| | When symptomatic hypoglycemia is achieved (laboratory blood glucose <40 mg/dL or 2.2 mmol/L), additional blood samples are collected to measure glucose and GH (+/− cortisol if the HPA axis is assessed simultaneously) levels at 20, 25, 30, 35, 40, 60, and 90 min |
| | The *patient* can begin drinking orange juice and eat to raise his/her blood glucose levels (IV 100 mL of 5 % dextrose can be administered if the patient cannot tolerate oral intake due to nausea or vomiting) |
| *At the end of the test* | |
| | Blood glucose levels measured from the glucometer should increase to levels >70 mg/dL (3.9 mmol/L) before the patient is discharged from the testing unit |
| *Interpretation*: | |
| | If adequate (symptomatic) hypoglycemia is not achieved (<40 mg/dL or 2.2 mmol/L), then GHD cannot be diagnosed |
| | Peak serum GH levels <5 μg/L at any time point during the hypoglycemic phase of the test is diagnostic of adult GHD |

*ACTH* adrenocorticotropic hormone, *HPA* hypothalamic-pituitary-adrenal, *IV* intravenous

[a]Two IV lines are placed because one IV line is used for the administration of insulin bolus and possibly for administration of IV 5 % dextrose if the patient requires resuscitation from hypoglycemia, while the other IV line is used for repeated blood draws

[b]In certain patients with BMIs >30 kg/m$^2$ who appear muscular with enhanced insulin sensitivity, clinical discretion is required in deciding the insulin dose for these patients. A lower dose may be more appropriate in preventing severe hypoglycemia

## Glucagon Stimulation Test (Table 9.2)

The use of the GST for the assessment of GH reserve was first described in 1969 by Mitchell et al. [16]. Since then, the GST has been shown by several investigators to have a GH secretory potency that is similar to or slightly less than the ITT, suggesting that it is more reliable than other classic agents such as arginine or clonidine for differentiating GH-deficient patients from normal subjects [17–22]. The GST has been validated with the ITT in assessing GH reserve [18, 23, 24] and hypothalamic-pituitary-adrenal (HPA) [25, 26] axes in children, but the true mechanism(s) of how glucagon stimulates GH release remains unclear. With the unavailability of the GHRH-arginine test due to the discontinuation of Geref® (a GHRH analogue) in the United States since 2008, the GST has since been increasingly used because of its availability, reproducibility, safety, and lack of influence by gender and hypothalamic cause of GHD [5, 6, 27].

The rate of nausea, vomiting, and headaches during GST ranges from less than 10 % [18] to 34 % [28]. In our experience of 425 GSTs performed at five academic centers in the United States, the main side effects reported were nausea (37.2 %), vomiting (2.4 %), hunger, headaches, sleepiness, body chills, lightheadedness, and abdominal cramping that occurred mainly between 60 and 210 min and that most of these events were mild or moderate in severity that resolved by 240 min of the test [29]. However, in this study, we also found a substantial number of patients with glucose intolerance and high body mass index (BMI) who failed the GST compared to those with normoglycemia and BMIs less than 30 kg/m$^2$ [29]. This raises the question of the reliability of the GST in assessing GH reserve in patients with underlying glucose intolerance and/or obesity. To address this question, Dichtel et al. [30] recently examined the GH response to glucagon in adult men with BMIs of 25 kg/m$^2$ or more and found that using the traditional peak GH cut-point value of 3 ng/mL on GST in otherwise healthy overweight and obese individuals led to significant overdiagnosis of adult GHD. Consequently, these investigators proposed a lower GH cut point of 1 ng/mL and demonstrated that this cut point significantly increases the specificity and preserves the sensitivity of the GST for diagnosing adult GHD in this population.

The diagnosis of secondary adrenal insufficiency can also be challenging, particularly in patients with recent pituitary surgery or cranial irradiation when the adrenal cortex may still be responsive to stress but the hypothalamic-pituitary function is compromised. A number of studies have investigated the utility of GST in evaluating the HPA axis [28, 31, 32], but to date, there is no accurate validation on the peak cortisol cut points that can reliably diagnose secondary adrenal insufficiency. In patients where there is a possibility of secondary adrenal insufficiency, I propose measuring cortisol levels during the GST. If peak cortisol levels during the GST exceed 20 µg/dL, then no further testing of the HPA axis is necessary, but if peak cortisol levels are 20 µg/dL or less, further testing of the HPA axis with either an ITT or an ACTH stimulation test is required to confirm the diagnosis of adrenal insufficiency.

**Table 9.2** Recommended protocol for performing the GST

| | |
|---|---|
| *Contraindications*: | |
| Malnourished patients or patients who have not eaten for >48 h | |
| *Precautions*: | |
| Patients may feel nauseous during and after the test (administration of IV antiemetics can be considered) | |
| Late hypoglycemia may occur (patients should be advised to eat small and frequent meals after completion of the test) | |
| No peak GH responses have been studied using the GST in normal subjects >70 years, and none of the previous studies included patients with diabetes mellitus. Therefore, caution should be exercised when interpreting normal GST results in these patients. If the suspicion of GHD remains high in these patients, it is reasonable to consider using a second GH stimulatory test | |
| *Procedure*: | |
| Ensure patient is fasted from midnight for 8–10 h from solids and liquids (except water) | |
| Withhold all morning medications (if the HPA axis is simultaneously assessed; glucocorticoids should be withheld ≥12 h before testing) | |
| Weigh patient | |
| Place IV cannula in one forearm | |
| Administer glucagon 1 mg (1.5 mg if patient weighs more than 90 kg) as an IM bolus | |
| *Sampling and measurements*: | |
| Serum GH (+/− ACTH at baseline and cortisol at all time points if the HPA axis is assessed simultaneously) and capillary blood glucose levels are measured at baseline, 30, 60, 90, 120, 150, 180, 210, and 240 min[a] | |
| *Interpretation*: | |
| Peak serum GH levels tend to occur between 120 and 180 min | |
| Peak GH levels <3 μg/L at any time point during testing is diagnostic of adult GHD | |

*IM* intramuscular
[a]Blood glucose levels are monitored for late hypoglycemia and not used to interpret the test. While the lowest blood glucose level with the GST in the literature was reported at 37 mg/dL [16], in our experience, we did not observe blood glucose levels below 40 mg/dL with this test [29]

## *GHRH-Arginine Test (Table 9.3)*

The GHRH-arginine test has been validated in several studies as a reliable alternative test when the ITT is contraindicated or impractical [8, 9] and is endorsed by the Endocrine Society [6], the American Association of Clinical Endocrinologists [5], and the GRS [4]. Arginine potentiates and reduces variability in GHRH-stimulated GH secretion by inhibiting release of somatostatin from the hypothalamus. In 2008, EMD Serono, the sole distributor of Geref® (a GHRH analogue) in the United States, discontinued its production leaving a need for an alternative test [11, 27]. Stratum Medical Corporation (San Diego, CA, USA) is currently developing GHRH Diagnostic, which is chemically identical to Geref®. However, GHRH Diagnostic is currently only available for investigational use under its

**Table 9.3** Recommended protocol for performing the GHRH-arginine test

| | |
|---|---|
| *Contraindications*: | |
| Allergy to GHRH analogue and arginine | |
| *Precautions*: | |
| Transient sensation of body warmth and/or flushing due to GHRH | |
| Other side effects of GHRH are nausea, headache, experiencing a strange taste in the mouth, and transient hypotension | |
| *Procedure*: | |
| Ensure patient is fasted from midnight for 8–10 h from solids and liquids (except water) | |
| Withhold all morning medications | |
| Weigh patient | |
| Place IV cannula in one forearm | |
| Administer GHRH analogue (1 µg/kg) [GHRH 1-29 (Geref®, Serono, Inc., Norwell, MA, USA)] as an IV bolus and arginine hydrochloride 30 g simultaneously as an IV infusion from 0 to 30 min | |
| *Sampling and measurements*: | |
| Baseline | |
| Blood is drawn for laboratory measurements of GH and IGF-I levels | |
| *During the test* | |
| Serum GH levels are measured at 30, 60, 90, and 120 min | |
| *Interpretation*: | |
| Two important factors must be taken into consideration when interpreting the GHRH-arginine test: | |
| 1. Because GHRH directly stimulates somatotroph cells, this test can yield misleadingly normal responses in patients with a hypothalamic GHD (e.g., patients with previous cranial radiotherapy or hypothalamic tumors) [43] | |
| 2. Cut points to diagnose adult GHD are BMI-dependent. Peak serum GH levels <11.0 µg/L, 8.0 µg/L, and 4.0 µL at any time point during testing in patients with BMIs ≥30 kg/m$^2$, 25–30 kg/m$^2$, and <25 kg/m$^2$, respectively, are diagnostic of adult GHD [5] | |

Investigational New Drug registration with the US Food and Drug Administration (PIND 106, 573) [33].

## *Arginine Test (Table 9.4)*

The diagnostic reliability of arginine alone has been previously questioned [8, 17]. Arginine alone is less reliable than the ITT or GHRH-arginine test [8] because the mean peak GH response to arginine alone is lower compared with the ITT in adults with GHD [34] and in normal lean subjects [22]. Thus, the Endocrine Society [6] and the American Association of Clinical Endocrinologist [5] guidelines recommend utilizing this test only when the ITT and the GST are contraindicated or if glucagon is unavailable. If this test is to be used, appropriately low peak GH cut points should be employed (for 95 % sensitivity, 1.4 µg/L; for 95 % specificity, 0.21 µg/L, and to minimize misclassification in either direction, 0.4 µg/L) [8].

**Table 9.4** Recommended protocol for performing the arginine test

| | |
|---|---|
| *Contraindications*: | |
| | Allergy to arginine |
| *Precautions*: | |
| | Nausea, vomiting, headache, and flushing |
| | If the solution extravasates, local skin irritation may occur |
| *Procedure*: | |
| | Ensure patient is fasted from midnight for 8–10 h from solids and liquids (except water) |
| | Withhold all morning medications |
| | Weigh patient |
| | Place IV cannula in one forearm |
| | Administer arginine 0.5 g/kg (maximum 30 g) as an IV infusion over 30 min |
| *Sampling and measurements*: | |
| *Baseline* | |
| | Blood is drawn for laboratory measurements of GH and IGF-I levels |
| *During the test* | |
| | Serum GH levels are measured at 30, 60, 90, and 120 min |
| *Interpretation*: | |
| | Peak GH levels <0.4 µg/L at any time point during testing is diagnostic of adult GHD [8] |

## *Ghrelin Mimetics*

The reliability of testing with GH secretagogues such as GH-releasing peptide-2 alone [35], GH-releasing peptide-6 alone, and combined GH-releasing peptide-6 plus GHRH [36] in comparison with the ITT has been previously evaluated. These agents work on the same concept as the GHRH-arginine test in stimulating pituitary GH release by mimicking the activity of the natural GH secretagogue receptor ligand (i.e., ghrelin) to stimulate endogenous GHRH and to block somatostatin action. The limitation of these agents is that they are more likely to explore the pituitary somatotroph releasable pool and might potentially induce misleadingly normal peak GH responses in patients with hypothalamic causes of GHD [37]. Previous studies have reported that GHRP-6 has been tested alone and in combination with GHRH as a provocative test for adult GHD [36–38], and these studies have demonstrated its accuracy comparable to ITT, although with varying cut points. The only notable side effect observed was flushing. In these studies, GHRP-6 was administered as an IV injection, and peak GH levels occur at 15–30 min, significantly earlier than in other GH provocative tests. Peak GH levels in the GHRH-GHRP-6 test are unaffected by age, sex, or increased BMI [38]. In addition, the GHRP-6 test is highly specific [39], but less sensitive than the ITT for the diagnosis of adult GHD, and is of little utility in the diagnosis of adrenal insufficiency [40]. In another study comparing GHRP-2 with ITT in adults with GHD and controls, a diagnostic cut point of 15 µg/L with GHRP-2 corresponded to a cut point of 3 µg/L with the ITT [35]. The results were reproducible on repeated testing, and the GH peak after GHRP-2 typically occurred within 1 h. Other GH secretagogues such as acylated ghrelin [41] and macimorelin [42] in assessing for adult GHD have also been recently reported. These agents utilize the same concept as the GHRH-arginine test in stimulating pituitary GH release by mimicking the activity of the natural GH secretagogue receptor ligand (i.e., ghrelin) and appear to demonstrate a good safety profile with relatively few contraindications. However, none of these GH secretagogue agents are currently available commercially in the United States.

## Future Perspectives

Recent studies have indicated that further refinements to the GST are still necessary to improve the sensitivity and specificity of this test. We reported a 2-year experience of fixed and weight-based dosing of 515 GSTs conducted at five academic centers in the United States and explored the potential of the GST in testing the HPA axis [29]. In this study, we found that the weight-based dosing regimen induced higher peak and nadir glucose levels, with peak GH and peak cortisol levels occurring later in the test compared to the fixed dosing regimen. Vomiting was more prevalent in the weight-based regimen, and age, BMI, and glucose tolerance may impact glucagon-induced GH and cortisol secretion. Overall, the GST was well tolerated and can be performed as an outpatient; however further studies are required to determine whether GSTs may falsely diagnose GHD in patients with fasting hyperglycemia and/or high BMIs. Thus, to improve the diagnostic reliability of the GST especially in patients with glucose intolerance and in those with high BMIs, a priming agent could be used to combine with the GST with appropriate cut points to improve its sensitivity and specificity, similar to the GHRH in priming the arginine test. Until such data becomes available, it may be necessary to consider repeating the GH stimulation test over time for such patients.

More recently, Garcia et al. [42] reported data of a multicenter study assessing the diagnostic efficacy of a novel oral GH secretagogue AEZS-130 (Macimorelin, Aeterna Zentaris, Inc., Basking Ridge, NJ, USA) compared to the GHRH-arginine test in 50 adults with GHD and 48 healthy controls [42]. The optimal GH cut point was 6.8 µg/L for patients with BMIs less than 30 kg/m$^2$ and 2.7 µg/L for patients with BMI of 30 kg/m$^2$ or more. These cut points yielded 82 % sensitivity, 92 %

specificity, and 87 % accuracy at the 60 min time point of the test. These results are promising as they demonstrate the safety, convenience, and comparable efficacy of oral macimorelin to the GHRH-arginine test in diagnosing adult GHD, but further studies involving larger numbers are needed to compare its diagnostic accuracy with that of the ITT.

## Conclusions

Laboratory testing for adult GHD should only be undertaken when GH replacement is considered in patients with an appropriate clinical context. In line with recently published consensus guidelines [4–6], the ITT should remain as the test of reference due to its greatest diagnostic accuracy, even in patients with suspected hypothalamic GHD. However, due to the inherent drawbacks of the ITT, the GST, with its current available evidence of its diagnostic accuracy, should remain as the alternative test to the ITT for diagnosing adult GHD. For the time being, the traditional peak GH cut-point value of 3 ng/mL should be employed until larger studies are performed to further validate the use of lower GH cut points of the GST in patients with underlying glucose intolerance and/or obesity. In addition, despite some studies demonstrating the comparability of the GST to the ITT in assessing the HPA axis [25, 26], further refinements to the cortisol cut points for the GST are still needed to improve the diagnostic accuracy of the GST in assessing the HPA axis in adults. If the GST can be shown to reliably distinguish adrenal sufficiency from insufficiency, then the ability of assessing both the GH and cortisol reserve simultaneously, just as in the ITT, would make this test more attractive. While previous studies have shown that the GST could be shortened from 4 to 3 h and yet maintain its diagnostic utility [28, 32], until further prospective data becomes available, the GST should be conducted over 4 h to ensure that delayed peak GH responses and late hypoglycemia are not missed. Recent GH stimulation studies using newly formulated GH secretagogue ghrelin mimetics appear promising as these tests are simple, effective, and well tolerated. With further validation and when they eventually become available commercially, these agents may potentially become the test of choice for evaluating adult GHD.

## References

1. Veldhuis JD, Bowers CY. Regulated recovery of pulsatile growth hormone secretion from negative feedback: a preclinical investigation. Am J Physiol Regul Integr Comp Physiol. 2011;301:R1143–52.
2. Giustina A, Veldhuis JD. Pathophysiology of the neuroregulation of growth hormone secretion in experimental animals and the human. Endocr Rev. 1998;19:717–97.
3. Bidlingmaier M, Freda PU. Measurement of human growth hormone by immunoassays: current status, unsolved problems and clinical consequences. Growth Horm IGF Res. 2010;20:19–25.

4. Ho KK. Consensus guidelines for the diagnosis and treatment of adults with GH deficiency II: a statement of the GH Research Society in association with the European Society for Pediatric Endocrinology, Lawson Wilkins Society, European Society of Endocrinology, Japan Endocrine Society, and Endocrine Society of Australia. Eur J Endocrinol. 2007;157:695–700.
5. Cook DM, Yuen KC, Biller BM, Kemp SF, Vance ML. American Association of Clinical Endocrinologists medical guidelines for clinical practice for growth hormone use in growth hormone-deficient adults and transition patients – 2009 update. Endocr Pract. 2009;15 Suppl 2:1–29.
6. Molitch ME, Clemmons DR, Malozowski S, Merriam GR, Vance ML. Evaluation and treatment of adult growth hormone deficiency: an endocrine society clinical practice guideline. J Clin Endocrinol Metab. 2011;96:1587–609.
7. Aimaretti G, Corneli G, Razzore P, Bellone S, Baffoni C, Arvat E, Camanni F, Ghigo E. Comparison between insulin-induced hypoglycemia and growth hormone (GH)-releasing hormone + arginine as provocative tests for the diagnosis of GH deficiency in adults. J Clin Endocrinol Metab. 1998;83:1615–8.
8. Biller BM, Samuels MH, Zagar A, Cook DM, Arafah BM, Bonert V, Stavrou S, Kleinberg DL, Chipman JJ, Hartman ML. Sensitivity and specificity of six tests for the diagnosis of adult GH deficiency. J Clin Endocrinol Metab. 2002;87:2067–79.
9. Corneli G, Di Somma C, Prodam F, Bellone J, Bellone S, Gasco V, Baldelli R, Rovere S, Schneider HJ, Gargantini L, Gastaldi R, Ghizzoni L, Valle D, Salerno M, Colao A, Bona G, Ghigo E, Maghnie M, Aimaretti G. Cut-off limits of the GH response to GHRH plus arginine test and IGF-I levels for the diagnosis of GH deficiency in late adolescents and young adults. Eur J Endocrinol. 2007;157:701–8.
10. Maghnie M, Salati B, Bianchi S, Rallo M, Tinelli C, Autelli M, Aimaretti G, Ghigo E. Relationship between the morphological evaluation of the pituitary and the growth hormone (GH) response to GH-releasing hormone Plus arginine in children and adults with congenital hypopituitarism. J Clin Endocrinol Metab. 2001;86:1574–9.
11. Serono E. http://www.fda.gov/cder/drug/shortages/GerefDiagnosticDiscontinuationLetter.pdf. July 2008.
12. Plumpton FS, Besser GM. The adrenocortical response to surgery and insulin-induced hypoglycaemia in corticosteroid-treated and normal subjects. Br J Surg. 1969;56:216–9.
13. Gabellieri E, Chiovato L, Lage M, Castro AI, Casanueva FF. Testing growth hormone deficiency in adults. Front Horm Res. 2010;38:139–44.
14. Hoeck HC, Vestergaard P, Jakobsen PE, Laurberg P. Test of growth hormone secretion in adults: poor reproducibility of the insulin tolerance test. Eur J Endocrinol. 1995;133:305–12.
15. Vestergaard P, Hoeck HC, Jakobsen PE, Laurberg P. Reproducibility of growth hormone and cortisol responses to the insulin tolerance test and the short ACTH test in normal adults. Horm Metab Res. 1997;29:106–10.
16. Mitchell ML, Byrne MJ, Silver J. Growth-hormone release by glucagon. Lancet. 1969;1: 289–90.
17. Aimaretti G, Baffoni C, DiVito L, Bellone S, Grottoli S, Maccario M, Arvat E, Camanni F, Ghigo E. Comparisons among old and new provocative tests of GH secretion in 178 normal adults. Eur J Endocrinol. 2000;142:347–52.
18. Berg C, Meinel T, Lahner H, Yuece A, Mann K, Petersenn S. Diagnostic utility of the glucagon stimulation test in comparison to the insulin tolerance test in patients following pituitary surgery. Eur J Endocrinol. 2010;162:477–82.
19. Conceicao FL, da Costa e Silva A, Leal Costa AJ, Vaisman M. Glucagon stimulation test for the diagnosis of GH deficiency in adults. J Endocrinol Invest. 2003;26:1065–70.
20. Ghigo E, Bartolotta E, Imperiale E, Bellone J, Cardinale G, Aimaretti G, Valetto MR, Cherubini V, Maccario M, Cocchi D, et al. Glucagon stimulates GH secretion after intramuscular but not intravenous administration. Evidence against the assumption that glucagon per se has a GH-releasing activity. J Endocrinol Invest. 1994;17:849–54.
21. Gomez JM, Espadero RM, Escobar-Jimenez F, Hawkins F, Pico A, Herrera-Pombo JL, Vilardell E, Duran A, Mesa J, Faure E, Sanmarti A. Growth hormone release after glucagon as a reliable test of growth hormone assessment in adults. Clin Endocrinol (Oxf). 2002;56:329–34.

22. Rahim A, Toogood AA, Shalet SM. The assessment of growth hormone status in normal young adult males using a variety of provocative agents. Clin Endocrinol (Oxf). 1996;45:557–62.
23. Micmacher E, Assumpcao RP, Redorat RG, Spina LD, Cruz IC, Silva CA, Vaisman M, Conceicao FL. Growth hormone secretion in response to glucagon stimulation test in healthy middle-aged men. Arq Bras Endocrinol Metabol. 2009;53:853–8.
24. Secco A, di Iorgi N, Napoli F, Calandra E, Ghezzi M, Frassinetti C, Parodi S, Casini MR, Lorini R, Loche S, Maghnie M. The glucagon test in the diagnosis of growth hormone deficiency in children with short stature younger than 6 years. J Clin Endocrinol Metab. 2009;94:4251–7.
25. Bottner A, Kratzsch J, Liebermann S, Keller A, Pfaffle RW, Kiess W, Keller E. Comparison of adrenal function tests in children–the glucagon stimulation test allows the simultaneous assessment of adrenal function and growth hormone response in children. J Pediatr Endocrinol Metab. 2005;18:433–42.
26. di Iorgi N, Napoli F, Allegri A, Secco A, Calandra E, Calcagno A, Frassinetti C, Ghezzi M, Ambrosini L, Parodi S, Gastaldi R, Loche S, Maghnie M. The accuracy of the glucagon test compared to the insulin tolerance test in the diagnosis of adrenal insufficiency in young children with growth hormone deficiency. J Clin Endocrinol Metab. 2010;95:2132–9.
27. Yuen KC, Biller BM, Molitch ME, Cook DM. Clinical review: is lack of recombinant growth hormone (GH)-releasing hormone in the United States a setback or time to consider glucagon testing for adult GH deficiency? J Clin Endocrinol Metab. 2009;94:2702–7.
28. Leong KS, Walker AB, Martin I, Wile D, Wilding J, MacFarlane IA. An audit of 500 subcutaneous glucagon stimulation tests to assess growth hormone and ACTH secretion in patients with hypothalamic-pituitary disease. Clin Endocrinol (Oxf). 2001;54:463–8.
29. Yuen KC, Biller BM, Katznelson L, Rhoads SA, Gurel MH, Chu O, Corazzini V, Spiller K, Gordon MB, Salvatori R, Cook DM. Clinical characteristics, timing of peak responses and safety aspects of two dosing regimens of the glucagon stimulation test in evaluating growth hormone and cortisol secretion in adults. Pituitary. 2013;16:220–30.
30. Dichtel LE, Yuen KC, Bredella MA, Gerweck AV, Russell BM, Riccio AD, Gurel MH, Sluss PM, Biller BM, Miller KK. Overweight/obese adults with pituitary disorders require lower peak growth hormone cutoff values on glucagon stimulation testing to avoid overdiagnosis of growth hormone deficiency. J Clin Endocrinol Metab. 2014;99:4712–9.
31. Arvat E, Maccagno B, Ramunni J, Maccario M, Giordano R, Broglio F, Camanni F, Ghigo E. Interaction between glucagon and human corticotropin-releasing hormone or vasopressin on ACTH and cortisol secretion in humans. Eur J Endocrinol. 2000;143:99–104.
32. Orme SM, Price A, Weetman AP, Ross RJ. Comparison of the diagnostic utility of the simplified and standard i.m. glucagon stimulation test (IMGST). Clin Endocrinol (Oxf). 1998;49:773–8.
33. Tschopp JF. www.StratumMedical.com. Accessed 27 April 2015.
34. Kinoshita Y, Tominaga A, Usui S, Arita K, Sakoguchi T, Sugiyama K, Kurisu K. The arginine and GHRP-2 tests as alternatives to the insulin tolerance test for the diagnosis of adult GH deficiency in Japanese patients: a comparison. Endocr J. 2013;60:97–105.
35. Chihara K, Shimatsu A, Hizuka N, Tanaka T, Seino Y, Katofor Y. A simple diagnostic test using GH-releasing peptide-2 in adult GH deficiency. Eur J Endocrinol. 2007;157:19–27.
36. Petersenn S, Jung R, Beil FU. Diagnosis of growth hormone deficiency in adults by testing with GHRP-6 alone or in combination with GHRH: comparison with the insulin tolerance test. Eur J Endocrinol. 2002;146:667–72.
37. Popovic V, Pekic S, Golubicic I, Doknic M, Dieguez C, Casanueva FF. The impact of cranial irradiation on GH responsiveness to GHRH plus GH-releasing peptide-6. J Clin Endocrinol Metab. 2002;87:2095–9.
38. Popovic V, Leal A, Micic D, Koppeschaar HP, Torres E, Paramo C, Obradovic S, Dieguez C, Casanueva FF. GH-releasing hormone and GH-releasing peptide-6 for diagnostic testing in GH-deficient adults. Lancet. 2000;356:1137–42.
39. Alaioubi B, Mann K, Petersenn S. Diagnosis of growth hormone deficiency in adults: provocative testing with GHRP6 in comparison to the insulin tolerance test. Horm Metab Res. 2009;41:238–43.

40. Alaioubi B, Mann K, Petersenn S. Diagnosis of adrenal insufficiency using the GHRP-6 test: comparison with the insulin tolerance test in patients with hypothalamic-pituitary-adrenal disease. Horm Metab Res. 2010;42:198–203.
41. Gasco V, Beccuti G, Baldini C, Prencipe N, Di Giacomo S, Berton A, Guaraldi F, Tabaro I, Maccario M, Ghigo E, Grottoli S. Acylated ghrelin as a provocative test for the diagnosis of GH deficiency in adults. Eur J Endocrinol. 2013;168:23–30.
42. Garcia JM, Swerdloff R, Wang C, Kyle M, Kipnes M, Biller BM, Cook D, Yuen KC, Bonert V, Dobs A, Molitch ME, Merriam GR. Macimorelin (AEZS-130)-stimulated growth hormone (GH) test: validation of a novel oral stimulation test for the diagnosis of adult GH deficiency. J Clin Endocrinol Metab. 2013;98:2422–9.
43. Darzy KH, Aimaretti G, Wieringa G, Gattamaneni HR, Ghigo E, Shalet SM. The usefulness of the combined growth hormone (GH)-releasing hormone and arginine stimulation test in the diagnosis of radiation-induced GH deficiency is dependent on the post-irradiation time interval. J Clin Endocrinol Metab. 2003;88:95–102.

# Chapter 10
# Pituitary Gland Imaging

**Natascia Di Iorgi, Giovanni Morana, Flavia Napoli, Andrea Rossi, and Mohamad Maghnie**

## Introduction

Establishing endocrine and magnetic resonance imaging (MRI) phenotypes is extremely helpful in the selection and management of patients with growth hormone deficiency (GHD), both in terms of the early diagnosis of evolving anterior pituitary hormone deficiencies and possible genetic counseling. Indeed, modern neuroimaging techniques represent an essential tool in the evaluation of the hypothalamic–pituitary area and brain structures, and the advent of MRI has significantly enhanced overall diagnostic accuracy. The use of MRI has led to an enormous increase in our comprehensive knowledge of pituitary morphology, improving, in particular, a differential diagnosis of hypopituitarism [1, 2].

Today there is convincing evidence to support the hypothesis that marked MRI differences in pituitary morphology with or without additional central nervous system abnormalities indicate a range of disorders which affect the organogenesis and function of the anterior pituitary gland with different prognoses. Specifically, MRI allows a detailed and precise anatomical study of the pituitary gland by differentiating between the anterior and posterior pituitary lobes. The MRI identification of pituitary hyperintensity in the posterior part of the sella, now commonly considered a marker of neurohypophyseal functional integrity, has been the most striking finding for the diagnosis and understanding of anterior and posterior pituitary diseases including idiopathic GHD, as well as hypopituitarism associated with permanent GHD [3–14].

---

N. Di Iorgi • F. Napoli • M. Maghnie (✉)
Department of Pediatrics, IRCCS Giannina Gaslini, University of Genova,
Largo Gerolamo Gaslini 5, 16147 Genoa, Italy
e-mail: mohamadmaghnie@gaslini.org; Mohamad.Maghnie@unige.it

G. Morana • A. Rossi
Department of Pediatric Neuroradiology, Instituto Giannina Gaslini, Genoa, Italy

These neuroimaging developments have inevitably raised some important questions. Is there a gold standard for the diagnosis of GHD and what then is the ultimate goal of MRI examination? Is MRI phenotype imaging informative? Does a diagnosis of MRI phenotype affect the evaluation of patients with GHD? Can MRI phenotype predict the outcome of patients with GHD? And, finally, what is the contribution of these MRI findings to overall GHD management? MRI is certainly an important benchmark, but several questions remain unanswered and others clearly represent a challenge.

This chapter will discuss the current state of knowledge in our understanding of the etiology of hypopituitarism associated with structural hypothalamic–pituitary abnormalities and the most relevant impact of MRI findings in the current management and outcome of diseases involving the hypothalamic–pituitary area.

## Imaging Techniques

MRI is the radiological examination method of choice for evaluating the hypothalamic–pituitary region. Most information is provided by 2–3 mm thick, high-resolution spin-echo (SE) T1- and turbo/fast spin-echo (TSE) T2-weighted images on sagittal and coronal planes. Additionally, heavily T2-weighted images [i.e., driven equilibrium (DRIVE), constructive interference in steady state (CISS), or fast imaging employing steady-state acquisition (FIESTA) sequences] obtained at submillimeter thickness are highly recommended, since they can provide more detailed information of the anatomy of the suprasellar compartment (Fig. 10.1). In particular, the evaluation of the pituitary stalk is significantly improved, while, in our experience, sensitivity is similar to that of post-contrast T1-weighted images; therefore, post-contrast imaging can be safely omitted in patients with an isolated growth hormone (GH) defect, provided that T2-DRIVE has been performed. These 3D sequences also allow a better and more reproducible evaluation of the pituitary stalk on serial studies, as they may be reformatted so as to obtain identical slice orientation when compared to prior studies. Additional midline structures, such as the median eminence, tuber cinereum, mammillary bodies, and the pineal gland, are also extremely well depicted; the main limitation of these sequences is the homogeneously low signal intensity of the pituitary gland that cannot thus be confidently separated into the anterior and posterior lobe [15].

When MRI is unavailable or contraindicated, computerized tomography (CT) remains a valuable alternative for the study of the sellar and parasellar region. Current multislice helical CT provides high-quality coronal and sagittal reformatted images from axial acquisitions. Helical imaging is also useful for minimizing imaging time and radiation dose. CT also has a complementary role in the identification of intralesional calcifications or to better evaluate bone structures (i.e., in the study of the skull base before transsphenoidal surgery or in the case of suspected bone lesions).

# 10 Pituitary Gland Imaging

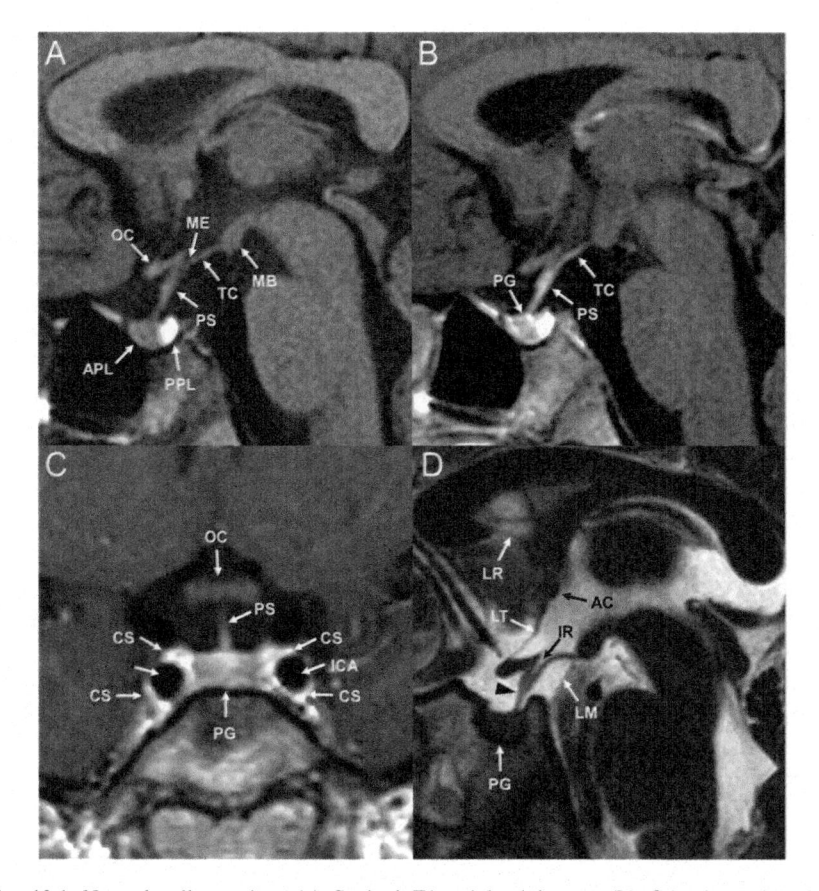

**Fig. 10.1** Normal sellar region. (**a**) Sagittal T1-weighted image; (**b**) Gd-enhanced sagittal T1-weighted image; (**c**) Gd-enhanced coronal T1-weighted image; (**d**) sagittal T2-DRIVE image (different subject). (**a**) The posterior pituitary lobe (PPL), physiologically bright on T1-weighted image, anterior pituitary lobe (APL), pituitary stalk (PS), median eminence (ME), optic chiasm (OC), tuber cinereum (TC), and mammillary bodies (MB) are clearly visible. (**b, c**) Following gadolinium injection, the pituitary gland (PG), stalk (PS), and tuber cinereum (TC) enhance, as well as the cavernous sinuses (CS). The internal carotid arteries (ICA) are recognizable within the cavernous sinuses (CS). On the coronal plane (C), the pituitary stalk (PS) is clearly visible in its midline position, generating a T-shape together with the overlying optic chiasm (OC). (**d**) The pituitary stalk (*arrowhead*) is optimally depicted with sharp delineation of the infundibular recess of the third ventricle (IR). Additional midline structure such as the lamina rostralis (LR), anterior commissure (AC), and lamina terminalis (LT), as well as the Liliequist membrane (LM), are clearly recognizable. Note the homogeneously low signal intensity of the pituitary gland (PG) that cannot thus be confidently separated into the anterior and posterior lobe

In addition to high-resolution sellar MR imaging, one or more survey sequences of the entire brain should also be performed. At least a fluid attenuation inversion recovery (FLAIR) and a diffusion-weighted imaging (DWI) sequence on the axial plane should be acquired to rule out additional brain abnormalities.

DWI provides information regarding diffusion of water molecules in the section studied, from which quantitative values, the so-called apparent diffusion coefficient (ADC), can be calculated. DWI is quick and easy to obtain and, in less than 1 min scan time, provides noninvasive estimation of differences in cell density and tissue structure that may be extremely helpful in characterizing sellar and extrasellar lesions.

Among advanced MR techniques, diffusion tensor imaging (DTI) can add valuable information in the evaluation and characterization of brain malformations that can be associated with hypothalamic–pituitary axis developmental defects. DTI provides information about both the rate and the direction of water motion through the measure of anisotropy, which is the tendency for water molecules to diffuse in some directions rather than equally in all directions. Water diffusion in white matter tends to be more facilitated in the direction of myelinated axons than in the orthogonal direction, and therefore, DTI is a sensitive method to assess normal white matter pathways (tractography) and their alterations in disease states that disrupt tract integrity [16].

MR spectroscopy (MRS) is another advanced MRI technique that can be used in selected cases, in particular in the evaluation and characterization of sellar–suprasellar mass lesions.

This imaging technique allows noninvasive detection and estimation of normal and abnormal metabolites within brain tissue. Different patterns of metabolite concentrations are associated with increased cellular growth, neuronal loss, necrosis, or normal tissue. MRS is presently largely available on clinical MRI scanners and can be performed automatically in most conditions [17]. Of note, the abovementioned advanced MR techniques are not part of the standard examination of the sellar region and should be performed on a case-by-case basis (Table 10.1).

## Neuroimaging of Pituitary Gland

The correct interpretation of MRI scans requires a detailed knowledge of the normal features of the pituitary gland (Fig. 10.1) and of its changes within the same individual over time. The assessment of the pituitary gland includes the evaluation of signal intensity, shape, size, position, and connection with surrounding tissues. The evaluation of central nervous system (CNS) structures, particularly the corpus callosum, septum pellucidum, optic chiasm, olfactory tracts, brain stem, and cerebellum is also mandatory.

### *Normal Pituitary Appearance During Childhood*

The pituitary gland undergoes dynamic changes [18] throughout life, reflecting its complex hormonal environment. In newborns, the gland is typically convex, sometimes pear-shaped, with very high signal intensity on T1-weighted images (Fig. 10.2).

# 10 Pituitary Gland Imaging

**Table 10.1** Standard and advanced MRI protocol in GHD

| | | |
|---|---|---|
| Conventional MRI | Sagittal SE T1 | Anterior and posterior pituitary discrimination. Midline structures and cranio-cervical junction evaluation. Absent bright spot in CDI. High-protein content cysts in craniopharyngiomas and Rathke cleft cysts |
| | Sagittal T2 DRIVE | Pituitary stalk and midline structures evaluation. Optic chiasm and nerves morphology |
| | | Pineal gland evaluation. Pituitary stalk thickness analysis on follow-up |
| | Coronal TSE T2 | Pituitary width evaluation. Pituitary stalk orientation. Optic nerves and chiasm depiction |
| | Axial FLAIR | Screening sequence to evaluate the whole brain. Additional structural sequences (i.e., 3D T1, axial T2) can be performed on a case-by-case basis |
| | Coronal, sagittal, and axial post-contrast T1 | Can be omitted. Pituitary stalk evaluation. Mass lesions characterization. Secondary dissemination |
| Advanced MRI (performed on a case-by-case basis) | Axial DWI | Estimation of differences in cell density and tissue structure (i.e., sellar–extrasellar mass lesions). Highly recommended in standard protocol |
| | DTI | Measurement of the location, orientation, and anisotropy of white matter tracts (i.e., brain malformations) |
| | MRS | Detection and estimation of normal and abnormal metabolites within brain tissue (i.e., sellar–suprasellar mass lesion characterization) |

*MRI* magnetic resonance imaging, *SE* spin echo, *CDI* central diabetes insipidus, *DRIVE* driven equilibrium, *TSE* turbo spin echo, *FLAIR* fluid attenuation inversion recovery, *DWI* diffusion-weighted imaging, *DTI* diffusion tensor imaging, *MRS* magnetic resonance spectroscopy

This morphology and signal intensity correlates with the intense endocrine activity, lactotroph hyperplasia, and protein synthesis known to occur in the gland during the neonatal period. This appearance gradually changes during the first and second months, until the infant configuration, with a flat or slightly concave superior surface and isointensity of the anterior lobe to the white matter on T1- and T2-weighted images, is achieved. During puberty, the anterior pituitary undergoes dramatic changes [19] in size and shape, basically represented by marked enlargement (Fig. 10.3).

By the second month of life, the posterior neural lobe of the gland becomes progressively recognizable next to the dorsum sellae as the "bright spot," because of its marked hyperintensity on T1-weighted images (Fig. 10.2). This finding has been demonstrated to specifically result from the storage of vasopressin, a hormone synthesized by the hypothalamus [20]. The vasopressin-associated carrier protein, neurophysin II, is a very high molecular weight glycoprotein that complexes with vasopressin to form insoluble crystal aggregates and typically shortens the T1 signal.

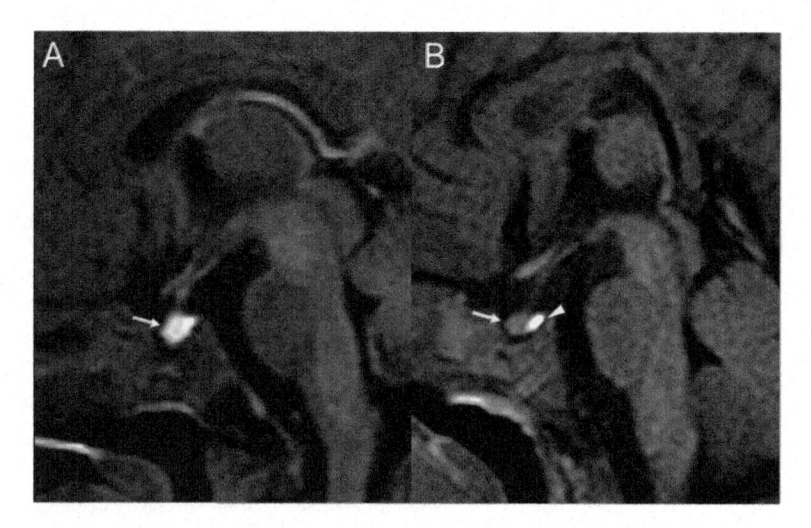

**Fig. 10.2** Postnatal appearance of the pituitary gland on sagittal T1-weighted images obtained in two different children. (**a**) Newborn. Typical pear-shaped configuration of the anterior pituitary lobe that appears spontaneously bright (*arrow*). (**b**) 2 months of age. The pituitary gland shows the typical adult pattern with isointensity of the anterior lobe (*arrow*) to the white matter and hyperintensity of the posterior lobe (*arrowhead*)

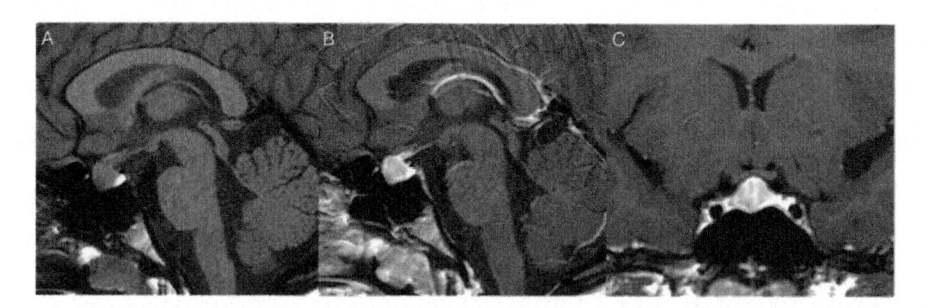

**Fig. 10.3** Pubertal hyperplasia of the pituitary gland in a 14-year-old girl. (**a**) Sagittal T1-weighted image; (**b**) gadolinium-enhanced sagittal T1-weighted image; (**c**) gadolinium-enhanced coronal T1-weighted image. Marked and symmetrical increase in size of the anterior pituitary lobe that appears nearly spherical, with homogeneous enhancement following gadolinium injection. The height of the gland is about 10 mm

Regardless of its chemical origin, the bright spot serves as an important marker of neurohypophyseal function and, when present, documents integrity of the hypothalamic neurohypophyseal tract. However, it is important to remember that the bright spot may be absent in 10 % of normal individuals. The posterior pituitary does not undergo physiological variations in either size or signal intensity during childhood.

Following gadopentetate dimeglumine (gadolinium, Gd-DTPA) administration, marked enhancement of the adenohypophysis and of the infundibulo-tuberal region

**Table 10.2** Hypothalamic–pituitary axis MRI

| Signal intensity | Anterior pituitary | Signal intensity equivalent to that of the white matter on precontrast T1 images (hyperintense at age 0–6 weeks) | |
|---|---|---|---|
| | Posterior pituitary | Bright spot next to the dorsum sellae on precontrast T1 images | |
| | Pituitary stalk | 3 mm near the optic chiasm—2 mm where it inserts into the gland (best seen on T2 DRIVE images) | |
| Size/height | Pituitary height: | 0–6 weeks: 2.6–5 mm | Measurement in the sagittal section on a plane perpendicular to the sella turcica floor |
| | | >2 years: 3–6 mm | |
| | | Puberty: up to 10–11 mm girls | |
| | | 7–8 mm boys | |
| | Pituitary volume: | $V = (\text{length} \times \text{height} \times \text{width})/2$ (Di Chiro formula: underestimation) | |
| | | $V = \text{area} \times \text{width}$ (overestimation) | |
| | | 3D volumetric MRI | |

is clearly evident (Fig. 10.1). The appearance of the posterior lobe blends with the anterior lobe because of its spontaneous hyperintensity.

A normal pituitary stalk usually tapers smoothly along its course. It is approximately 3 mm in diameter near the optic chiasm and 2 mm where it inserts into the gland. The pituitary stalk is divided into two parts: one is the neuronal component made up of the track of axons extending from the hypothalamic nuclei down to the axon terminals in the posterior pituitary pouch, while the other is the vascular component that provides blood supply to the anterior pituitary gland from the superior hypophyseal arteries through the pituitary portal system [21] (Table 10.2).

## *Normal Pituitary Size*

Pediatric pituitary gland size and shape change physiologically throughout life depending on age and sex. Furthermore, even among children of identical age and gender, there is wide morphological and dimensional variability [22, 23]; the morphology of the gland may also vary from side to side reflecting a physiological asymmetric development of the pituitary fossa, which in turn may be influenced by the variable degree of pneumatization of the underlying sphenoid sinus throughout infancy. With this in mind, a simple measure of a single dimension (i.e., height) should not be considered a reliable indicator of the size of a tridimensional structure such as the pituitary gland. Nevertheless, measurement of the pituitary gland height is still the most widely used method to obtain a quick, indirect determination of the gland size. Normal pituitary gland height values range between 3 and 6 mm in prepubertal children. In particular, in newborns, the gland typically presents an upward convex margin with a mean height (about 4–5 mm) slightly higher when compared to the gland height of the following months of age. In general, the height of the pituitary gland slightly decreases or remains stable during the first 2 years of life, whereas its width (transverse measurement) and depth (anterior–posterior measurement) slightly increase; then, a mild but progressive increase in height occurs until puberty, when the pituitary gland undergoes rapid and profound changes in size and shape, with marked enlargement. In girls, the gland may swell symmetrically to a height of 10–11 mm, appearing nearly spherical, whereas in pubertal boys it may reach 7–8 mm [2, 24]. Indirect pituitary volume assessment has been calculated using formulas adapted from the formula for the volume of an ellipsoid (i.e., the Di Chiro formula: $V = 1/2$ length × height × width). Because glands are usually not spherical, these methods do not allow a precise calculation of the real size of the gland [25]. To overcome the abovementioned computational bias, volumetric data, based on a direct calculation of pituitary volumes from 3D MRI sequences, represent a significant advance over the information collected using prior methods. A 3D data set of T1-weighted images can be reformatted on sagittal or coronal planes, and the entire volume is calculated adding the volume of the gland on each slice [26, 27]. Unfortunately, this method is time consuming and of limited practical use in daily work. Furthermore, a careful comparison of the results obtained by three [25–27] prior different studies shows a relative discrepancy among results, with wide variations of normal ranges; for instance, in one study [25] in which the volume of the gland included the posterior pituitary, the average volume of the entire gland resulted smaller at a given age, when compared to another study in which only the volume of the adenohypophysis was taken into account [26]. A better standardization of the computation method and larger series is awaited to better elucidate the clinical significance and reproducibility of volumetric results that, at present, appear somewhat incomplete.

## MRI Phenotypes in GHD

Patients with idiopathic or genetically determined GHD can present with (a) normal or hypoplastic pituitary gland without anatomical abnormalities of the hypothalamus or pituitary stalk, (b) moderate to severe hypoplastic pituitary gland with ectopic posterior pituitary (EPP) located anywhere from the median eminence to the distal stalk (pituitary dystopia), or (c) agenesis of the pituitary gland. Isolated GHD (IGHD) is more commonly observed in the first category, while multiple pituitary hormone deficits (MPHD) occur in the last two. An empty sella is reported in about 10 % of IGHD.

In a large cohort of patients from a post-marketing observational study [28], the analysis of MRI findings in 1844 patients—that had been previously classified as "idiopathic short stature" (ISS) and small for gestational age (SGA)—showed 151

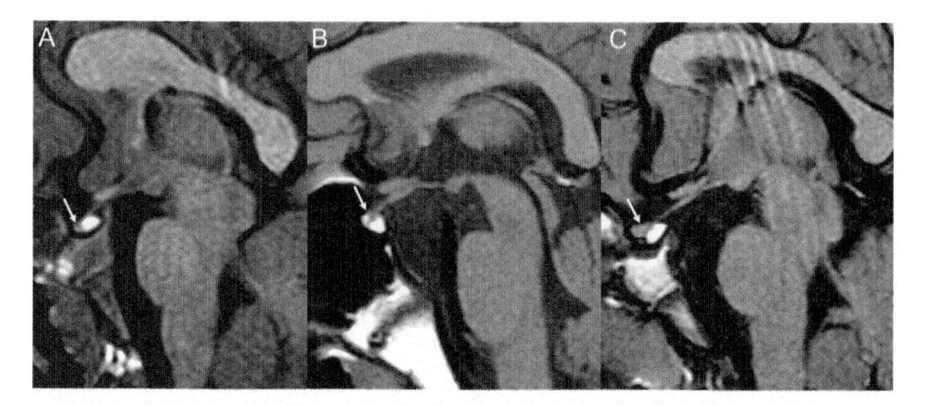

**Fig. 10.4** Pituitary hypoplasia. (**a–c**) Sagittal T1-weighted images. Different degrees of anterior pituitary hypoplasia (*arrows*) in three different children, ranging from severe (**a**) to mild (**c**). The pituitary stalk and posterior lobe are normal

patients (8 %) with pituitary area abnormalities, with pituitary hypoplasia and EPP associated with pituitary hypoplasia and missing pituitary stalk being the most common ones. These anomalies were equally distributed between ISS and SGA patients. This raises the question about the misclassification bias based on GH response to stimulation tests, where false-negative results have been reported in patients with structural hypothalamic–pituitary abnormalities [29].

## Pituitary Gland Hypoplasia

Pituitary hypoplasia (Fig. 10.4) is defined as a small anterior pituitary housed within a small or normal pituitary fossa. It may either be isolated or as a part of complex syndromes, such as Kallmann syndrome, Pallister–Hall syndrome, CHARGE (coloboma, heart anomaly, choanal atresia, retardation, genital, and ear anomalies) (Fig. 10.5), and Coffin–Siris syndrome. It may also be associated with other CNS malformations, such as septo-optic dysplasia (SOD), holoprosencephaly, corpus callosum dysgenesis, and Chiari malformation.

## Pituitary Dystopia

Pituitary dystopia consists of failed conjunction between the anterior and the posterior lobe. Morphologically, it is characterized by:

1. Hypoplasia of the anterior pituitary lobe, which is housed within a small pituitary fossa.
2. Absence or marked thinning of the pituitary stalk. The stalk is usually not identifiable on baseline MRI, although, when present, it may be seen after gadolinium

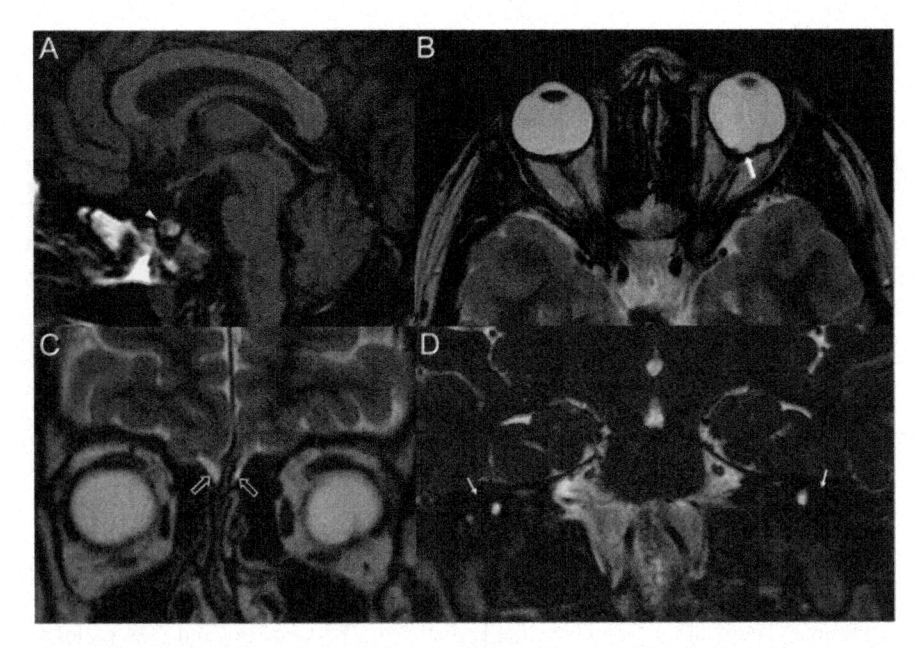

**Fig. 10.5** Pituitary hypoplasia in CHARGE syndrome. (**a**) Sagittal T1-weighted image; (**b**) axial T2-weighted image; (**c**) coronal T2-weighted image; (**d**) coronal T2 DRIVE image. Small anterior pituitary (*arrowhead*, **a**). Left optic nerve head coloboma (*thick arrow*, **b**). Bilateral absence of the olfactory bulbs (*open arrows*, **c**). Coronal view of the inner ear structures at the level of the vestibule shows bilateral agenesis of the semicircular canals (*thin arrows*, **d**)

administration (Fig. 10.6) or using high-resolution, heavily T2-weighted sequences (CISS, DRIVE, or FIESTA) (Fig. 10.7).
3. EPP ("ectopic bright spot"). The ectopic posterior lobe is usually located at level of the infundibular recess of the third ventricle, but it may be found anywhere along the infundibular axis (Fig. 10.8).

Pituitary dystopia can be an isolated condition or associated with other central nervous system (CNS) malformations, similar to pituitary hypoplasia (i.e., SOD (Fig. 10.9), holoprosencephaly, corpus callosum dysgenesis, Chiari malformation).

In particular, IGHD is more commonly observed in association with normal or hypoplastic anterior pituitary gland, whereas MPHD occurs more frequently in the presence of EPP. In addition, MPHD may be associated with a spectrum of cerebral malformations (Fig. 10.9) such as Arnold–Chiari I and II, agenesis of the septum pellucidum, SOD, vermis dysplasia, syringomyelia, absence of the internal carotid artery, dysgenesis of the corpus callosum, arachnoid cysts, and tentorium anomalies with basilar impression [2, 7]. The frequency of these radiological findings and their spectrum of pituitary hormone deficiencies are variable. In particular, MPHD is more frequently associated than IGHD with EPP and with anterior pituitary

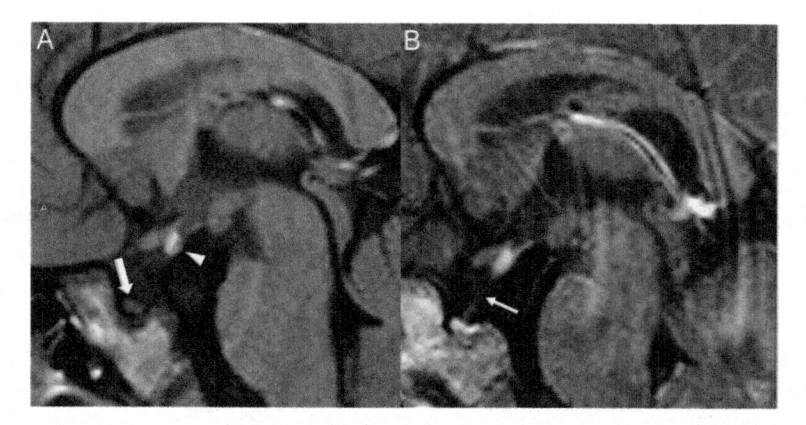

**Fig. 10.6** Pituitary dystopia. (**a**) Sagittal T1-weighted image; (**b**) gadolinium-enhanced sagittal T1-weighted image. The ectopic posterior lobe is located at the level of the median eminence (*arrowhead*, **a**) and the hypoplastic anterior lobe is located in a small pituitary fossa (*thick arrow*, **a**). The pituitary stalk is not identifiable on baseline sagittal T1-weighted image (**a**). Following gadolinium injection, a very thin pituitary stalk is seen (*thin arrow*, **b**)

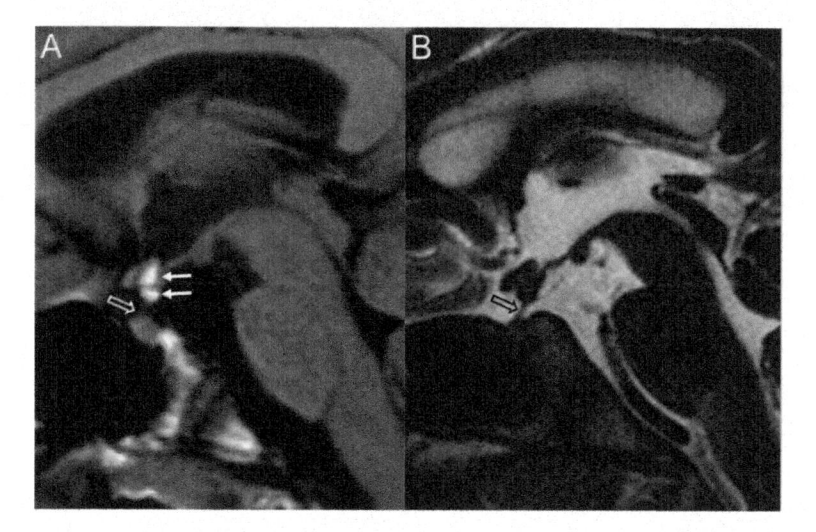

**Fig. 10.7** Pituitary dystopia. (**a**) Sagittal T1-weighted image; (**b**) sagittal T2 DRIVE image. There is a bulky ectopic posterior lobe with bilobated appearance located at the level of the median eminence and within the proximal third of the infundibulum (*thin arrows*, **a**). The pituitary stalk is barely recognizable on T1-weighted image (*open white arrow*, **a**), whereas it is confidently demonstrated on T2 DRIVE image (*open black arrow*, **b**)

hypoplasia [1–14, 22–24, 30] (Table 10.3). The variability between different studies can be attributed to the degree of restriction in diagnostic criteria, to the diagnostic limits of GHD itself (transitory deficits, recovery, false positives, etc.), and/or to the lack of a convincing standard for a normal-size pituitary gland among the prepubertal

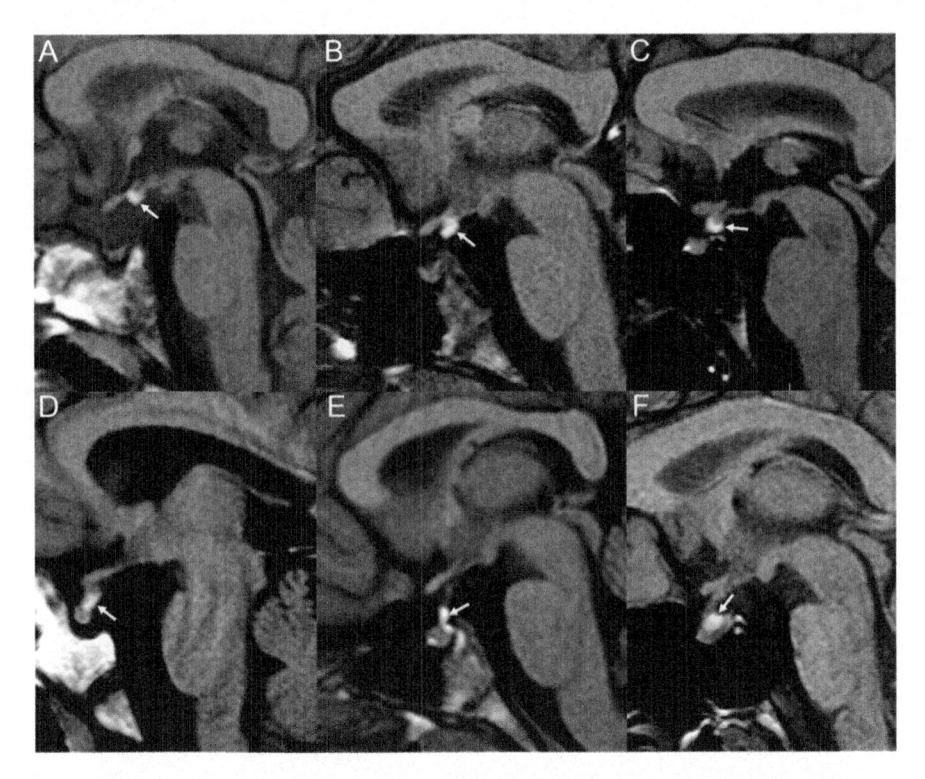

**Fig. 10.8** Posterior lobe ectopia in different children. (**a–f**) Sagittal T1-weighted images. Different locations of the ectopic posterior lobe from the median eminence (*arrows*, **a**, **b**), to mid-(*arrows*, **c**, **d**) and distal stalk (*arrows*, **e**, **f**)

pediatric population. The high frequency of sporadic forms of idiopathic GHD associated with EPP in the absence of genetic identification remains intriguing, suggesting that other factors may play a role as well.

The identification of EPP or pituitary stalk agenesis itself is helpful in the diagnosis and prognosis of patients with GHD, and the size of EPP may vary considerably between patients, ranging from small EPP to large EPP and even huge EPP. In particular, the *size* and the *location* of EPP are early markers of evolving pituitary hormone deficiencies as reported in studies showing that small EPP surface area and/or hypothalamic-sited EPP are predictive of the development of MPHD [14, 15]. On the other hand, it is worth pointing out that a hypothalamic location of EPP is generally associated with complete pituitary stalk agenesis and that a huge EPP was misdiagnosed as a subhypothalamic tumor in a patient subsequently subjected to unnecessary neurosurgery [49].

The presence of a vascular component of the stalk has prognostic significance since patients with agenesis of the pituitary stalk run a greater risk of developing

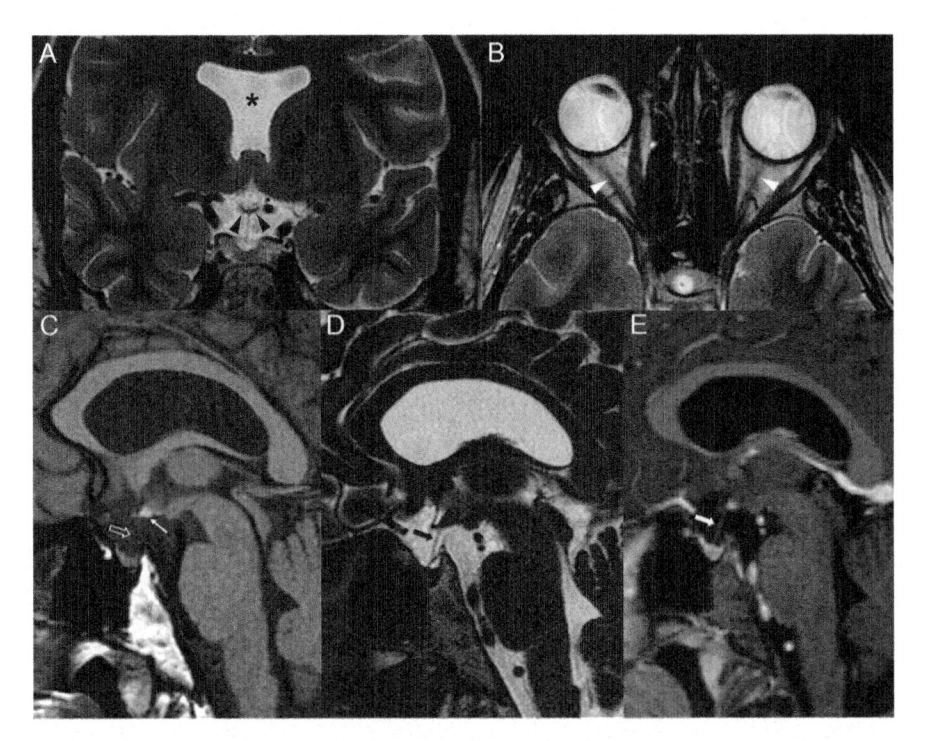

**Fig. 10.9** Pituitary dystopia and septo-optic dysplasia. (**a**) Coronal T2-weighted image; (**b**) axial T2-weighted image; (**c**) sagittal T1-weighted image; (**d**) sagittal T2 DRIVE image; (**e**) gadolinium-enhanced sagittal T1-weighted image. There is absence of the septum pellucidum (*asterisk*, **a**) with marked thinning of the optic chiasm (*black arrowheads*, **a**) and of the optic nerves (*white arrowheads*, **b**). Typical pituitary dystopia with an ectopic posterior lobe at the level of the median eminence (*thin arrow*, **c**). The pituitary stalk is not visible on the sagittal T1-weighted image (*open arrow*, **c**), whereas it is clearly demonstrated both on the 3D DRIVE sequence (*black thick arrow*, **d**) and post-contrast T1-weighted image (*white thick arrow*, **e**)

MPHD than those who show a vascular residue of the stalk. Patients in whom a pituitary stalk cannot be identified after Gd-DTPA administration have a risk of developing MPHD evolving to MPHD that is 27 times greater than those with a residual vascular pituitary stalk [9, 50].

A detailed study of the pituitary stalk with administration of Gd-DTPA is no longer recommended provided that T2-DRIVE has been performed. T2-DRIVE obtained at submillimetric thickness allows for an excellent and detailed representation of the anatomy of the suprasellar compartment, and in particular of the pituitary stalk; pituitary stalk thickness is better evaluated than with conventional precontrast T1- and T2-weighted images and, in our experience, the sensitivity is similar to that of post-contrast T1-weighted images.

**Table 10.3** Reports from the literature on MRI features in subjects with idiopathic GHD (number ≥35) [28, 31–47]

| Reference | Year | Patients | MRI (%) EPP | HA | NA | Presenting pituitary functions (%) IGHD (EPP) | MPHD (EPP) |
|---|---|---|---|---|---|---|---|
| Bressani | 1990 | 57 | 34 (59) | 23 (40) | 0 | 36 (37) | 21 (95) |
| Maghnie | 1991 | 45 | 20 (44) | 13 (29) | 12 (26) | 33 (24) | 8 (100) |
| Abrahams | 1991 | 35 | 15 (43) | 20 (57) | 15 (43) | 2 (10) | 13 (87) |
| Argyropoulou | 1992 | 46 | 29 (63) | 10 (21) | 7 (15) | 26 (38) | 20 (95) |
| Triulzi | 1994 | 101 | 59 (48) | ND | ND | 67 (44) | 34 (85) |
| Pinto | 1997 | 51 | 51 (100) | 41 (83) | 6 (13) | 16 (100) | 35 (100) |
| Nagel | 1997 | 56 | 24 (42) | 11 (19) | 17 (30) | 43 (27) | 13 (92) |
| Kornreich | 1997 | 51 | 41 (80) | 0 | 10 (20) | 23 (56) | 28 (100) |
| Hamilton | 1998 | 35 | 25 (71) | 3 (<1) | 2 (<1) | 20 (70) | 15 (73) |
| Arifa | 1999 | 100 | 20 (20) | 28 (28) | 41 (41) | 79 (ND) | 19 (ND) |
| Bozzola | 2000 | 93 | 30 (32) | 69 (65) | 24 (35) | 5 (8) | 25 (76) |
| Osorio | 2002 | 76 | 54 (71) | 36 (84) | ND | 33 (55)[a] | 43 (57)[b] |
| Arends | 2002 | 39 | 24 (61) | 22 (56) | 17 (44) | 11 (44) | 13 (87) |
| Melo | 2007 | 62 | 48 (100)[c] | 0 | 0 | 10 (100)[c] | 38 (100)[c] |
| Mehta | 2009 | 137 | 63 (46) | 113 (82) | 24 (18) | 44 (34) | 93 (52) |
| Acharya | 2011 | 44 | 14 (32) | 27 (61) | ND | 30 (27) | 14 (43) |
| Jagtap | 2012 | 103 | 25 (24) | 62 (60) | 39 (38) | 72 (14) | 31 (48) |
| Maghnie | 2013 | 13,616[d] | 1018 (8) | 1178 (9) | 10,917 (80) | 11,358 (5) | 2258 (23) |
| Deal | 2013 | 8230 | 312 (4) | 342 (4) | 7039 (86) | 7516 (ND) | 714 (ND) |
| Naderi | 2015 | 40 | ND | 4 (10) | ND | 33 (ND) | 7 (ND) |
| Deillon | 2015 | 63 | 7 (11) | 12 (19) | 43 (68) | 58 (7) | 5 (60) |

Adapted from Argente et al. [48]
*EPP* ectopic posterior pituitary, *HA* hypoplastic anterior pituitary with normal located posterior pituitary, *NA* normal anatomy, *ND* not determined
[a]One patient with GH-1 deletion
[b]5 Prop1 and 1 Pit1 defects
[c]Posterior pituitary position not evaluated in 14 subjects
[d]Eight percent of ISS and SGA patients showed pituitary anomalies at MRI

## *Agenesis of the Pituitary Gland*

Congenital pituitary gland absence (aplasia) is an extremely rare anomaly that involves variably the anterior pituitary, both the anterior and the posterior pituitary lobes, and, in many cases, the pituitary stalk. The characteristic imaging finding of pituitary aplasia is the absence of an identifiable pituitary gland. In addition, the sella is small and flat, and it is sometimes covered by a layer of dura. The differential diagnosis includes severe hypoplasia of the pituitary gland. In patients with

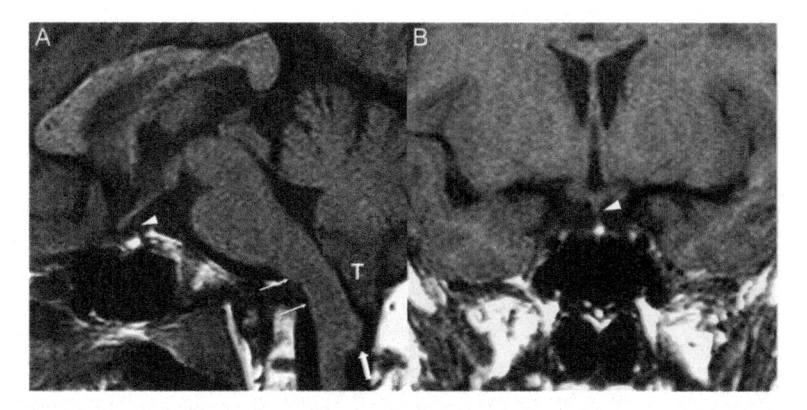

**Fig. 10.10** Anterior pituitary gland aplasia and Chiari I malformation. (**a**) Sagittal T1-weighted image; (**b**) coronal T1-weighted image. Small pituitary fossa containing the posterior pituitary lobe, physiologically bright, without evidence of the adenohypophysis. The pituitary stalk is barely visible (*arrowheads*, **a**, **b**). There is concomitant downward displacement of the cerebellar tonsils (*T*). Note elongation of the medulla oblongata (*thin arrows*, **a**) and cervicomedullary kinking (*thick arrow*, **a**)

neonatal panhypopituitarism, severe symptoms of hypoglycemia may appear during the first hours of life. Symptoms include seizures, apnea, and cardiovascular collapse and arrest.

Congenital absence of the pituitary gland can be isolated (rarer) or associated with other major brain anomalies, such as craniofacial defects, SOD, arhinencephaly, holoprosencephaly, anencephaly, and Chiari I malformation (Fig. 10.10) [51].

## *Empty Sella*

The so-called empty sella is a misnomer, as the sella almost never is really empty. This term had been introduced in the pre-CT, pre-MRI era, when neurosurgeons used to operate on a suspected pituitary mass lesion on the basis of an expanded sella turcica on plain radiography and, in many cases, the sella was found to be filled only with cerebrospinal fluid (CSF) instead of a tumor, with a pituitary gland flattened along the sellar floor. At present, the term empty sella basically indicates an intrasellar herniation of the subarachnoid spaces through an incompetent sellar diaphragm (arachnoidal diverticulum) [52]. Rhythmic CSF pulsations contribute to chronic compression of the pituitary gland and enlargement of the pituitary fossa (so-called primary empty sella). MRI clearly demonstrates the presence of a deep and enlarged pituitary fossa mainly filled with CSF, containing an anterior pituitary lobe that appears as a thin layer along its floor. The posterior lobe is flattened against

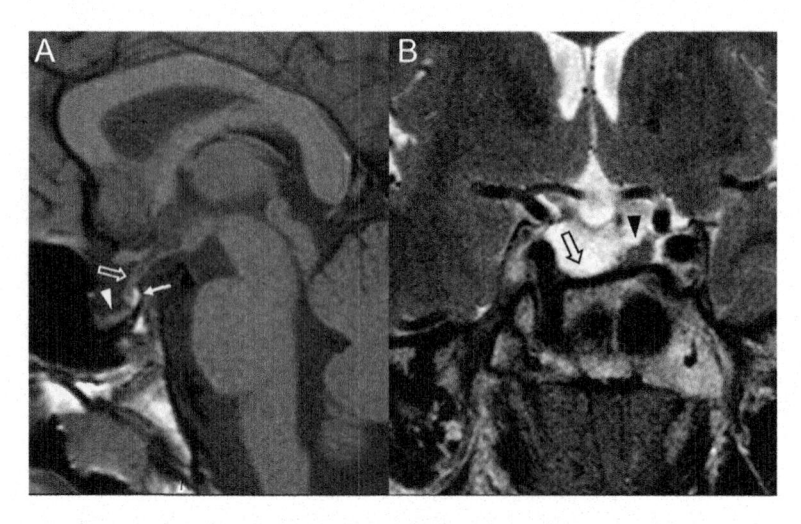

**Fig. 10.11** Empty sella in two different patients. (**a**) Primary empty sella. Sagittal T1-weighted image shows a deep pituitary fossa containing an anterior pituitary lobe that appears as a thin layer (*arrowhead*). The posterior lobe is flattened against the dorsum sellae (*arrow*). The pituitary fossa is mainly filled with CSF. The pituitary stalk is thinned and displaced posteriorly (*open arrow*). (**b**) Secondary empty sella. Coronal T2-weighted image shows a pituitary fossa mainly filled with CSF (*open arrow*) secondary to surgical resection of a pituitary adenoma. Residual pituitary parenchyma is visible in the left lateral portion of the sella (*arrowhead*)

the dorsum sellae, with a thin and stretched pituitary stalk (Fig. 10.11). An intrasellar arachnoid expansion can also occur secondary to a reduced intrasellar tissue volume due to such causes as surgical resection, radiation necrosis, pituitary atrophy, or infarction (secondary empty sella). In such cases, it is essentially an "ex vacuo" phenomenon where intracranial subarachnoid space secondarily extends into the sella (Fig. 10.11).

Previous studies have reported the prevalence of primary empty sella to be about 5–9 % for all ages, with an increase in prevalence with age [53]. Most frequently, this anomaly is an incidental finding, the only exceptions being patients with pseudotumor cerebri (benign intracranial hypertension) in which clinical symptoms and additional MRI findings may orient the diagnosis [54] or in children with anterior pituitary deficiency [55].

Semantic problems can also arise with the so-called partially empty sella, in which only part of the intrasellar space (less than 50 %) is filled with an arachnoid diverticulum; in this case, the height of the gland is reduced on the midline, but gland tissue is seen to extend to the full height along the bilateral sellar margins. The presence of a small pituitary fossa may help in distinguishing pituitary hypoplasia from a partially empty sella.

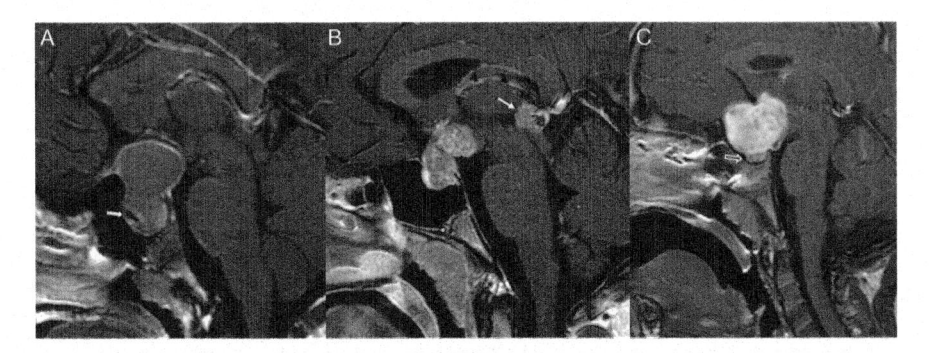

**Fig. 10.12** Sellar suprasellar mass lesions. (**a–c**) Gadolinium-enhanced sagittal T1-weighted images. (**a**) Craniopharyngioma. Predominantly cystic sellar–suprasellar mass lesion with wall enhancement. A small hypointense area is visible within the lesion (*thick arrow*) in keeping with calcification. The pituitary gland is not recognizable. (**b**) Germinoma. Contrast-enhancing solid mass lesion involving the hypothalamic–hypophyseal region. There is also pathologic involvement and enlargement of the pineal gland (*thin arrow*) in keeping with a bifocal lesion. (**c**) Pilocytic astrocytoma. Suprasellar solid mass lesion of the chiasmatic–hypothalamic region with marked enhancement. The pituitary gland is normal (*open arrow*)

## MRI Phenotypes in Secondary GHD

Acquired GHD is commonly due to classic lesions leading to a pattern of secondary empty sella or may be the consequence of a sellar–suprasellar mass lesion, mainly including craniopharyngiomas, suprasellar germinomas, Langerhans cell histiocytosis (LCH), lymphocytic hypophysitis, and chiasmatic–hypothalamic gliomas (Fig.10.12).

Craniopharyngiomas are benign, predominantly cystic and contrast-enhancing mass lesions, more commonly located in the suprasellar compartment. The cysts may contain various amounts of cholesterol, methemoglobin, protein, and desquamated epithelium, resulting in increased signal intensity on T1-weighted images. Calcifications represent a hallmark of craniopharyngiomas [56].

Suprasellar germinomas, LCH, and lymphocytic hypophysitis typically present with central diabetes insipidus, absence of the posterior pituitary bright spot, and thickening of the pituitary stalk [57, 58]. GHD can be variably associated. Concomitant involvement of the pineal gland or basal ganglia is highly suggestive of a germinoma. Germinomas are highly cellular tumors and typically appear iso- to hypointense on T2-weighted images and can show restricted diffusion on DWI. Contrast enhancement is usually moderate to mark. They can also give secondary CSF dissemination with typical involvement of the subependymal regions.

Brain MRI evidence of soft tissue or skull lesions, as well as areas of T2 hyperintensity involving the brainstem and deep cerebellar white matter, is diagnostic clue suggestive of LCH, a rare reactive disorder of the reticuloendothelial system characterized by abnormal proliferation of Langerhans-type histiocytes. A high frequency of pineal cysts and enlarged pineal glands has been reported in patients with LCH; however, this finding remains nonspecific.

Volumetric increase in the size of the stalk and anterior pituitary on follow-up studies supports the diagnosis of infiltrative/neoplastic disorders, particularly germinoma. On the other hand, the association of anterior pituitary hormone deficiency with MRI evidence of progressive reduction in size of the anterior pituitary is suggestive of an inflammatory cause such as lymphocytic infundibulo-hypophysitis [59]. On the whole, the MRI appearance of lymphocytic hypophysitis is similar to that of suprasellar germinomas or LCH, with which it may be confused. The gold standard for unequivocal diagnosis remains pituitary biopsy; however, follow-up studies are fundamental and can usually clear the view [60].

Children with chiasmatic–hypothalamic gliomas usually present with visual loss; endocrine dysfunction is seen in around 20 % of cases. Histologically, most of these tumors are pilocytic astrocytomas, but pilomyxoid astrocytomas, fibrillary, and anaplastic variants are also possible. MRI depicts these tumors as multilobular or oval masses that are usually well marginated. The pituitary gland is typically not involved, and the epicenter of the lesion, as well the pattern of growth along the visual pathways, can confidently allow a differential diagnosis from other sellar–suprasellar mass lesions [21].

## MRI Findings and Pituitary Genes

Our understanding of the genetic regulation of pituitary gland development in humans and the mouse has also increased considerably, and mutations in a number of genes have been associated with pituitary dysfunction and abnormal pituitary gland development. Animal and human studies, along with the correlation of a particular genetic profile to certain endocrine and MRI phenotypes, have yielded great insights into pituitary development [2]. MRI findings include normal pituitary gland in patients with mutations in GH1, GHRHR, and RNPC3 and IGHD or with hypoplastic pituitary gland with additional pituitary defects associated with or without pituitary stalk abnormalities including POU1F1, PROP1, LHX3, LHX4, HESX1, OTX2, SOX2, SOX3, GLI2, GLI3, FGFR1, FGF8, and PROKR2 (Table 10.4).

## Conclusions

Pituitary gland morphology on MRI may suggest the etiology of GHD, as well as the prognosis, in an individual. Thus, MRI is informative and should be used in the evaluation of patients with GHD.

**Table 10.4** Endocrine/pituitary phenotypes and associated features linked with mutations responsible for congenital GHD with structural hypothalamic–pituitary abnormalities [42, 45, 48, 61–66]

| Genes | Inheritance | Locus | Hormone deficiencies GH | PRL | TSH | LH/FSH | ACTH | Pituitary phenotypes | Associated features |
|---|---|---|---|---|---|---|---|---|---|
| GH-1 (IGHD IA) | AR | 17q22-q24 | ■ | □ | □ | □ | □ | Normal AP/EPP | No |
| GH1 (IGHD II) | AD | 17q22-q24 | ■ | □ | ■[b] | □ | ■ | Normal AP/APH | Evolutive endocrinopathy |
| GHRHR (IGHD IB) | AR | 7p15-p14 | ■ | ? | □ | □ | □ | Normal AP/APH | Chiari I malformation, arachnoid cyst, dysmorphic anterior pituitary |
| POU1F1 | AR/AD | 3p11 | ■ | ■ | ■/□ | □ | □ | Normal AP/APH | No |
| PROP1 | AR | 5q | ■ | ■ | ■[b] | ■ | ■/□ | Normal/large AP/APH/EPP | ACTH deficiency in 1/3 of cases Risk of evolutive endocrinopathy |
| HESX1 | AR/AD | 3p21.2-p21.1 | ■ | ■/□ | ■/□ | ■/□ | ■/□ | Normal AP/AP aplasia/APH+EPP/isolated APH | SOD–SOD variants Coloboma—CC agenesis or hypoplasia |
| LHX3 | AR | 9q34.3 | ■ | ■ | ■ | ■ | □ | APH/large AP | Stubby neck—anomalies of cervical vertebrae (including atlantic spina bifida occulta) Elevated and anteverted shoulders Limited head rotation in most cases Psychomotor delay—short arms |
| LHX4 | AD | 1q25 | ■ | □ | □ | ■ | ■ | Normal AP/large AP/APH/EPP | Chiari I—CC hypoplasia—neonatal hypoglycemia, cardiac insufficiency, and respiratory distress |
| GLI2 | AD | 2q14 | ■ | ? | ■/□ | ■/□ | ■/□ | APH/AP aplasia/EPP | Holoprosencephaly-like features |
| SOX3 | X linked | Xq27 | ■ | ? | ■/□ | ■/□ | ■/□ | APH/EPP | Intellectual disability +/− holoprosencephaly-like features |

(continued)

Table 10.4 (continued)

| Genes | Inheritance | Locus | Hormone deficiencies GH | PRL | TSH | LH/FSH | ACTH | Pituitary phenotypes | Associated features |
|---|---|---|---|---|---|---|---|---|---|
| SOX2 | AD | 3q26.3-q27 | ■/□ | □ | ■/□ | ■ | ■ | APH/EPP/normal AP | Microphthalmia/anophthalmia, ONH, CNS abnormalities, micropenis, cryptorchidism[a] |
| OTX2 | AD | 14q22-23 | ■ | □ | ■ | ■ | ■/□ | Normal AP/APH/EPP/PSA | Bilateral anophthalmia, ONH, retinal dystrophy, seizures, Chiari I, cleft palate, short stature. Neonatal hypoglycemia, jaundice, and respiratory distress |
| Kallmann syndrome genes (FGFR1, FGF8, PROKR2) | X linked, AD, AR | | | □ | | | ■/□ | APH/EPP/PSA | Olfactory bulbs agenesis or hypoplasia, CNS abnormalities |
| RNPC3 | AR | | ■ | □ | □ | □ | □ | APH | No |

Adapted from Argente et al. [48]

*AD* autosomal dominant, *AR* autosomal recessive, ■ hormone deficiency, □ no hormone deficiency, *AP* anterior pituitary, *EPP* ectopic posterior pituitary, *APH* anterior pituitary hypoplasia, *SOD* septo-optic dysplasia, *CC* corpus callosum, *ONH* optic nerve hypoplasia, *CNS* central nervous system, *PS* pituitary stalk, *PSA* pituitary stalk agenesis

[a]Hippocampal abnormalities, partial agenesis of the corpus callosum, absence of septum pellucidum, hypothalamic hamartoma, reduction of white matter
[b]Exceptionally reported (one patient) [45]

# References

1. Maghnie M, Ghirardello S, Genovese E. Magnetic resonance imaging of the hypothalamus-pituitary unit in children suspected of hypopituitarism: who, how and when to investigate. J Endocrinol Invest. 2004;27:496–509.
2. Di Iorgi N, Allegri AE, Napoli F, Bertelli E, Olivieri I, Rossi A, Maghnie M. The use of neuroimaging for assessing disorders of pituitary development. Clin Endocrinol (Oxf). 2012;76:161–76.
3. Fujisawa I, Kikchi K, Nishimura K, Togashi K, Itoh K, Noma S, Minami S, Sagoh T, Hiraoka T, Momoi T. Transection of the pituitary stalk: development of an ectopic posterior lobe associated with MR imaging. Radiology. 1987;165:487–9.
4. Kikuchi K, Fujisawa I, Momoi T, Yamanaka C, Kaji M, Nakano Y, Konishi J, Mikawa H, Sudo M. Hypothalamic-pituitary function in growth hormone-deficient patients with pituitary transection. J Clin Endocrinol Metab. 1988;67:817–23.
5. Maghnie M, Triulzi F, Larizza D, Scotti G, Beluffi G, Cecchini A, Severi F. Hypothalamic-pituitary dwarfism: comparison between MR imaging and CT findings. Pediatr Radiol. 1990;20:229–35.
6. Maghnie M, Triulzi F, Larizza D, Preti P, Priora C, Scotti G, Severi F. Hypothalamic-pituitary dysfunction in growth hormone-deficient patients with pituitary abnormalities. J Clin Endocrinol Metab. 1991;72:79–83.
7. Triulzi F, Scotti G, di Natale B, Pellini C, Lukezic M, Scognamiglio M, Chiumello G. Evidence of a congenital midline brain anomaly in pituitary dwarfs: a magnetic resonance imaging study in 101 patients. Pediatrics. 1994;93:409–16.
8. Pinto G, Netchine I, Sobrier ML, Brunelle F, Souberbielle JC, Brauner R. Pituitary stalk interruption syndrome: a clinical-biological-genetic assessment of its pathogenesis. J Clin Endocrinol Metab. 1997;82:3450–4.
9. Maghnie M, Genovese E, Villa A, Spagnolo L, Campan R, Severi F. Dynamic MRI in the congenital agenesis of the neural pituitary stalk syndrome: the role of the vascular pituitary stalk in predicting residual anterior pituitary function. Clin Endocrinol (Oxf). 1996;45:281–90.
10. Arrigo T, De Luca F, Maghnie M, Blandino A, Lombardo F, Messina MF, Wasniewska M, Ghizzoni L, Bozzola M. Relationships between neuroradiological and clinical features in apparently idiopathic hypopituitarism. Eur J Endocrinol. 1998;139:84–8.
11. Chen S, Leger J, Garel C, Hassan M, Czernichow P. Growth hormone deficiency with ectopic neurohypophysis: anatomical variations and relationship between the visibility of the pituitary stalk asserted by magnetic resonance imaging and anterior pituitary function. J Clin Endocrinol Metab. 1999;84:2408–13.
12. Maghnie M, Ambrosini L, Cappa M, Pozzobon G, Ghizzoni L, Ubertini MG, di Iorgi N, Tinelli C, Pilia S, Chiumello G, Lorini R, Loche S. Adult height in patients with permanent growth hormone deficiency with and without multiple pituitary hormone deficiencies. J Clin Endocrinol Metab. 2006;91:2900–5.
13. Maghnie M, Strigazzi C, Tinelli C, Autelli M, Cisternino M, Loche S, Severi F. Growth hormone (GH) deficiency (GHD) of childhood onset: reassessment of GH status and evaluation of the predictive criteria for permanent GHD in young adults. J Clin Endocrinol Metab. 1999;84:1324–8.
14. Murray PG, Hague C, Fafoula O, Gleeson H, Patel L, Banerjee I, Raabe AL, Hall CM, Wright NB, Amin R, Clayton PE. Likelihood of persistent GH deficiency into late adolescence: relationship to the presence of an ectopic or normally sited posterior pituitary gland. Clin Endocrinol (Oxf). 2009;71:215–9.
15. Di Iorgi N, Morana G, Gallizia AL, Maghnie M. Pituitary gland imaging and outcome. Endocr Dev. 2012;23:16–29.
16. Vossough A, Nabavizadeh SA. Functional imaging based diagnostic strategy: intra-axial brain masses. In: Scott HF, Feroze BM, editors. Functional neuroradiology, principles and clinical application. New York: Springer; 2011. p. 197–220.

17. Rossi A, Gandolfo C, Morana G, Severino M, Garrè ML, Cama A. New MR sequences (diffusion, perfusion, spectroscopy) in brain tumours. Pediatr Radiol. 2010;40:999–1009.
18. Elster AD. Modern imaging of the pituitary. Radiology. 1993;187:1–14.
19. Elster AD, Chen MTM, Williams III DW, Key LL. Pituitary gland: MR imaging of physiologic hypertrophy in adolescence. Radiology. 1990;174:681–5.
20. Bonneville F, Cattin F, Marsot-Dupuch K, Dormonnt D, Bonneville JF, Chiras J. T1 signal hyperintensity in the sellar region: spectrum of findings. Radiographics. 2006;26:93–113.
21. Tortori-Donati P, Rossi A, Biancheri R. Sellar and suprasellar disorders. In: Tortori-Donati P, editor. Pediatric neuroradiology. Berlin: Springer; 2005. p. 855–91.
22. Cox TD, Elster AD. Normal pituitary gland: changes in shape, size, and signal intensity during the 1st year of life at MR imaging. Radiology. 1991;179:721–4.
23. Dietrich RB, Lis LE, Greensite FS, Duane P. Normal MR appearance of the pituitary gland in the first 2 years of life. AJNR Am J Neuroradiol. 1995;16:1413–9.
24. Tsunoda A, Okuda O, Sato K. MR height of the pituitary gland as a function of age and sex: especially physiological hypertrophy in adolescence and in climacterium. AJNR Am J Neuroradiol. 1997;18:551–4.
25. Fink AM, Vidmar S, Kumbla S, Pedreira CC, Kanumakala S, Williams C, Carlin JB, Cameron FJ. Age-related pituitary volumes in prepubertal children with normal endocrine function: volumetric magnetic resonance data. J Clin Endocrinol Metabol. 2005;90:3274–8.
26. Marziali S, Gaudiello F, Bozzao A, Scirè G, Ferone E, Colangelo V, Simonetti A, Boscherini B, Floris R, Simonetti G. Evaluation of anterior pituitary gland volume in childhood using three-dimensional MRI. Pediatr Radiol. 2004;34:547–51.
27. Takano K, Utsunomiya H, Ono H, Ohfu M, Okazaki M. Normal development of the pituitary gland: assessment with three-dimensional MR volumetry. AJNR Am J Neuroradiol. 2004;20:312–5.
28. Maghnie M, Lindberg A, Koltowska-Häggström M, Ranke MB. Magnetic resonance imaging of CNS in 15,043 children with GH deficiency in KIGS (Pfizer International Growth Database). Eur J Endocrinol. 2013;168(2):211–7.
29. Secco A, di Iorgi N, Napoli F, Calandra E, Ghezzi M, Frassinetti C, Parodi S, Casini MR, Lorini R, Loche S, et al. The glucagon test in the diagnosis of growth hormone deficiency in children with short stature younger than 6 years. J Clin Endocrinol Metabol. 2009;94: 4251–7.
30. Argyropoulou M, Perignon F, Brunelle F, Brauner R, Rappaport R. Height of normal pituitary gland as a function of age evaluated by magnetic resonance imaging in children. Pediatr Radiol. 1991;21:247–9.
31. Bressani N, di Natale B, Pellini C, Triulzi F, Scotti G, Chiumello G. Evidence of morphological and functional abnormalities in the hypothalamus of growth-hormone-deficient children: a combined magnetic resonance imaging and endocrine study. Horm Res. 1990;34:189–92.
32. Abrahams JJ, Trefelner E, Boulware SD. Idiopathic growth hormone deficiency: MR findings in 35 patients. Am J Neuroradiol. 1991;12:155–60.
33. Melo ME, Marui S, Carvalho LR, Arnhold IJ, Leite CC, Mendonca BB, Knoepfelmacher M. Hormonal, pituitary magnetic resonance, LHX4 and HESX1 evaluation in patients with hypopituitarism and ectopic posterior pituitary lobe. Clin Endocrinol (Oxf). 2007;66:95–102.
34. Argyropoulou M, Perignon F, Brauner R, Brunelle F. Magnetic resonance imaging in the diagnosis of growth hormone deficiency. J Pediatr. 1992;120:886–91.
35. Nagel BH, Palmbach M, Petersen D, Ranke MB. Magnetic resonance images of 91 children with different causes of short stature: pituitary size reflects growth hormone secretion. Eur J Pediatr. 1997;156:758–63.
36. Kornreich L, Horev G, Lazar L, Josefsberg Z, Pertzelan A. MR findings in hereditary isolated growth hormone deficiency. Am J Neuroradiol. 1997;18:1743–7.
37. Hamilton J, Chitayat D, Blaser S, Cohen LE, Phillips 3rd JA, Daneman D. Familial growth hormone deficiency associated with MRI abnormalities. Am J Med Genet. 1998;80:128–32.
38. Arifa N, Leger J, Garel C, Czernichow P, Hassan M. Cerebral anomalies associated with growth hormone insufficiency in children: major markers for diagnosis? Arch Pediatr. 1999;6:14–21.

39. Bozzola M, Mengarda F, Sartirana P, Tato L, Chaussain JL. Long-term follow-up evaluation of magnetic resonance imaging in the prognosis of permanent GH deficiency. Eur J Endocrinol. 2000;143:493–6.
40. Osorio MG, Marui S, Jorge AA, Latronico AC, Lo LS, Leite CC, Estefan V, Mendonca BB, Arnhold IJ. Pituitary magnetic resonance imaging and function in patients with growth hormone deficiency with and without mutations in GHRH-R, GH-1, or PROP-1 genes. J Clin Endocrinol Metab. 2002;87(11):5076–84.
41. Arends NJ, V d Lip W, Robben SG, Hokken-Koelega AC. MRI findings of the pituitary gland in short children born small for gestational age (SGA) in comparison with growth hormone-deficient (GHD) children and children with normal stature. Clin Endocrinol (Oxf). 2002;57: 719–24.
42. Mehta A, Hindmarsh PC, Mehta H, Turton JP, Russell-Eggitt I, Taylor D, Chong WK, Dattani MT. Congenital hypopituitarism: clinical, molecular and neuroradiological correlates. Clin Endocrinol (Oxf). 2009;71(3):376–82.
43. Acharya SV, Gopal RA, Lila A, Sanghvi DS, Menon PS, Bandgar TR, Shah NS. Phenotype and radiological correlation in patients with growth hormone deficiency. Indian J Pediatr. 2011;78(1):49–54.
44. Jagtap VS, Acharya SV, Sarathi V, Lila AR, Budyal SR, Kasaliwal R, Sankhe SS, Bandgar TR, Menon PS, Shah NS. Ectopic posterior pituitary and stalk abnormality predicts severity and coexisting hormone deficiencies in patients with congenital growth hormone deficiency. Pituitary. 2012;15(2):243–50.
45. Deal C, Hasselmann C, Pfäffle RW, Zimmermann AG, Quigley CA, Child CJ, Shavrikova EP, Cutler Jr GB, Blum WF. Associations between pituitary imaging abnormalities and clinical and biochemical phenotypes in children with congenital growth hormone deficiency: data from an international observational study. Horm Res Paediatr. 2013;79(5):283–92.
46. Naderi F, Eslami SR, Mirak SA, Khak M, Amiri J, Beyrami B, Shekarchi B, Poureisa M. Effect of growth hormone deficiency on brain MRI findings among children with growth restrictions. J Pediatr Endocrinol Metab. 2015;28(1–2):117–23.
47. Deillon E, Hauschild M, Faouzi M, Stoppa-Vaucher S, Elowe-Gruau E, Dwyer A, Theintz GE, Dubuis JM, Mullis PE, Pitteloud N, Phan-Hug F. Natural history of growth hormone deficiency in a pediatric cohort. Horm Res Paediatr. 2015;83(4):252–61.
48. Argente J, Flores R, Gutiérrez-Arumí A, Verma B, Martos-Moreno GÁ, Cuscó I, Oghabian A, Chowen JA, Frilander MJ, Pérez-Jurado LA. Defective minor spliceosome mRNA processing results in isolated familial growth hormone deficiency. EMBO Mol Med. 2014;6(3):299–306.
49. Werder EA, Zachmann M, Wichmann W, Valavanis A. Neurohypophyseal ectopy in growth hormone insufficiency. Horm Res. 1989;31:210–2.
50. Genovese E, Maghnie M, Beluffi G, Villa A, Sammarchi L, Severi F, Campani R. Hypothalamic-pituitary vascularization in pituitary stalk transection syndrome: is the pituitary stalk really transected? The role of gadolinium-DTPA with spin-echo T1 imaging and turbo-FLASH technique. Pediatr Radiol. 1997;27:48–53.
51. Cervantes LF, Altman NR, Medina LS. Case 102: pituitary aplasia. Radiology. 2006;241: 936–8.
52. Seeger JF. Normal variations of the skull and its content. In: Zimmerman RA, Gibby WA, Carmody RF, editors. Neuroimaging, clinical and physical principles. New York: Springer; 2000. p. 415–89.
53. Cacciari E, Zucchini S, Ambrosetto P, et al. Empty sella in children and adolescents with possible hypothalamic-pituitary disorders. J Clin Endocrinol Metab. 1994;78:767–71.
54. Degnan AJ, Levy LM. Pseudotumor cerebri: brief review of clinical syndrome and imaging findings. AJNR Am J Neuroradiol. 2011;32:1986–93.
55. Lenz AM, Root AW. Empty sella syndrome. Pediatr Endocrinol Rev. 2012;9:710–5.
56. Morana G, Maghnie M, Rossi A. Pituitary tumors: advances in neuroimaging. Endocr Dev. 2010;17:160–74.
57. Di Iorgi N, Morana G, Napoli F, Allegri AE, Rossi A, Maghnie M. Management of diabetes insipidus and adipsia in the child. Best Pract Res Clin Endocrinol Metab. 2015;29:415–36.

58. Di Iorgi N, Morana G, Maghnie M. Pituitary stalk thickening on MRI: when is the best time to re-scan and how long should we continue re-scanning for? Clin Endocrinol (Oxf). 2015. doi:10.1111/cen.12769. (Epub ahead of print)
59. Maghnie M, Cosi G, Genovese E, Manca-Bitti ML, Cohen A, Zecca S, Tinelli C, Gallucci M, Bernasconi S, Boscherini B, Severi F, Aricò M. Central diabetes insipidus in children and young adults. N Engl J Med. 2000;343:998–1007.
60. Di Iorgi N, Allegri AE, Napoli F, Calcagno A, Calandra E, Fratangeli N, Vannati M, Rossi A, Bagnasco F, Haupt R, Maghnie M. Central diabetes insipidus in children and young adults: etiological diagnosis and long-term outcome of idiopathic cases. J Clin Endocrinol Metab. 2014;99:1264–72.
61. Alatzoglou KS, Dattani MT. Genetic causes and treatment of isolated growth hormone deficiency-an update. Nat Rev Endocrinol. 2010;6:562–76.
62. Correa FA, Trarbach EB, Tusset C, Latronico AC, Montenegro LR, Carvalho LR, Franca MM, Otto AP, Costalonga EF, Brito VN, Abreu AP, Nishi MN, Jorge AAL, Arnhold IJP, Sidis Y, Pitteloud N, Mendonca BB. FGFR1 and PROKR2 rare variants found in patients with combined pituitary hormone deficiencies. Endocr Connect. 2015;4(2):100–7.
63. Li G, Shao P, Sun X, Wang Q, Zhang L. Magnetic resonance imaging and pituitary function in children with panhypopituitarism. Horm Res Paediatr. 2010;73(3):205–9.
64. Pfaeffle RW, Hunter CS, Savage JJ, Duran-Prado M, Mullen RD, Neeb ZP, Eiholzer U, Hesse V, Haddad NG, Stobbe HM, Blum WF, Weigel JF, Rhodes SJ. Three novel missense mutations within the LHX4 gene are associated with variable pituitary hormone deficiencies. J Clin Endocrinol Metab. 2008;93(3):1062–71.
65. Hilal L, Hajaji Y, Vie-Luton MP, Ajaltouni Z, Benazzouz B, Chana M, Chraïbi A, Kadiri A, Amselem S, Sobrier ML. Unusual phenotypic features in a patient with a novel splice mutation in the GHRHR gene. Mol Med. 2008;14(5–6):286–92.
66. Secco A, Di Iorgi N, Maghnie M. Structural abnormalities in congenital growth hormone deficiency. In: Ho K, editor. Growth hormone related diseases and therapy: a molecular and physiological perspective for the clinician. New York: Springer; 2011. p. 103–35.

# Part III
# Etiologies of Human Growth Hormone Deficiency

# Chapter 11
# Growth Hormone-Releasing Hormone Receptor and Growth Hormone Gene Abnormalities

Jan M. Wit, Monique Losekoot, and Gerhard Baumann

## Introduction

It is assumed that the incidence of congenital isolated growth hormone deficiency (IGHD) is in the order of 1 in 4000 to 1 in 10,000 [1, 2]. In most cases this is sporadic, but 3–30 % of cases are familial, depending on the cohort screened [3, 4].

The classical way to classify familial IGHD is to distinguish four types, according to the inheritance pattern: autosomal recessive inheritance (IGHD types 1A and 1B), autosomal dominant (IGHD type II), and X-linked inheritance (IGHD type III) [3, 4]. Patients with IGHD type IA have severe growth retardation which usually becomes apparent in the first 6 months of life and is caused by deletions, insertions, frameshift, or nonsense mutations in *GH1* (encoding growth hormone, GH). In patients with IGHD type IB, serum GH levels are low but detectable and the phenotype is more heterogeneous. In most cases, splice site, frameshift, missense, or nonsense mutations in *GH1* or *GHRHR* (encoding the GH-releasing hormone receptor) are found, but mutations in other genes, like *HESX1* (homeobox gene expressed in ES cells), *SOX3* (SRY-related HMGbox gene 3), *GHSR* (ghrelin receptor), retinoic receptor-α, or mAchR (muscarinic acetylcholine receptor) have been described as well [4–7]. Apparent IGHD can also be the first presentation of mutations in genes encoding early and late transcription factors playing a role in pituitary ontogeny [4]. A recent report showed that IGHD can also be caused by biallelic mutations in the *RNPC3* gene,

---

J.M. Wit (✉)
Department of Pediatrics, Leiden University Medical Center, Leiden, The Netherlands
e-mail: j.m.wit@lumc.nl

M. Losekoot
Department of Clinical Genetics, Leiden University Medical Center, Leiden, The Netherlands

G. Baumann
Division of Endocrinology, Metabolism and Molecular Medicine, Department of Medicine, Northwestern University Feinberg School of Medicine, Chicago, IL, USA

which codes for a minor spliceosome protein required for U11/U12 small nuclear ribonucleoprotein (snRNP) formation and splicing of U12-type introns [8].

In IGHD type II, with autosomal dominant inheritance, GH secretion is very low but usually still detectable, and in most cases, it is associated with heterozygous splice site, missense, splice enhancer mutations, or intronic deletions in *GH1* [4–6]. In the classical classification, bioactive GH syndrome is considered part of IGHD type II, because it usually has an autosomal dominant pattern of inheritance, but the biochemical presentation is quite different.

There is also an X-linked type III IGHD, which was observed in only few families [9–11] and is considered extremely rare [4, 12]. In one study, it was suggested that the long arm of X chromosome may be involved and that the disorder may be caused by mutations and/or deletions of a portion of the X chromosome containing two loci, one necessary for normal immunoglobulin production and the other for GH expression [13, 14]. In another report, an association was found with an exon-skipping mutation in *BTK* (Bruton tyrosine kinase) gene [11]. However, in other patients with *BTK* mutations, no GHD was noticed, so that the genetic etiology of this condition has remained unknown.

We believe that, given the results from genetic studies in IGHD in the last few decades, this classification may deserve revision. The heterogeneity of genetic causes of GHD type IB makes this diagnostic label questionable, and lumping heterozygous GH mutations which cause real GHD and those with bioactive GH syndrome into one group (type II) may also be confusing for clinicians. In our opinion a classification based primarily on the genetic origin, and further subclassified according to phenotype and type of inheritance, would be preferable. In this chapter we shall describe the various presentations of abnormalities of *GHRHR* and *GH1* according to this principle.

## GHRHR Mutations

*GHRHR*, the gene encoding the receptor for the hypothalamic hormone GHRH, is located on chromosome 7p14. The GHRHR is a 423-amino acid protein belonging to the class B of G protein-coupled 7-transmembrane domain receptors. It is primarily expressed in pituitary somatotrophs. A key regulator of *GHRHR* expression is the transcription factor POU1F1 (Pit-1), and there are two Pit-1-binding elements in the promoter region of *GHRHR*. The GHRHR signals primarily through the Gsα-cAMP pathway, although other minor pathways (calmodulin, protein kinase C (PKC), and eicosanoid) have also been implicated. GHRH is the main driver of GH production and has three major roles subserving this function: it is critical to proliferative expansion of the somatotroph population late in pituitary ontogeny, it stimulates GH synthesis, and it triggers GH release from storage granules [15–18]. In the absence of a functional GHRH signaling system, all three functions are severely curtailed (see below), but there remains a residual complement of somatotrophs and production of very low amounts of GH. Therefore, the phenotype of GHRHR deficiency presents as GHD type IB.

## Inactivating GHRHR Mutations

After the discovery that a spontaneously occurring dwarf mouse model (the little mouse) had a homozygous missense mutation in *Ghrhr* [19, 20], it was not until 1996 that the first homozygous loss-of-function *GHRHR* mutation was reported in two patients from a consanguineous Indian family [21]. Independently, the same mutation (p.Glu72*) was described in a cohort of short-statured people in Pakistan [22, 23] and in two Tamil patients from southern India [24]. Since then, as recently summarized [4], more than 30 pathogenic mutations have been reported, including nonsense, missense, and splice site mutations, in addition to deletions and regulatory mutations affecting the POU1F1-binding sites in the promoter region. For a detailed list of these mutations, the reader is referred to the recent review by Alatzoglou et al. [4]. These mutations, and a few more since described [25–27], are shown in Fig. 11.1. In addition, a number of polymorphisms and functionally silent variants have been reported; these are not depicted in Fig. 11.1. Also not shown are variants for which the evidence for pathogenicity is weak or equivocal (e.g., p.Thr257Ala, p.Lys264Glu) or undetermined because they are only seen in heterozygous form (e.g., p.Ser317Thr).

In general, the mode of inheritance of GHRHR deficiency is autosomal recessive. Haploinsufficiency of *GHRHR* shows no growth phenotype and either no or only a minimal growth-related biochemical phenotype (e.g., mildly decreased insulin-like growth factor-1 (IGF-I) levels) [22, 23, 28, 29], although there is a lower body weight and increased insulin sensitivity [29]. To date, with one potential exception, no case of a dominant-negative mutation has been described, so that simple heterozygosity is not associated with GHD. In contrast, loss of biallelic function (homozygosity or compound heterozygosity) causes severe GHD with very high or complete penetrance starting in infancy. Despite the foregoing, Fig. 11.1 includes three mutations that have been described only in heterozygous form (c.-166t>c, c.-164t>c, and p.Val10Gly). The reason is that for these mutations, there is strong experimental in vitro evidence that they are deleterious. The first two impair the P2-binding site for POU1F1 in the promoter region, and the third has been shown to prevent signal peptide cleavage and normal receptor trafficking to the plasma membrane [30, 31].

The mutations are dispersed throughout the *GHRHR* gene, and no particular clustering is evident. Some (c.57+1G>A, p.Arg161Trp, p.Ala176Val, p.Ser330Leu, and p.Arg357Cys) are located in mutational CpG hotspots. The majority of these mutations have been described in a single to a few patients belonging to geographically and otherwise distinct families, often with a consanguineous background; sporadic mutations appear to be uncommon. Both homozygosity and compound heterozygosity contribute to the affected patient population, with the latter accounting for about a third of the occurrences. There are, however, two large cohorts of affected patients where founder mutations are thought to be responsible: the Pakistani cohort ("dwarfs of Sindh") bearing the p.Glu72* mutation and the Brazilian cohort (Itabaianinha people) bearing the c.57+1G>A mutation. The former kindred is composed of over 20 affected subjects, the latter of approximately

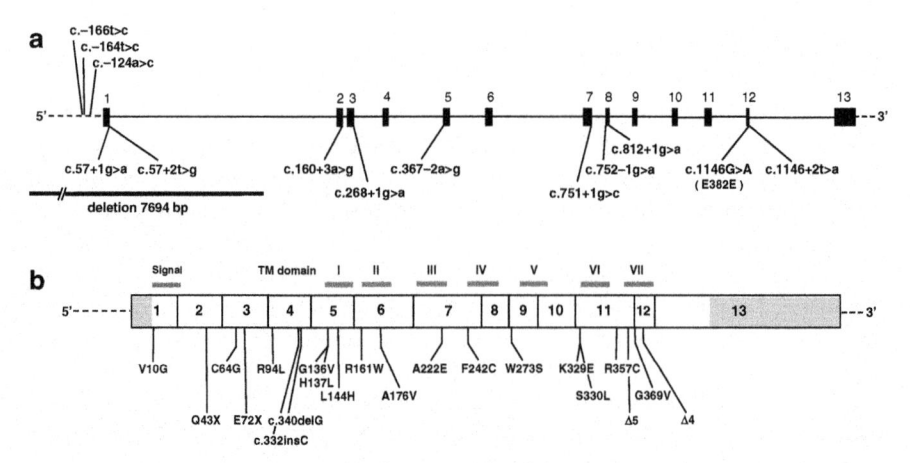

**Fig. 11.1** Pathogenic mutations described in the human GHRHR gene. (**a**) Genomic organization of GHRHR. The 13 exons are shown as *boxes*, introns as *lines*, and flanking regions as *dashed lines*. The locations of splice site mutations (n=9; seven in donor splice sites, two in acceptor splice sites) are shown. Also shown are three mutations in the promoter region, a mutation in the last base of exon 12 acting as a disruptor of an exonic splice enhancer, and a large deletion encompassing 4434 bp of the 5′-flanking region (counting from the A of the start codon), exon 1, and 68 % of intron 1. The deleted fragment is replaced by a 9 bp insert, thus rendering the mutation an indel. Bases located in introns or flanking regions are denoted in *lowercase letters*. For comparison of nomenclatures used in the literature, c.57+1g>a=IVS1+1G>A, c.57+2t>g=IVS1+2T>G, c.160+3a>g=IVS2+3A>G, c.268+1g>a=IVS3+1G>A, c.367−2a>g=IVS4−2A>G, c.751+1g>c=IVS7+1G>C, c.752−1g>a=IVS7−1G>A, c.812+1g>a=IVS8+1G>A, and c.1146+2t>a=IVS12+2T>A. (**b**) cDNA organization of GHRHR. The *shaded areas* denote untranslated regions. Shown above the cDNA are the regions coding for the signal peptide and the seven transmembrane domains. The locations of missense mutations (n=15), nonsense mutations (n=2), microdeletions (n=3), and microinsertions (n=1) are depicted. Δ5 and Δ4 denote 5 and 4 base deletions c.1089-1093del (also known as del1140-1144) and c.1120-1123del, respectively. The c.332insC is also reported as c.380insC. For clarity, the nomenclature for missense mutation is abbreviated without the prefix "p." Criteria for pathogenicity and thus inclusion in the figure were (*a*) clear-cut clinical and/or biochemical evidence for GHD, (*b*) severely disruptive nature of mutation (truncation, splice aberration, frameshift, deletion), and (*c*) experimental in vitro evidence for significant dysfunction. For missense mutations, mere in silico prediction of a deleterious nature, in the absence of other evidence, was not considered sufficient for inclusion

100 affected individuals. The p.Glu72* mutation has been found to be quite prevalent in the western part of the Indian subcontinent [32]; haplotype analysis is consistent with a founder mutation occurring about 2000 years ago [33]. The c.57+1G>A mutation prevalent in Brazil is also a founder mutation, presumably of more recent origin [34, 35].

The mechanism of pathogenicity has been directly examined for some mutations and inferred for others. For those that severely disrupt mRNA and protein generation, such as large deletions, nonsense, frameshift, and splice site mutations, the inferred mechanism is absence of a gene product, premature truncation/nonsense mRNA decay, and aberrant splicing products. For some of the splice site mutations, in vitro functional analysis has directly revealed the abnormal splice products: intron readthrough and whole or partial intron retention has been shown for c.57+2T>G, c.160+3A>G, and c.812+1G>A; exon skipping (whole or partial) for c.812+1G>A and c.1146G>A [30, 36–38]. The latter is a synonymous exonic mutation (p.Glu382Glu) of the last base in exon 12 that affects the adjacent splice site directly or via exonic splice enhancer or suppressor motifs to weaken the intron 12 splice donor site. For the other splice site mutations, in silico analysis predicts aberrant splicing with or without speculation about the nature of the products. Of note, several different abnormal splice products can result from a mutated splice site, as illustrated by the examples cited. The three mutations in the P1- and P2-binding elements for POU1F1 (Pit-1) in the promoter region have been shown to substantially impair binding of POU1F1 and *GHRHR* transactivation [30, 39]. Among the missense mutations, p.Val10Gly affects preprotein processing and prevents receptor trafficking to the plasma membrane [31], while eight others that were functionally examined are present at the cell surface but do not respond to GHRH with cAMP production. For p.His137Leu, p.Leu144His, p.Ala176Val, p.Ala222Glu, and p.Phe242Cys, the defect has been shown to reside in their inability to bind GHRH, with p.Lys329Glu showing reduced ligand binding [40].

The phenotype of patients with biallelic inactivating *GHRHR* mutations is IGHD type IB, with some distinctive features. Postnatal growth retardation is severe and progressive, with adult height reaching −7 to −9 SDS. Birth size is normal. Dysmorphic features are either absent or relatively mild; there is generally no microphallus. Many, but not all patients, have increased abdominal adiposity. Puberty is delayed, fertility and lactation are normal, and menopause occurs at the expected age. Childhood hypoglycemia is extremely rare and has been reported in only one case. The biochemical phenotype includes low basal and stimulated serum GH, very low IGF-I, low IGF-II, low IGFBP-3, low ALS, and high IGFBP-2 levels. Cardiovascular risk factors, including low-density lipoprotein (LDL) cholesterol and C-reactive protein, are elevated. The diurnal rhythm of GH secretion and spontaneous GH production rates have been studied in four young adult male patients with the p.Glu72* mutation and two young adults (one male, one female) with the c.751+1G>C mutation (both null mutations) [41, 42]. Both studies showed that the amplitude of GH pulses was severely attenuated, but peak frequency was normal, indicating that GHRH is not involved in the regulation of GH secretory rhythmicity. Therefore, somatostatin is the likely pacesetter for GH pulsatility. The daily GH production rates ranged from 4 to 16 % of normal.

In children, bone age is delayed. In adults, bone density is normal when expressed as volumetric bone density to correct for small bone size [43, 44]. This finding is surprising as it differs from adult-onset acquired GHD, where bone density is diminished. Hypoplasia of the anterior pituitary, first described in the Pakistani Sindh cohort [45], is a common but not universal finding. In part, the apparent absence of pituitary hypoplasia may be due to the difficulty to differentiate, on MRI scans, normal from hypoplastic pituitary size in very young children. The little mouse has significant pituitary hypoplasia because of a drastically reduced somatotroph population, which normally accounts for at least 50 % of anterior pituitary mass in both mouse and humans [16, 20]. Thus, pituitary hypoplasia in GHRHR deficiency would be expected as part of the phenotype. Nevertheless, there is variability in pituitary size even among first-degree family members bearing the same mutation [46].

An interesting feature described in the Pakistani Sindh patients is relative microcephaly (mean head circumference −4 SDS), which is different from the more typical −2 SDS for other types of GHD. This relatively small head explains the normal (miniaturized adult) aspect of these patients, in contrast with the more "dwarf-like" aspect due to a comparatively large head in other forms of GHD. The little mouse also has relative microcephaly, which has been attributed to the deficient role of GHRH in normal brain development and glial proliferation [47]. It is unknown whether "proportionate microcephaly" is a general feature of GHRHR deficiency as this issue has not been systematically examined in patients other than the Sindh cohort. There is currently insufficient information to answer the question whether there is a genotype–phenotype relationship in patients with *GHRHR* mutations, as most mutations are reported in one or a few patients of varying ages studied under different protocols.

Therapy with GH is very effective in patients with GHRHR deficiency, and there are no reports of neutralizing anti-GH antibody generation. The possibility that ghrelin analogues (GH secretagogues [GHS] or GH-releasing peptides [GHRPs]), which signal through their own receptor, may be of therapeutic benefit was considered though deemed unlikely in view of the somatotroph depletion and the fact that GHS have very limited potency in vitro in the absence of GHRH input. Acute treatment with GHS showed indeed that there is a small GH response but that without a functioning GHRH signaling system, GH secretion is insufficient to be of therapeutic value [48, 49]. The same conclusion has been reached with chronic GHS treatment of a GHRH knockout mouse [50].

## *Activating GHRHR Mutations?*

The possibility of gain-of-function GHRHR mutations as a potential etiology of somatotroph tumors has been evaluated in 80 GH-producing pituitary adenomas. To date, no activating mutation in the *GHRHR* gene has been identified [51, 52].

## *Contribution of GHRHR Variants to Normal Height Variation*

The *GHRHR* gene has been identified as a locus that controls adult height in a Sami and another population in Northern Sweden [53]. Specific haplotypes within and in the 3′-flanking region of *GHRHR* were linked to adult height in those populations. More recently, a variation resulting in a conservative amino acid substitution (c.363G>T, p.Glu121Asp) in exon 4 of *GHRHR* has been identified as playing a role in normal height determination of a population in Spain [54]. It is possible that *GHRHR* is one of the genes in the GH-IGF axis implicated in height determination, although its contribution is quite small and may depend on the population studied. It is noteworthy that in more comprehensive searches for genes associated with height determination, *GHRHR* was not among those identified [55, 56], so that this possibility needs further study.

For additional details on *GHRHR* mutations, the reader is referred to the website of the Growth Genetics Consortium (http://growthgenetics.com).

## *GH1* Mutations Causing GHD or a Syndrome of Bioinactive GH

*GH1* is located on chromosome 17q22-24 within a cluster of five homologous genes and has a highly polymorphic proximal promoter [57]. The pituitary-specific expression of *GH1* is regulated by the binding of POU1F1 (Pit-1) to conserved sequences of the *GH1* proximal promoter, but the interaction of POU1F1 (Pit-1) with response elements in two locus control regions (LCRI and LCRII) located approximately 14.5 to 32 kb upstream of *GH1* is required for an appropriate level of *GH1* expression [58–62]. An association was found between adult height and the mean in vitro expression value corresponding to an individual's *GH1* promoter haplotype combination, and 3.3 % of the variance in adult height was explained by this parameter [57].

*GH1* consists of five exons and four introns (intervening sequences, IVSs). Exon 3 is flanked by weak acceptor and donor splice sites, compared with the strong acceptor site in exon 4. The correct splicing of this gene results in the generation of the mature, full-length 22-kDa peptide, which constitutes almost 75 % of the total circulating GH. Use of the cryptic splice site in exon 3 will result in the 20-kDa isoform that lacks amino acids 32–46, which corresponds to 5–10 % of transcripts. Complete skipping of exon 3 results in the generation of a 17.5-kDa product that lacks amino acids 32 to 71 and corresponds with 1–5 % of transcripts [4, 63], but the corresponding protein product has not been demonstrated to be produced in detectable amounts in normal people. The 17.5-kDa product does not have biological activity and disturbs wild-type GH secretion. Several areas in and around exon 3 have been identified as being important for correct splicing of exon 3, such as two exonic splice enhancers (ESE1 and ESE2) and a cryptic splice site within exon 3, and intronic elements such as the first 6 nucleotides of intron 3, the intronic splice enhancer (ISE), and branching point site (BPS) (for schematic representation, see [4]).

Sequencing of the promoter region, and particularly of the locus control regions (LCRs), suggested a possible association of two variants with IGHD [64], and there may also be an association between a functional common polymorphism in the vitamin D-responsive element and isolated GHD [65]. However, in two later studies, no abnormalities were found in the *LCR-GH1* region in patients with IGHD [61, 66].

From a clinical perspective, we believe that the following subclassification of abnormalities of *GH1* is more informative than the classical one: (1) autosomal recessive form with complete lack of circulating GH and severe short stature (with or without the development of anti-GH antibodies on GH treatment), (2) autosomal recessive form with low but detectable GH concentrations and less severe short stature, (3) autosomal dominant GHD, and (4) bioinactive GH syndrome.

Tables 11.1, 11.2, 11.3, and 11.4 show the mutations in *GH1* as they have been published until February 2015, based on a recent review [4] and a literature search

Table 11.1 Autosomal recessive *GH1* mutations with complete lack of circulating GH (classical type IA)

| *GH1* mutation (HGVS) | Reported as | Location | Zygosity | Other allele | Comments | References |
|---|---|---|---|---|---|---|
| 6.7 kb deletion | | *GH1* | HM | n.a. | | [67, 68] |
| 7.0 kb deletion | | *GH1* | HM | n.a | | [69, 70] |
| 7.6 kb deletion | | *GH1* | HM | n.a | | [71, 72] |
| 45 kb deletion | | *GH1, GH2, CSH, CSHL1* | HM | n.a | Normal birth size, probably because of retention of *CSH2* | [68, 73–75] |
| Double deletions/complex chromosomal rearrangements (40 kb) | | *GH1, GH2, CSH1, CSH2* | HM | n.a. | | [76] |
| c.43delC | GGCcTGC, codon-12 | | HM | n.a. | | [5] |
| c.52delC | c.50delC (codon-11) | Exon 2; SP | CHT | 6.7 kb deletion | | [77] |
| c.59G>A, p.Trp20* | p.W-7X | Exon 2; SP | HM | n.a. | G→A in 20th codon of SP. Termination of translation after residu 19 of SP | [78, 79] |
| c.67G>T, p.Glu23* | p.E-4X | Exon 2; SP | HM | n.a. | CAG→TAG gives stopcodon 23 of SP | [68] |
| c.39_64dup, (p.Gln22Leufs*87) | c.64-65ins26 | Exon 2 | HM | n.a. | Introduces frameshift that introduces 86 novel aas before premature stop codon | [80] |

| GH1 mutation (HGVS) | Reported as | Location | Zygosity | Other allele | Comments | References |
|---|---|---|---|---|---|---|
| c.245_246delAG, (p.Glu82Valfs*51) | c.243-244delAG | Exon 3 | CHT | 6.7 kb deletion | Predicted to introduce a termination codon after aa residu 131 in exon 4. Considered as type1B by Phillips and Cogan (1994) | [81] |
| c.270_285del16, (p.Glu91Asnfs*4) | | Exon 3 | CHT | c.291+4A>T (IVS3+4,A>T) | Predicted to cause nonsense-mediated mRNA decay. Point mutation mosaicism (father's sperm) | [82] |
| c.280_281delCA, (p.Gln94fs*132) | (p.Q68fsX106) | Exon 3 | CHT | c.426C>G p.Asp142Glu | Predicted to cause nonsense-mediated mRNA decay | [83] |

The transcript that was used for HGVS nomenclature was NM_000515.4, and the Protein reference sequence was NP_000506.2. Predicted protein sequences are in bracket

*aa* amino acid, *CHT* compound heterozygous, *HGVS* Human Genome Variation Society, *HM* homozygous, *n.a.* not applicable, *SP* signal peptide, *c.* denotes nucleotide position on cDNA, with the A of the translation start site (ATG) of the cDNA numbered +1

Table 11.2 Autosomal recessive GH1 mutations with low but detectable GH concentrations (part of classical type IB)

| GH1 mutation (HGVS) | Reported as | Location | Zygosity | Age at dg (years) | Height SDS at dg | GH peak (μg/L) | IGF-I SDS | Comments | References |
|---|---|---|---|---|---|---|---|---|---|
| c.1A>G, p.Met1Val | p.M-26V | Initiation codon | CHT 7.6 kb del | 3.3 | −6.5 | 1.8 | – | | [86] |
| c.115G>T, p.Ala39Ser | c.177G>T, p.A13S | Exon 2 | HM | 11.8 | −3.2 | 3.4 | <−2 | No functional studies | [79] |
| c.291+1G>C | IVS3+1,G>C | Intron 3 | HM | 11, 9 and 0.8 | −2.5, −2.9, −5.2 | <0.2[a] | – | Activates a cryptic donor splice site 73 bases upstream. Loss of aa 103–126 in exon 4 and frameshift of exon 5, which normally encodes aa127–191 | [78, 87] |
| c.426C>G, p.Asp142Glu | p.D116E | Exon 4 | CHT p.Q68fsX106 | 7.1 | −3.0 | 2.9 | – | Functionality uncertain | [83] |
| c.437G>T, p.Gly146Val | p.G120V | Exon 4 | HM | 9.8 | −5.0 | 0.1 | −2.0 | No in vitro studies, likely antagonistic action | [61] |
| c.456+1G>T | IVS4+1,G>T | Intron 4 | HM | – | – | – | – | Loss of aa 103–126 in exon 4; frameshift in 5 | [88] |

158  J.M. Wit et al.

| GHI mutation (HGVS) | Reported as | Location | Zygosity | Age at dg (years) | Height SDS at dg | GH peak (μg/L) | IGF-I SDS | Comments | References |
|---|---|---|---|---|---|---|---|---|---|
| c.456+5G>C | IVS4+5,G>C | Intron 4 | HM | 5–13 years (n=4) | −3.6 to −5.2 | <0.6–1.3 | – | Destruction of the splice site and use of a cryptic splice site in exon 4; loss of aa 103–126 in exon 4; frameshift in 5. The predicted 196-aa final protein product shares 1–102 with GH, and has 29 aa from exon 5 and 65 aa from the frameshift. Heterozygotes are shorter than homozygous WT | [89, 90] |
| c.624C>A, p.Cys208* | p.C182X | Exon 5 | HM | 8.1 | −5.7 | 0.16 | <−3.5 | Truncated protein; disulfide bond disruption | [61] |

The transcript that was used for HGVS nomenclature was NM_000515.4, and the protein reference sequence was NP_000506.2

[a]Despite the low serum GH, this mutation was considered type 1B instead of type 1A, based on mild growth faltering and absence of anti-GH antibodies

*aa* amino acid, *CHT* compound heterozygous, *dg* diagnosis, *HM* homozygous, *SDS* standard deviation score, *WT* wild type, *c.* denotes nucleotide position on cDNA with the A of the translation start site (ATG) of the cDNA numbered +1

**Table 11.3** Autosomal dominant GHD (all heterozygous)

| GH1 mutation (HGVS) | Reported as | Location | Comments[a] | References |
|---|---|---|---|---|
| *Single bp mutations within the coding region and in ESEs* | | | | |
| c.47T>C, p.Leu16Pro | p.L-11P | Exon 2; SP | In expression studies, not secreted in the medium | [64] |
| c.75T>G, p.Ser25Arg | p.S-1R | Exon 2; SP | No parental DNA, no functional studies | [66] |
| c.172G>A, p.Glu58Lys | E3+1 G/A | Exon 3 | ESE1; loss of exon 3 | [92] |
| c.172G>T, p.Glu32* | E3+1 | Exon 3 | ESE1; loss of exon 3 | [93] |
| c.172G>A, p.Glu32Lys | E3+1 | Exon 3 | ESE1; alters splice site strength and splicing enhancer function; loss exon 3 | [92, 94] |
| c.173A>C, p.Glu32Ala | E3+2 | Exon 3 | ESE1: % 17.5 kDa and 20 kDa increased. Mutant less secreted | [95] |
| c.176A>G, p.Glu33Gly | E3+5 | Exon 3 | ESE1: % 17.5 kDa and 20 kDa increased | [79, 96, 97] |
| c.199A>T, p.Lys67* | p.L41X; E3+28 | Exon 3 | ESE2; prediction of truncated product, effect on splicing and bioactivity | [98] |
| c.255G>A, p.Pro85Pro | c.255G>A | Exon 3 | In splicing regulatory element | [99] |
| c.272A>T, p.E91V | c.272A>T | Exon 3 | In splicing regulatory element | [99] |
| c.344C>T, p.Pro115Leu | p.P89L | Exon 4 | Affects trafficking in the secretory pathway | [5, 100] |
| c.305T>C, p.Leu102Pro | c.305T>C | Exon 4 | Predicted damaging. Father carrier very short | [101] |
| c.400A>T, p.Ser134Cys | p.S108C | Exon 4 | Reduced secretion in vitro | [64] |
| c.406G>T, p.Val136Phe | p.V110F | Exon 4 | Likely to result in steric hindrance (beginning third α-helix) | [102] |
| c.406G>A, p.Val136Ile | p.V110I | Exon 4 | Considered functional polymorphism by Millar et al. | [64, 101] |
| c.574_576delTTC, p.Phe192del | c.del636-638, p.ΔF166 | Exon 5 | No functional studies | [79] |
| c.601A>G, p.Thr201Ala | p.T175A | Exon 5 | Reduced ability to activate JAK/STAT pathway | [64] |
| c.626G>A, p.Arg209His | p.R183H | Exon 5 | Impaired GH secretion | [97, 101, 103, 104] |

(continued)

**Table 11.3** (continued)

| GH1 mutation (HGVS) | Reported as | Location | Comments[a] | References |
|---|---|---|---|---|
| *Splice site mutations* | | | | |
| | IVS1, insertion of GAAA to +178A | Intron 1 | May create (GAA) ESE motif in the intron 1 region affecting intron splicing | [79] |
| c.171+5G>C | c.171+5G>C | Intron 2 | Abolition of splice donor site | [105] |
| c.172-1G>A | IVS2-1,G>A | Intron 2 | 3′-Acceptor splice site, skipping exon 3 | [64] |
| c.172-1G>C | IVS2-1G>C | Intron 2 | 3′-Acceptor splice site, skipping exon 3 | [7] |
| c.172-2A>T | IVS2-2,A>T | Intron 2 | 3′-Acceptor splice site, skipping exon 3 | [106] |
| c.291+1G>A | IVS3+1,G>A | Intron 3 | Skipping exon 3 | [7, 97, 107] |
| c.291+1G>C | IVS3+1,G>C | Intron 3 | Skipping exon 3 | [97, 108] |
| c.291+1G>T | IVS3+1, G>T | Intron 3 | Skipping exon 3 | [97, 105] |
| c.291+2T>A | IVS3+2, T>A | Intron 3 | Skipping exon 3 | [61] |
| c.291+2T>C | IVS3+2,T>C | Intron 3 | Skipping exon 3 | [97, 106] |
| c.291+4A>T | IVS3+4,A>T | Intron 3 | In silico prediction of exon 3 skipping. Paternal mosaicism for the mutation | [61, 82] |
| c.291+5G>A | IVS3+5,G>A | Intron 3 | Skipping exon 3 | [97, 109, 110] |
| c.291+5G>C | IVS3+5,G>C | Intron 3 | Skipping exon 3 | [97, 111] |
| c.291+6T>C | IVS3+6,T>C | Intron 3 | Skipping exon3 | [87, 88] |
| c.291+6T>G | IVS3+6,T>G | Intron 3 | Skipping exon 3. Apparent de novo but arose in father's germ cells | [112] |
| c.291+28G>A | IVS3+28, G>A | Intron, ISEm1 | Disrupts ISE; abnormal splicing; skipping exon 3 | [113, 114] |
| c.291+29_291+46del | IVSdel+28_45 | Intron 3, ISEm2 | 18-bp deletion; disrupts ISE; skipping exon 3 | [113, 114] |
| c.292-37_292-16del | IVS3del+56_77 | Intron 3 | Removes BPS in intron 3; skipping exon 3 and partial or total exon 4 skipping | [115] |
| c.456G>A | IVS4-1,G>A | Intron 4 | No aa change; assumed to affect splicing | [116] |
| c.456+1G>C | IVS4+1, G>C | Intron 4 | First base of donor splice site of intron 4; unstable or bioinactive protein | [78] |

(continued)

**Table 11.3** (continued)

| GH1 mutation (HGVS) | Reported as | Location | Comments[a] | References |
|---|---|---|---|---|
| c.456+1G>T | IVS4+1, G>T | Intron 4 | First base of donor splice site of intron 4; unstable or bioactive protein | [88] |
| c.456+5G>C | IVS4+5, G>C | Intron 4 | Protein shares 1-102 with GH, has 29 aa from exon 5 and 65 aa from frameshift | [89] |
| c.456+8delT | IVS4'del+7 | Intron 4 | Interferes with splicing process | [117] |

The transcript that was used for HGVS nomenclature was NM_000515.4, and the protein reference sequence was NP_000506.2

[a]Loss of exon 3 leads to a del32-71 GH protein (17.5 kD)

*aa* amino acid, *BPS* branch point sequence (branching point site), *ESE* exon splice enhancer, *ISE* intron splice enhancer, *IVS* intervening sequence, intron, *SP* signal peptide, *c*. denotes nucleotide position on cDNA with the A of the translation start site (ATG) of the cDNA numbered +1

and screening of the Human Gene Mutation Database (HGMD) in February 2015. We chose to use the Human Genome Variation Society (HGVS) nomenclature, where in a coding DNA reference sequence nucleotide "1" is the A of the ATG translation initiation codon. We also show the nomenclature used in the various reports, in most of which the 26 amino acids corresponding to the signal peptide were not included.

## *Autosomal Recessive Form with Complete Lack of Circulating GH*

This condition, type IA according to the classical definition, was first described in pedigrees with homozygous *GH1* deletions, particularly of 6.7, 7.0, or 7.6 kb. These deletions are thought to result from unequal crossing over events between homologous regions that flank the *GH1* gene [69]. The 6.7 kb deletion is the most frequent one [14]. Typically, such patients present with severe growth failure by the first 6 months of life (length SD score [SDS] < −4.5) and undetectable GH concentrations. On GH treatment, many children, but not all [71], develop GH antibodies, presumably because GH protein is seen as a foreign molecule, unknown to the body's immune tolerance system. Besides *GH1* deletions, this form can also be caused by homozygous or compound heterozygous mutations resulting in frameshift or nonsense mutations affecting the signal peptide or exon 3 that result in a severely truncated or absent GH molecule. Table 11.1 shows a list of the genetic findings associated with this clinical presentation [5, 67–83].

11 Growth Hormone-Releasing Hormone Receptor and Growth... 163

Table 11.4 Genetic, clinical, and biochemical characteristics of patients with bioinactive GH syndrome

| GH1 mutation (HGVS) | Reported as | Location | Zygosity | Age at dg (year) | Height SDS at dg | GHmax (ng/mL) | IGF-I SDS | GH therapy response | Comments | References |
|---|---|---|---|---|---|---|---|---|---|---|
| c.236G>C, p.Cys79Ser | p.Cys53Ser | Exon 3 | HM | | −3.6 | 44.7 | −3.4 | +/good | Absence of disulfide bridge (Cys-53 to Cys-165); reduced affinity for GHR | [130] |
| c.253C>T, p.Pro85Ser | p.Pro59Ser | Exon 3 | HT | 9.9 | −4.6 | 17 | −2.8 | − | Lower affinity for binding to GHR and Jak2/Stat5 signaling | [131] |
| | | | | 8.0 | −5.5 | 11 | −3.0 | − | | |
| c.254C>T, p.Pro85Leu | p.Pro59Leu | Exon 3 | HT | 7.7 | −2.5 | 6.9; 5.6 | −2.4 | +/good | Lower affinity for binding to GHR and JAK2/STAT5 signaling | [132] |
| | | | | 13.6 | −2.0 | 4.7; 4.8 | − | +/good | | |
| | | | | Ad | −4.2 | − | − | − | | |
| c.290C>T, p.Ser97Phe | p.Ser71Phe | Exon 3 | HT | 13.5 | −3.8 | 27.2 | − | − | No data on segregation. Reduces ability to activate JAK2/STAT | [64] |
| c.307C>T, p.Arg103Cys | p.Arg77Cys | Exon 4 | HT | 5.6 | −6.1 | 38; 15; 35 | −2.1 | +/poor | Inhibition of binding of WT GH. Mutant not expressed in father | [133] |
| | | | | 37 | −0.2 | 23.7 | −1 | − | | |

(continued)

**Table 11.4** (continued)

| GH1 mutation (HGVS) | Reported as | Location | Zygosity | Age at dg (year) | Height SDS at dg | GHmax (ng/mL) | IGF-I SDS | GH therapy response | Comments | References |
|---|---|---|---|---|---|---|---|---|---|---|
| c.307C>T, p.Arg103Cys | p.Arg77Cys | Exon 4 | HT | 6-20 | −2.5 to −1.9 | 253 | −3.1 to −2.2 | − | Less induction of GHR/GHBP | [134, 135] |
|  |  |  |  | 32 | −1.4 | 261 | −2.1 | − |  |  |
|  |  |  |  | 64 | −1.7 | 242 | −2.3 | − |  |  |
| c.400A>C, p.Ser134Arg | p.Ser108Arg | Exon 4 | HT | − | − | − | − | − | Reduced signal transduction | [64] |
| c.413A>G, p.Asp138Gly | p.Asp112Gly | Exon 4 | HT | 3 | −3.6 | 26; 41; 51 | −2.5 | +/good | Mutant prevents dimerization | [136] |
| c.601A>G, p.Thr201Ala | p.Thr175Ala | Exon 5 | HT | − | − | − | − | − | Reduced signal transduction | [64] |
| c.611G>A, p.Arg204His | p.Arg178His | Exon 5 | HT | 5.1 | −5.4 | 3.9 | <−3.5 | ? |  | [61] |
| c.611G>A, p.Arg204His | p.Arg178His | Exon 5 | HT |  | −6.0 to −7.2 | 3.9 | −2.3 | +/moderate (+3.2 SD) | Affects GH secretion, binding, and signaling | [137] |
| c.615C>G, p.Ile205Met | p.Ile179Met | Exon 5 | HT | 6.9 | −2.7 | 10.4 | −1.2 | − | Affects GH signal transduction; activation of ERK reduced to half | [138] |
| c.615C>G, p.Ile205Met | p.Ile179Met | Exon 5 | HT | 4.7 | −2.0 | 5.9 | − | +/good | No functional studies; segregation with phenotype | [66] |

The transcript that was used for HGVS nomenclature was NM_000515.4, and the Protein reference sequence was NP_000506.2. Adapted from [4, 139]
*HT* heterozygous, *c.* denotes nucleotide position on cDNA with the A of the translation start site (ATG) of the cDNA numbered +1

When the clinician is confronted with a child with such severe phenotype, *GH1* testing yields a defect in almost all cases.

In two siblings with a 26-bp insertion [80], type I Arnold–Chiari malformation was demonstrated and in one of them also pituitary hypoplasia and mild hydrocephalus. Interestingly, several cases of hypopituitarism associated with Arnold–Chiari malformation have been reported [84], as well as cases with POU1F1 mutation [85].

## *Autosomal Recessive Form with Low But Detectable GH Concentrations*

This condition, which is part of the classical type IB GHD, can be caused by homozygous splice site, frameshift, and nonsense GH1 mutations (Table 11.2) [61, 78, 79, 83, 86–90]. On GH treatment, no antibody formation has been observed. Most patients are the product of consanguineous pedigrees or specific ethnic background (for details, see [4]). Confronted with such clinical presentation, the first two genes to test include *GH1* and *GHRHR*, but many other gene defects (though all rare) can be associated with this phenotype as well. Therefore, whole exome sequencing might be a more cost-effective approach [91] or a gene panel encompassing all known gene defects associated with recessive isolated GHD.

## *Autosomal Dominant GHD*

*GH1* mutations associated with this form, classically labeled type II GHD, are shown in Table 11.3 [5, 7, 61, 64, 66, 78, 79, 82, 87–89, 92–110, 112–117]. This condition is mostly caused by heterozygous *GH1* mutations that affect *GH1* splicing, resulting in skipping of exon 3. This results in the production of the 17.5-kDa isoform, which lacks amino acids 32–71 and, hence, the loop that connects helix 1 and helix 2 in the tertiary structure of GH. This isoform exerts a dominant-negative effect on the secretion of the wild-type 22-kDa molecule in neuroendocrine cells containing secretory granules [4, 110, 118, 119]. The decrease in wild-type GH secretion is probably associated with the accumulation of the 17.5-kD isoform in the endoplasmic reticulum (ER) causing ER stress and apoptosis in somatotrophs [120]. Ratios of 17.5-/22-kDa *GH1* transcripts in cultured lymphocytes from family members with the same *GH1* mutation (c.172G>A, reported as E3+1 G/A) correlated with differences in their height SD scores, suggesting that expression levels of both the mutant and normal *GH1* allele are important in the pathogenesis of this condition [94].

Exon skipping can also result from mutations in ESE1 (Table 11.3), which strengthens the use of the upstream weak 3' splice site and suppresses a downstream cryptic splice site [4, 121]. ESE1 mutations result in abnormal splicing and complete or partial exon 3 skipping and the generation of the 17.5-kDa and 20-kDa isoforms at various concentrations [4]. Translationally silent mutations can also affect splicing and lead to GH deficiency [4, 96, 121]. Also, mutations within exon 3 in ESE2 can lead to exon skipping, but the effects on growth are more variable [64, 122]. Recently two other splicing regulatory elements in exon 3 were discovered associated with positions c.255 and c.272 [99]. Furthermore, various mutations in intron 3, which affect ISEs [113, 114] or the branching point site [115], can also result in exon 3 skipping.

Besides through exon 3 skipping, heterozygous missense mutations can also affect GH secretion through other mechanisms. For example, the p.Arg209His mutation (reported as p.Arg183His) results in defects of exocytosis of secretory granules [104, 123], and the p.Pro115Leu mutation (reported as p.Pro89Leu) disturbs the secretory pathway by altering the orientation of the GH helices and affecting the correct folding of the molecule [4, 100]. Other mutations affect GH secretion as well as its affinity for the GH receptor; these will be discussed in the next section.

While this dominant form of GHD is usually not associated with other pituitary deficiencies, it is now clear that these can develop over time, probably related to progressive pituitary degeneration (perhaps due to collateral damage of somatotroph death) [100, 124, 125]. Subjects presenting with a splice site mutation within the first 2 bp of intron 3 leading to skipping exon 3 appear more likely to present with other pituitary hormone deficiencies [124].

Even if patients with this phenotype have no defect identified at first testing [126], it is still worthwhile to repeat the test with more advanced technology if the phenotype and family history are strongly suggestive for a genetic syndrome, as we recently showed for two pedigrees [7]. Identification of pathogenic mutations has important clinical implications for surveillance and genetic counseling.

Children with this type of GH treatment show a sustained catch-up growth over a period as long as 6 years and usually reach their target height range [97]. However, several attempts are underway to develop a genetic approach to treat this condition [4, 127–129].

## Bioinactive GH Syndrome

A list of presently known *GH1* mutations associated with bioinactive GH syndrome is shown in Table 11.4 [61, 64, 66, 130–138]. Most cases with this syndrome do, at first sight, not present as IGHD, because GH secretion appears normal or even increased, but in some cases, the *GH1* mutation causes a combination of decreased GH secretion in combination with decreased GH bioactivity (Table 11.4). A severe short stature and very low serum IGF-I and IGFBP-3, in contrast with apparently normal (or low or high) GH secretion, would be a good reason to sequence *GH1*, particularly if more than one case is found in the same family.

## Prevalence of GH1 Abnormalities

In several studies, the prevalence of the various forms of *GH1* defects was investigated. In a study by the London group on 190 pedigrees with IGHD [61], *GH1* mutations were identified in 7.4 %, with a higher prevalence among familial cases (22.7 %; 10 of 44 pedigrees) compared with sporadic (2.7 %; four patients out of 146 pedigrees). Most mutations in *GH1* (78.6 %) led to an autosomal dominant type of GHD as a result of splice site and missense mutations, in contrast with low percentages of type 1A (7.1 %) and type 1B (14.3 %). Patients with type II IGHD due to splice site mutations had a lower peak GH upon provocation compared with those with missense mutations. The anterior pituitary was reported as hypoplastic in 60 % of patients with splice site mutations (6 of 10) and in 25 % (1 of 4) of those with missense mutations. The authors concluded that IGHD patients with severe growth failure and a positive family history should be screened for genetic mutations.

In an earlier study on 151 subjects with severe growth retardation originating from many different countries and analyzed in Switzerland, mutations in *GH1* were detected in 12.5 % of familial and 10 % of sporadic IGHD [68]. Recently, the results of a specific screening strategy in a Moroccan cohort of patients with isolated GHD were reported [66]. Genetic screening was first based on MRI findings and then on the endocrine phenotype, associated abnormalities and gender. Patients with IGHD and a eutopic posterior pituitary were screened for mutations in *GH1*, *GHRHR*, *GHRH*, *GHSR*, *HESX1*, and the locus control region (LCR) of *GH1*. *GH1* deletions were tested for all patients with a GH peak undetectable or below 1 ng/mL. *GH1* was analyzed in 49 index cases; among them 11 were tested for a *GH1* deletion. Three distinct molecular defects were identified: two mutations known as deleterious (*GH1* 67-kb deletion and p.Ile205Met) and one variation (p.Ser25Arg). No mutation was detected in the three POU1F1-binding sites of the LCR-GH1 region. In this study, 12.2 % (6/49) of IGHD patients with a eutopic posterior pituitary had a genetic defect in *GH1* or *GHRHR* genes, in keeping with other studies [61, 140]. In a study in Turkey, a *GH1* defect was found in 12 % patients [79]. In the northwestern region of India, 17.5 % had a 6.7 kb or 7.6 kb deletion of *GH1* [141]. Twenty-two percent in Argentina [101] and 6 % in Brazil 6 % had *GH1* mutations [105], most of whom had *GH1* deletions.

## Contribution of GH1 Variants to Normal Height Variation

In general, heterozygous carriers of a *GH1* mutation that is associated with a recessive type of GHD do not have lower body stature, but there appears to be one exception. In an Israeli study [89] in an extended, consanguineous Arab–Bedouin family, carriers of the mutant *GH1* allele were significantly shorter than noncarriers (−1.7 versus −0.4 SDS), suggesting that apparent idiopathic short stature may be caused by heterozygosity for a *GH1* mutation. Still, at a population level, variation in *GH1*, as well as other genes in the GH/IGF axis, has only a small effect on adult height variation [55].

## Conclusion

Screening for *GH1* defects in children with severe isolated GHD (strong growth faltering and very low GH peaks in a stimulation test) should be performed, particularly if there is a positive family history. In case of autosomal dominant inheritance, *GH1* should be tested; if an autosomal recessive pattern is suspected, *GH1* and *GHRHR* are the candidate genes. Phenotypic features can help in deciding which gene to test first, for example, head circumference which is smaller in *GHRHR* defects.

## References

1. Lacey KA, Parkin JM. Causes of short stature. A community study of children in Newcastle upon Tyne. Lancet. 1974;1:42–5.
2. Vimpani GV, Vimpani AF, Lidgard GP, Cameron EH, Farquhar JW. Prevalence of severe growth hormone deficiency. Br Med J. 1977;2:427–30.
3. Mullis PE. Genetics of GHRH, GHRH-receptor, GH and GH-receptor: its impact on pharmacogenetics. Best Pract Res Clin Endocrinol Metab. 2011;25:25–41.
4. Alatzoglou KS, Webb EA, Le Tissier P, Dattani MT. Isolated growth hormone deficiency (GHD) in childhood and adolescence: recent advances. Endocr Rev. 2014;35:376–432.
5. Mullis PE. Genetics of isolated growth hormone deficiency. J Clin Res Pediatr Endocrinol. 2010;2:52–62.
6. Wit JM, Kiess W, Mullis P. Genetic evaluation of short stature. Best Pract Res Clin Endocrinol Metab. 2011;25:1–17.
7. Kempers MJ, van der Crabben SN, de Vroede M, Alfen-van der Velden J, Netea-Maier RT, Duim RA, et al. Splice site mutations in GH1 detected in previously (Genetically) undiagnosed families with congenital isolated growth hormone deficiency type II. Horm Res Paediatr. 2013;80:390–6.
8. Argente J, Flores R, Gutierrez-Arumi A, Verma B, Martos-Moreno GA, Cusco I, et al. Defective minor spliceosome mRNA processing results in isolated familial growth hormone deficiency. EMBO Mol Med. 2014;6:299–306.
9. Fleisher TA, White RM, Broder S, Nissley SP, Blaese RM, Mulvihill JJ, et al. X-linked hypogammaglobulinemia and isolated growth hormone deficiency. N Engl J Med. 1980;302:1429–34.
10. Sitz KV, Burks AW, Williams LW, Kemp SF, Steele RW. Confirmation of X-linked hypogammaglobulinemia with isolated growth hormone deficiency as a disease entity. J Pediatr. 1990;116:292–4.
11. Duriez B, Duquesnoy P, Dastot F, Bougneres P, Amselem S, Goossens M. An exon-skipping mutation in the btk gene of a patient with X-linked agammaglobulinemia and isolated growth hormone deficiency. FEBS Lett. 1994;346:165–70.
12. Stewart DM, Tian L, Notarangelo LD, Nelson DL. X-linked hypogammaglobulinemia and isolated growth hormone deficiency: an update. Immunol Res. 2008;40:262–70.
13. Conley ME, Burks AW, Herrod HG, Puck JM. Molecular analysis of X-linked agammaglobulinemia with growth hormone deficiency. J Pediatr. 1991;119:392–7.
14. Mullis PE. Genetic control of growth. Eur J Endocrinol. 2005;152:11–31.
15. Billestrup N, Swanson LW, Vale W. Growth hormone-releasing factor stimulates proliferation of somatotrophs in vitro. Proc Natl Acad Sci U S A. 1986;83:6854–7.
16. Wilson DB, Wyatt DP, Gadler RM, Baker CA. Quantitative aspects of growth hormone cell maturation in the normal and little mutant mouse. Acta Anat (Basel). 1988;131:150–5.
17. Baringa M, Yamonoto G, Rivier C, Vale W, Evans R, Rosenfeld MG. Transcriptional regulation of growth hormone gene expression by growth hormone-releasing factor. Nature. 1983;306:84–5.

18. Cronin MJ, Hewlett EL, Evans WS, Thorner MO, Rogol AD. Human pancreatic tumor growth hormone (GH) – releasing factor and cyclic adenosine 3′,5′-monophosphate evoke GH release from anterior pituitary cells: the effects of pertussis toxin, cholera toxin, forskolin, and cycloheximide. Endocrinology. 1984;114:904–13.
19. Godfrey P, Rahal JO, Beamer WG, Copeland NG, Jenkins NA, Mayo KE. GHRH receptor of little mice contains a missense mutation in the extracellular domain that disrupts receptor function. Nat Genet. 1993;4:227–32.
20. Lin SC, Lin CR, Gukovsky I, Lusis AJ, Sawchenko PE, Rosenfeld MG. Molecular basis of the little mouse phenotype and implications for cell type-specific growth. Nature. 1993;364:208–13.
21. Wajnrajch MP, Gertner JM, Harbison MD, Chua Jr SC, Leibel RL. Nonsense mutation in the human growth hormone-releasing hormone receptor causes growth failure analogous to the little (lit) mouse. Nat Genet. 1996;12:88–90.
22. Baumann G, Maheshwari H. The Dwarfs of Sindh: severe growth hormone (GH) deficiency caused by a mutation in the GH-releasing hormone receptor gene. Acta Paediatr Suppl. 1997;423:33–8.
23. Maheshwari HG, Silverman BL, Dupuis J, Baumann G. Phenotype and genetic analysis of a syndrome caused by an inactivating mutation in the growth hormone-releasing hormone receptor: Dwarfism of Sindh. J Clin Endocrinol Metab. 1998;83:4065–74.
24. Netchine I, Talon P, Dastot F, Vitaux F, Goossens M, Amselem S. Extensive phenotypic analysis of a family with growth hormone (GH) deficiency caused by a mutation in the GH-releasing hormone receptor gene. J Clin Endocrinol Metab. 1998;83:432–6.
25. Demirbilek H, Tahir S, Baran RT, Sherif M, Shah P, Ozbek MN, et al. Familial isolated growth hormone deficiency due to a novel homozygous missense mutation in the growth hormone releasing hormone receptor gene: clinical presentation with hypoglycemia. J Clin Endocrinol Metab. 2014;99:E2730–4.
26. Kale S, Budyal S, Kasaliwal R, Shivane V, Raghavan V, Lila A, et al. A novel gross indel in the growth hormone releasing hormone receptor gene of Indian IGHD patients. Growth Horm IGF Res. 2014;24:227–32.
27. Arman A, Dundar BN, Cetinkaya E, Erzaim N, Buyukgebiz A. Novel growth hormone-releasing hormone receptor gene mutations in Turkish children with isolated growth hormone deficiency. J Clin Res Pediatr Endocrinol. 2014;6:202–8.
28. Hayashida CY, Gondo RG, Ferrari C, Toledo SP, Salvatori R, Levine MA, et al. Familial growth hormone deficiency with mutated GHRH receptor gene: clinical and hormonal findings in homozygous and heterozygous individuals from Itabaianinha. Eur J Endocrinol. 2000;142:557–63.
29. Pereira RM, Aguiar-Oliveira MH, Sagazio A, Oliveira CR, Oliveira FT, Campos VC, et al. Heterozygosity for a mutation in the growth hormone-releasing hormone receptor gene does not influence adult stature, but affects body composition. J Clin Endocrinol Metab. 2007;92:2353–7.
30. Inoue H, Kangawa N, Kinouchi A, Sakamoto Y, Kimura C, Horikawa R, et al. Identification and functional analysis of novel human growth hormone secretagogue receptor (GHSR) gene mutations in Japanese subjects with short stature. J Clin Endocrinol Metab. 2011;96:E373–8.
31. Godi M, Mellone S, Petri A, Arrigo T, Bardelli C, Corrado L, et al. A recurrent signal peptide mutation in the growth hormone releasing hormone receptor with defective translocation to the cell surface and isolated growth hormone deficiency. J Clin Endocrinol Metab. 2009;94:3939–47.
32. Desai MP, Upadhye PS, Kamijo T, Yamamoto M, Ogawa M, Hayashi Y, et al. Growth hormone releasing hormone receptor (GHRH-r) gene mutation in Indian children with familial isolated growth hormone deficiency: a study from western India. J Pediatr Endocrinol Metab. 2005;18:955–73.
33. Wajnrajch MP, Gertner JM, Sokoloff AS, Ten I, Harbison MD, Netchine I, et al. Haplotype analysis of the growth hormone releasing hormone receptor locus in three apparently unrelated kindreds from the indian subcontinent with the identical mutation in the GHRH receptor. Am J Med Genet A. 2003;120A:77–83.
34. Salvatori R, Hayashida CY, Aguiar-Oliveira MH, Phillips III JA, Souza AH, Gondo RG, et al. Familial dwarfism due to a novel mutation of the growth hormone-releasing hormone receptor gene. J Clin Endocrinol Metab. 1999;84:917–23.

35. Marui S, Trarbach EB, Boguszewski MC, Franca MM, Jorge AA, Inoue H, et al. GH-releasing hormone receptor gene: a novel splice-disrupting mutation and study of founder effects. Horm Res Paediatr. 2012;78:165–72.
36. Hilal L, Hajaji Y, Vie-Luton MP, Ajaltouni Z, Benazzouz B, Chana M, et al. Unusual phenotypic features in a patient with a novel splice mutation in the GHRHR gene. Mol Med. 2008;14:286–92.
37. Soneda A, Adachi M, Muroya K, Asakura Y, Takagi M, Hasegawa T, et al. Novel compound heterozygous mutations of the growth hormone-releasing hormone receptor gene in a case of isolated growth hormone deficiency. Growth Horm IGF Res. 2013;23:89–97.
38. Wang Q, Diao Y, Xu Z, Li X, Luo XP, Xu H, et al. Identification of a novel splicing mutation in the growth hormone (GH)-releasing hormone receptor gene in a Chinese family with pituitary dwarfism. Mol Cell Endocrinol. 2009;313:50–6.
39. Salvatori R, Fan X, Mullis PE, Haile A, Levine MA. Decreased expression of the GHRH receptor gene due to a mutation in a Pit-1 binding site. Mol Endocrinol. 2002;16:450–8.
40. Alba M, Salvatori R. Naturally-occurring missense mutations in the human growth hormone-releasing hormone receptor alter ligand binding. J Endocrinol. 2005;186:515–21.
41. Roelfsema F, Biermasz NR, Veldman RG, Veldhuis JD, Frolich M, Stokvis-Brantsma WH, et al. Growth hormone (GH) secretion in patients with an inactivating defect of the GH-releasing hormone (GHRH) receptor is pulsatile: evidence for a role for non-GHRH inputs into the generation of GH pulses. J Clin Endocrinol Metab. 2001;86:2459–64.
42. Maheshwari HG, Pezzoli SS, Rahim A, Shalet SM, Thorner MO, Baumann G. Pulsatile growth hormone secretion persists in genetic growth hormone-releasing hormone resistance. Am J Physiol Endocrinol Metab. 2002;282:E943–51.
43. Maheshwari HG, Bouillon R, Nijs J, Oganov VS, Bakulin AV, Baumann G. The Impact of congenital, severe, untreated growth hormone (GH) deficiency on bone size and density in young adults: insights from genetic GH-releasing hormone receptor deficiency. J Clin Endocrinol Metab. 2003;88:2614–8.
44. Epitacio-Pereira CC, Silva GM, Salvatori R, Santana JA, Pereira FA, Gois-Junior MB, et al. Isolated GH deficiency due to a GHRH receptor mutation causes hip joint problems and genu valgum, and reduces size but not density of trabecular and mixed bone. J Clin Endocrinol Metab. 2013;98:E1710–5.
45. Murray RA, Maheshwari HG, Russell EJ, Baumann G. Pituitary hypoplasia in patients with a mutation in the growth hormone-releasing hormone receptor gene. AJNR Am J Neuroradiol. 2000;21:685–9.
46. Alba M, Hall CM, Whatmore AJ, Clayton PE, Price DA, Salvatori R. Variability in anterior pituitary size within members of a family with GH deficiency due to a new splice mutation in the GHRH receptor gene. Clin Endocrinol (Oxf). 2004;60:470–5.
47. Morisawa K, Sugisaki T, Kanamatsu T, Aoki T, Noguchi T. Factors contributing to cerebral hypomyelination in the growth hormone-deficient little mouse. Neurochem Res. 1989;14:173–7.
48. Maheshwari HG, Rahim A, Shalet SM, Baumann G. Selective lack of growth hormone (GH) response to the GH-releasing peptide hexarelin in patients with GH-releasing hormone receptor deficiency. J Clin Endocrinol Metab. 1999;84:956–9.
49. Gondo RG, Aguiar-Oliveira MH, Hayashida CY, Toledo SP, Abelin N, Levine MA, et al. Growth hormone-releasing peptide-2 stimulates GH secretion in GH-deficient patients with mutated GH-releasing hormone receptor. J Clin Endocrinol Metab. 2001;86:3279–83.
50. Alba M, Fintini D, Bowers CY, Parlow AF, Salvatori R. Effects of long-term treatment with growth hormone-releasing peptide-2 in the GHRH knockout mouse. Am J Physiol Endocrinol Metab. 2005;289:E762–7.
51. Salvatori R, Thakker RV, Lopes MB, Fan X, Eswara JR, Ellison D, et al. Absence of mutations in the growth hormone (GH)-releasing hormone receptor gene in GH-secreting pituitary adenomas. Clin Endocrinol (Oxf). 2001;54:301–7.
52. Lee EJ, Kotlar TJ, Ciric I, Lee MK, Lim SK, Lee HC, et al. Absence of constitutively activating mutations in the GHRH receptor in GH-producing pituitary tumors. J Clin Endocrinol Metab. 2001;86:3989–95.

53. Johansson A, Jonasson I, Gyllensten U. Extended haplotypes in the growth hormone releasing hormone receptor gene (GHRHR) are associated with normal variation in height. PLoS One. 2009;4, e4464.
54. Camats N, Fernandez-Cancio M, Carrascosa A, Andaluz P, Albisu MA, Clemente M, et al. Contribution of human growth hormone-releasing hormone receptor (GHRHR) gene sequence variation to isolated severe growth hormone deficiency (ISGHD) and normal adult height. Clin Endocrinol (Oxf). 2012;77:564–74.
55. Lettre G, Butler JL, Ardlie KG, Hirschhorn JN. Common genetic variation in eight genes of the GH/IGF1 axis does not contribute to adult height variation. Hum Genet. 2007;122:129–39.
56. Wood AR, Esko T, Yang J, Vedantam S, Pers TH, Gustafsson S, et al. Defining the role of common variation in the genomic and biological architecture of adult human height. Nat Genet. 2014;46:1173–86.
57. Horan M, Millar DS, Hedderich J, Lewis G, Newsway V, Mo N, et al. Human growth hormone 1 (GH1) gene expression: complex haplotype-dependent influence of polymorphic variation in the proximal promoter and locus control region. Hum Mutat. 2003;21:408–23.
58. Jin Y, Surabhi RM, Fresnoza A, Lytras A, Cattini PA. A role for A/T-rich sequences and Pit-1/GHF-1 in a distal enhancer located in the human growth hormone locus control region with preferential pituitary activity in culture and transgenic mice. Mol Endocrinol. 1999;13:1249–66.
59. Shewchuk BM, Liebhaber SA, Cooke NE. Specification of unique Pit-1 activity in the hGH locus control region. Proc Natl Acad Sci U S A. 2002;99:11784–9.
60. Cattini PA, Yang X, Jin Y, Detillieux KA. Regulation of the human growth hormone gene family: possible role for Pit-1 in early stages of pituitary-specific expression and repression. Neuroendocrinology. 2006;83:145–53.
61. Alatzoglou KS, Turton JP, Kelberman D, Clayton PE, Mehta A, Buchanan C, et al. Expanding the spectrum of mutations in GH1 and GHRHR: genetic screening in a large cohort of patients with congenital isolated growth hormone deficiency. J Clin Endocrinol Metab. 2009;94:3191–9.
62. Yang X, Jin Y, Cattini PA. Appearance of the pituitary factor Pit-1 increases chromatin remodeling at hypersensitive site III in the human GH locus. J Mol Endocrinol. 2010;45:19–32.
63. Procter AM, Phillips III JA, Cooper DN. The molecular genetics of growth hormone deficiency. Hum Genet. 1998;103:255–72.
64. Millar DS, Lewis MD, Horan M, Newsway V, Easter TE, Gregory JW, et al. Novel mutations of the growth hormone 1 (GH1) gene disclosed by modulation of the clinical selection criteria for individuals with short stature. Hum Mutat. 2003;21:424–40.
65. Giordano M, Godi M, Mellone S, Petri A, Vivenza D, Tiradani L, et al. A functional common polymorphism in the vitamin D-responsive element of the GH1 promoter contributes to isolated growth hormone deficiency. J Clin Endocrinol Metab. 2008;93:1005–12.
66. Fritez N, Sobrier ML, Iraqi H, Vie-Luton MP, Netchine I, El Annas A, et al. Molecular screening of a large cohort of Moroccan patients with congenital hypopituitarism. Clin Endocrinol (Oxf). 2015;82:876–84.
67. Phillips III JA, Hjelle BL, Seeburg PH, Zachmann M. Molecular basis for familial isolated growth hormone deficiency. Proc Natl Acad Sci U S A. 1981;78:6372–5.
68. Wagner JK, Eble A, Hindmarsh PC, Mullis PE. Prevalence of human GH-1 gene alterations in patients with isolated growth hormone deficiency. Pediatr Res. 1998;43:105–10.
69. Kamijo T, Phillips III JA. Detection of molecular heterogeneity in GH-1 gene deletions by analysis of polymerase chain reaction amplification products. J Clin Endocrinol Metab. 1992;74:786–9.
70. He YA, Chen SS, Wang YX, Lin XY, Wang DF. A Chinese familial growth hormone deficiency with a deletion of 7.1 kb of DNA. J Med Genet. 1990;27:151–4.
71. Laron Z, Kelijman M, Pertzelan A, Keret R, Shoffner JM, Parks JS. Human growth hormone gene deletion without antibody formation or growth arrest during treatment–a new disease entity? Isr J Med Sci. 1985;21:999–1006.
72. Braga S, Phillips III JA, Joss E, Schwarz H, Zuppinger K. Familial growth hormone deficiency resulting from a 7.6 kb deletion within the growth hormone gene cluster. Am J Med Genet. 1986;25:443–52.

73. Akinci A, Kanaka C, Eble A, Akar N, Vidinlisan S, Mullis PE. Isolated growth hormone (GH) deficiency type IA associated with a 45-kilobase gene deletion within the human GH gene cluster. J Clin Endocrinol Metab. 1992;75:437–41.
74. Baroncini C, Baldazzi L, Pirazzoli P, Marchetti G, Capelli M, Cacciari E, et al. Deletion breakpoints in a 32 bp perfect repeat located 45.1 Kb apart in the human growth hormone gene cluster. Hum Mol Genet. 1993;2:2151–3.
75. Ghizzoni L, Duquesnoy P, Torresani T, Vottero A, Goossens M, Bernasconi S. Isolated growth hormone deficiency type IA associated with a 45-kilobase gene deletion within the human growth hormone gene cluster in an Italian family. Pediatr Res. 1994;36:654–9.
76. Goossens M, Brauner R, Czernichow P, Duquesnoy P, Rappaport R. Isolated growth hormone (GH) deficiency type 1A associated with a double deletion in the human GH gene cluster. J Clin Endocrinol Metab. 1986;62:712–6.
77. Duquesnoy P, Amselem S, Gourmelen M, Le Bouc Y, Goossens M. A frameshift mutation causing isolated growth hormone deficiency type 1A. Am J Hum Genet. 1990;47:A110.
78. Cogan JD, Phillips III JA, Sakati N, Frisch H, Schober E, Milner RD. Heterogeneous growth hormone (GH) gene mutations in familial GH deficiency. J Clin Endocrinol Metab. 1993;76:1224–8.
79. Coker A, Cetinkaya E, Dundar B, Siklar Z, Buyukgebiz A, Arman A. Characterization of GH-1 mutations in children with isolated growth hormone deficiency in the Turkish population. J Pediatr Endocrinol Metab. 2009;22:937–46.
80. Iughetti L, Sobrier ML, Predieri B, Netchine I, Carani C, Bernasconi S, et al. Complex disease phenotype revealed by GH deficiency associated with a novel and unusual defect in the GH-1 gene. Clin Endocrinol (Oxf). 2008;69:170–2.
81. Igarashi Y, Ogawa M, Kamijo T, Iwatani N, Nishi Y, Kohno H, et al. A new mutation causing inherited growth hormone deficiency: a compound heterozygote of a 6.7 kb deletion and a two base deletion in the third exon of the GH-1 gene. Hum Mol Genet. 1993;2:1073–4.
82. Tsubahara M, Hayashi Y, Niijima S, Yamamoto M, Kamijo T, Murata Y, et al. Isolated growth hormone deficiency in two siblings because of paternal mosaicism for a mutation in the GH1 gene. Clin Endocrinol (Oxf). 2012;76:420–4.
83. Dateki S, Hizukuri K, Tanaka T, Katsumata N, Katavetin P, Ogata T. An immunologically anomalous but considerably bioactive GH produced by a novel GH1 mutation (p.D116E). Eur J Endocrinol. 2009;161:301–6.
84. Maghnie M, Triulzi F, Larizza D, Preti P, Priora C, Scotti G, et al. Hypothalamic-pituitary dysfunction in growth hormone-deficient patients with pituitary abnormalities. J Clin Endocrinol Metab. 1991;73:79–83.
85. Pfaffle RW, DiMattia GE, Parks JS, Brown MR, Wit JM, Jansen M, et al. Mutation of the POU-specific domain of Pit-1 and hypopituitarism without pituitary hypoplasia. Science. 1992;257:1118–21.
86. Hayashi Y, Kamijo T, Yamamoto M, Murata Y, Phillips III JA, Ogawa M, et al. A case with isolated growth hormone deficiency caused by compound heterozygous mutations in GH-1: a novel missense mutation in the initiation codon and a 7.6kb deletion. Growth Horm IGF Res. 2007;17:249–53.
87. Cogan JD, Phillips III JA, Schenkman SS, Milner RD, Sakati N. Familial growth hormone deficiency: a model of dominant and recessive mutations affecting a monomeric protein. J Clin Endocrinol Metab. 1994;79:1261–5.
88. Phillips III JA, Cogan JD. Genetic basis of endocrine disease. 6. Molecular basis of familial human growth hormone deficiency. J Clin Endocrinol Metab. 1994;78:11–6.
89. Leiberman E, Pesler D, Parvari R, Elbedour K, Abdul-Latif H, Brown MR, et al. Short stature in carriers of recessive mutation causing familial isolated growth hormone deficiency. Am J Med Genet. 2000;90:188–92.
90. Abdul-Latif H, Leiberman E, Brown MR, Carmi R, Parks JS. Growth hormone deficiency type IB caused by cryptic splicing of the GH-1 gene. J Pediatr Endocrinol Metab. 2000;13:21–8.
91. Guo MH, Shen Y, Walvoord EC, Miller TC, Moon JE, Hirschhorn JN, et al. Whole exome sequencing to identify genetic causes of short stature. Horm Res Paediatr. 2014;82:44–52.

92. Shariat N, Holladay CD, Cleary RK, Phillips III JA, Patton JG. Isolated growth hormone deficiency type II caused by a point mutation that alters both splice site strength and splicing enhancer function. Clin Genet. 2008;74:539–45.
93. Takahashi I, Takahashi T, Komatsu M, Sato T, Takada G. An exonic mutation of the GH-1 gene causing familial isolated growth hormone deficiency type II. Clin Genet. 2002;61:222–5.
94. Hamid R, Phillips III JA, Holladay C, Cogan JD, Austin ED, Backeljauw PF, et al. A molecular basis for variation in clinical severity of isolated growth hormone deficiency type II. J Clin Endocrinol Metab. 2009;94:4728–34.
95. Petkovic V, Lochmatter D, Turton J, Clayton PE, Trainer PJ, Dattani MT, et al. Exon splice enhancer mutation (GH-E32A) causes autosomal dominant growth hormone deficiency. J Clin Endocrinol Metab. 2007;92:4427–35.
96. Moseley CT, Mullis PE, Prince MA, Phillips III JA. An exon splice enhancer mutation causes autosomal dominant GH deficiency. J Clin Endocrinol Metab. 2002;87:847–52.
97. Binder G, Iliev DI, Mullis PE, Ranke MB. Catch-up growth in autosomal dominant isolated growth hormone deficiency (IGHD type II). Growth Horm IGF Res. 2007;17:242–8.
98. Gucev Z, Tasic V, Saranac L, Stobbe H, Kratzsch J, Klammt J, et al. A novel GH1 mutation in a family with isolated growth hormone deficiency type II. Horm Res Paediatr. 2012;77:200–4.
99. Babu D, Mellone S, Fusco I, Petri A, Walker GE, Bellone S, et al. Novel mutations in the GH gene (GH1) uncover putative splicing regulatory elements. Endocrinology. 2014;155:1786–92.
100. Salemi S, Yousefi S, Baltensperger K, Robinson IC, Eble A, Simon D, et al. Variability of isolated autosomal dominant GH deficiency (IGHD II): impact of the P89L GH mutation on clinical follow-up and GH secretion. Eur J Endocrinol. 2005;153:791–802.
101. Juanes M, Marino R, Ciaccio M, Di Palma I, Ramirez P, Warman DM, et al. Presence of GH1 and absence of GHRHR gene mutations in a large cohort of Argentinian patients with severe short stature and isolated GH deficiency. Clin Endocrinol (Oxf). 2014;80:618–20.
102. Binder G, Keller E, Mix M, Massa GG, Stokvis-Brantsma WH, Wit JM, et al. Isolated GH deficiency with dominant inheritance: new mutations, new insights. J Clin Endocrinol Metab. 2001;86:3877–81.
103. Miyata I, Cogan JD, Prince MA, Kamijo T, Ogawa M, Phillips III JA. Detection of growth hormone gene defects by dideoxy fingerprinting (ddF). Endocr J. 1997;44:149–54.
104. Deladoey J, Stocker P, Mullis PE. Autosomal dominant GH deficiency due to an Arg183His GH-1 gene mutation: clinical and molecular evidence of impaired regulated GH secretion. J Clin Endocrinol Metab. 2001;86:3941–7.
105. Lido AC, Franca MM, Correa FA, Otto AP, Carvalho LR, Quedas EP, et al. Autosomal recessive form of isolated growth hormone deficiency is more frequent than the autosomal dominant form in a Brazilian cohort. Growth Horm IGF Res. 2014;24:180–6.
106. Fofanova OV, Evgrafov OV, Polyakov AV, Poltaraus AB, Peterkova VA, Dedov II. A novel IVS2–2A>T splicing mutation in the GH-1 gene in familial isolated growth hormone deficiency type II in the spectrum of other splicing mutations in the Russian population. J Clin Endocrinol Metab. 2003;88:820–6.
107. Cogan JD, Ramel B, Lehto M, Phillips III J, Prince M, Blizzard RM, et al. A recurring dominant negative mutation causes autosomal dominant growth hormone deficiency–a clinical research center study. J Clin Endocrinol Metab. 1995;80:3591–5.
108. Binder G, Ranke MB. Screening for growth hormone (GH) gene splice-site mutations in sporadic cases with severe isolated GH deficiency using ectopic transcript analysis. J Clin Endocrinol Metab. 1995;80:1247–52.
109. Missarelli C, Herrera L, Mericq V, Carvallo P. Two different 5′ splice site mutations in the growth hormone gene causing autosomal dominant growth hormone deficiency. Hum Genet. 1997;101:113–7.
110. Hayashi Y, Yamamoto M, Ohmori S, Kamijo T, Ogawa M, Seo H. Inhibition of growth hormone (GH) secretion by a mutant GH-I gene product in neuroendocrine cells containing secretory granules: an implication for isolated GH deficiency inherited in an autosomal dominant manner. J Clin Endocrinol Metab. 1999;84:2134–9.

111. Hayashi Y, Kamijo T, Yamamoto M, Ohmori S, Phillips III JA, Ogawa M, et al. A novel mutation at the donor splice site of intron 3 of the GH-I gene in a patient with isolated growth hormone deficiency. Growth Horm IGF Res. 1999;9:434–7.
112. Katsumata N, Matsuo S, Sato N, Tanaka T. A novel and de novo splice-donor site mutation in intron 3 of the GH-1 gene in a patient with isolated growth hormone deficiency. Growth Horm IGF Res. 2001;11:378–83.
113. Cogan JD, Prince MA, Lekhakula S, Bundey S, Futrakul A, McCarthy EM, et al. A novel mechanism of aberrant pre-mRNA splicing in humans. Hum Mol Genet. 1997;6:909–12.
114. McCarthy EM, Phillips III JA. Characterization of an intron splice enhancer that regulates alternative splicing of human GH pre-mRNA. Hum Mol Genet. 1998;7:1491–6.
115. Vivenza D, Guazzarotti L, Godi M, Frasca D, di Natale B, Momigliano-Richiardi P, et al. A novel deletion in the GH1 gene including the IVS3 branch site responsible for autosomal dominant isolated growth hormone deficiency. J Clin Endocrinol Metab. 2006;91:980–6.
116. Fofanova OV, Evgrafov OV, Polyakov AV, Peterkova VA, Dedov II. A novel splicing mutation in exon 4 (456G>A) of the GH1 gene in a patient with congenital isolated growth hormone deficiency. Hormones (Athens). 2006;5:288–94.
117. Rojas-Gil AP, Ziros PG, Kanetsis E, Papathanassopoulou V, Nikolakopoulou NM, He K, et al. Combined effect of mutations of the GH1 gene and its proximal promoter region in a child with growth hormone neurosecretory dysfunction (GHND). J Mol Med (Berl). 2007;85:1005–13.
118. Lee MS, Wajnrajch MP, Kim SS, Plotnick LP, Wang J, Gertner JM, et al. Autosomal dominant growth hormone (GH) deficiency type II: the Del32-71-GH deletion mutant suppresses secretion of wild-type GH. Endocrinology. 2000;141:883–90.
119. McGuinness L, Magoulas C, Sesay AK, Mathers K, Carmignac D, Manneville JB, et al. Autosomal dominant growth hormone deficiency disrupts secretory vesicles in vitro and in vivo in transgenic mice. Endocrinology. 2003;144:720–31.
120. Ariyasu D, Yoshida H, Yamada M, Hasegawa Y. Endoplasmic reticulum stress and apoptosis contribute to the pathogenesis of dominantly inherited isolated GH deficiency due to GH1 gene splice site mutations. Endocrinology. 2013;154:3228–39.
121. Ryther RC, McGuinness LM, Phillips III JA, Moseley CT, Magoulas CB, Robinson IC, et al. Disruption of exon definition produces a dominant-negative growth hormone isoform that causes somatotroph death and IGHD II. Hum Genet. 2003;113:140–8.
122. Ryther RC, Flynt AS, Harris BD, Phillips III JA, Patton JG. GH1 splicing is regulated by multiple enhancers whose mutation produces a dominant-negative GH isoform that can be degraded by allele-specific small interfering RNA (siRNA). Endocrinology. 2004;145:2988–96.
123. Zhu YL, Conway-Campbell B, Waters MJ, Dannies PS. Prolonged retention after aggregation into secretory granules of human R183H-growth hormone (GH), a mutant that causes autosomal dominant GH deficiency type II. Endocrinology. 2002;143:4243–8.
124. Mullis PE, Robinson IC, Salemi S, Eble A, Besson A, Vuissoz JM, et al. Isolated autosomal dominant growth hormone deficiency: an evolving pituitary deficit? A multicenter follow-up study. J Clin Endocrinol Metab. 2005;90:2089–96.
125. Turton JP, Buchanan CR, Robinson IC, Aylwin SJ, Dattani MT. Evolution of gonadotropin deficiency in a patient with type II autosomal dominant GH deficiency. Eur J Endocrinol. 2006;155:793–9.
126. Fintini D, Salvatori R, Salemi S, Otten B, Ubertini G, Cambiaso P, et al. Autosomal-dominant isolated growth hormone deficiency (IGHD type II) with normal GH-1 gene. Horm Res. 2006;65:76–82.
127. Shariat N, Ryther RC, Phillips III JA, Robinson IC, Patton JG. Rescue of pituitary function in a mouse model of isolated growth hormone deficiency type II by RNA interference. Endocrinology. 2008;149:580–6.
128. Lochmatter D, Strom M, Eble A, Petkovic V, Fluck CE, Bidlingmaier M, et al. Isolated GH deficiency type II: knockdown of the harmful Delta3GH recovers wt-GH secretion in rat tumor pituitary cells. Endocrinology. 2010;151:4400–9.
129. Poling JS, Phillips III JA, Cogan JD, Hamid R. Pharmacologic correction of dominant-negative GH1 deficiency causing mutations. Clin Transl Sci. 2011;4:175–9.

130. Besson A, Salemi S, Deladoey J, Vuissoz JM, Eble A, Bidlingmaier M, et al. Short stature caused by a biologically inactive mutant growth hormone (GH-C53S). J Clin Endocrinol Metab. 2005;90:2493–9.
131. Petkovic V, Miletta MC, Boot AM, Losekoot M, Fluck CE, Pandey AV, et al. Short stature in two siblings heterozygous for a novel bioinactive GH mutant (GH-P59S) suggesting that the mutant also affects secretion of the wild-type GH. Eur J Endocrinol. 2013;168:K35–43.
132. Petkovic V, Eble A, Pandey AV, Betta M, Mella P, Fluck CE, et al. A novel GH-1 gene mutation (GH-P59L) causes partial GH deficiency type II combined with bioinactive GH syndrome. Growth Horm IGF Res. 2011;21:160–6.
133. Takahashi Y, Kaji H, Okimura Y, Goji K, Abe H, Chihara K. Brief report: short stature caused by a mutant growth hormone [see comments]. N Engl J Med. 1996;334:432–6.
134. Petkovic V, Thevis M, Lochmatter D, Besson A, Eble A, Fluck CE, et al. GH mutant (R77C) in a pedigree presenting with the delay of growth and pubertal development: structural analysis of the mutant and evaluation of the biological activity. Eur J Endocrinol. 2007;157 Suppl 1:S67–74.
135. Petkovic V, Besson A, Thevis M, Lochmatter D, Eble A, Fluck CE, et al. Evaluation of the biological activity of a growth hormone (GH) mutant (R77C) and its impact on GH responsiveness and stature. J Clin Endocrinol Metab. 2007;92:2893–901.
136. Takahashi Y, Shirono H, Arisaka O, Takahashi K, Yagi T, Koga J, et al. Biologically inactive growth hormone caused by an amino acid substitution. J Clin Invest. 1997;100:1159–65.
137. Petkovic V, Godi M, Pandey AV, Lochmatter D, Buchanan CR, Dattani MT, et al. Growth hormone (GH) deficiency type II: a novel GH-1 gene mutation (GH-R178H) affecting secretion and action. J Clin Endocrinol Metab. 2010;95:731–9.
138. Lewis MD, Horan M, Millar DS, Newsway V, Easter TE, Fryklund L, et al. A novel dysfunctional growth hormone variant (Ile179Met) exhibits a decreased ability to activate the extracellular signal-regulated kinase pathway. J Clin Endocrinol Metab. 2004;89:1068–75.
139. Wit JM, Oostdijk W, Losekoot M. Spectrum of insulin-like growth factor deficiency. Endocr Dev. 2012;23:30–41.
140. Osorio MG, Marui S, Jorge AA, Latronico AC, Lo LS, Leite CC, et al. Pituitary magnetic resonance imaging and function in patients with growth hormone deficiency with and without mutations in GHRH-R, GH-1, or PROP-1 genes. J Clin Endocrinol Metab. 2002;87:5076–84.
141. Desai MP, Mithbawkar SM, Upadhye PS, Rao SC, Bhatia V, Vijaykumar M. Molecular genetic studies in isolated growth hormone deficiency (IGHD). Indian J Pediatr. 2013;80:623–30.

# Chapter 12
# Combined Pituitary Hormone Deficiency

Frédéric Castinetti and Thierry Brue

## The Murine Pituitary Development: A Useful Tool to Decode Human Pituitary Development

Human pituitary development is assumed to follow more or less closely the murine pituitary development, and this is why the murine model currently represents the most appropriate model to determine the major temporospatial interactions between signaling pathways and transcription factors leading to a mature endocrine organ [1, 2]. Pituitary development in humans is imperfectly known, and all the steps described in the following lines are based on our knowledge of murine pituitary development.

Anterior and posterior pituitary lobes have two different embryonic origins: the anterior lobe is derived from oral ectoderm, whereas the posterior lobe is derived from neurectoderm. Even if close connections exist between both structures, we will only focus on the development of the anterior lobe and the mature pituitary. No study to date on human pituitary deficiency has identified strong connections and phenotypic associations that include anterior pituitary deficiencies and congenital diabetes insipidus (except for the only reported aryl hydrocarbon receptor nuclear translocator (*ARNT2*) mutation, as described later).

Briefly, anterior pituitary ontogenesis begins early during brain neurogenesis, around embryonic day (e) 7.5 in the mouse, corresponding to the first visualization

---

F. Castinetti (✉) • T. Brue
Aix-Marseille Université, CNRS, Centre de Recherche en Neurobiologie et Neurophysiologie de Marseille CRN2M UMR 7286, 3344 Cedex 15, Marseille, France

APHM, Hôpital Conception, Service d'Endocrinologie,
Diabète et Maladies Métaboliques, 13385 Cedex 5, Marseille, France

Centre de Référence des Maladies Rares d'Origine Hypophysaire DEFHY,
13385 Cedex 15, Marseille, France
e-mail: Frédéric.castinetti@univ-amu.fr

© Springer International Publishing Switzerland 2016
L.E. Cohen (ed.), *Growth Hormone Deficiency*,
DOI 10.1007/978-3-319-28038-7_12

of the pituitary placode [3]. At e9, the placode forms the rudimentary Rathke's pouch, under the control of signaling molecules issued from the infundibulum (bone morphogenetic protein 4 (Bmp4) and fibroblast growth factor 8 (Fgf8)). Definitive Rathke's pouch is observed at e11.5 [4]. Progenitors around the lumen move progressively to the developing pituitary and differentiate under the control of several factors including SRY-box (Sox)2, Sox9, and Isl Lim homeobox (Isl)-1, among others; the majority of these have not been identified as causative factors for pituitary deficiencies, suggesting that they are either crucial (and would lead to early death if abnormal) or that other pathways can be used if they are abnormal [5–7]. This first step leading to terminal differentiation of the pituitary is possible due to a tightly controlled temporospatial gradient of morphogenic factors from different origins, the diencephalon (Bmp4, Fgf8, 10 and 18, Wnt5a), the ectoderm (Isl1, Bmp2, sonic hedgehog (Shh), Wnt 4), the ventral mesoderm (chordin, Bmp2) [8], or the pituitary cells (Table 12.1).

At e11.5, α-subunit is expressed in the rostral tip [9], followed by adrenocorticotropin (ACTH) (e12.5), thyrotropin (TSH)β (e14.5), proopiomelanocortin (Pomc)

**Table 12.1** Main differences between human and murine phenotypes and partial/complete loss of function of the major proteins encoded by genes involved in combined pituitary hormone deficiencies

|  | Murine phenotype | Human phenotype | Transmission |
|---|---|---|---|
| POU1F1 | GH, TSH, Prl deficiency | GH, TSH, Prl deficiency. Pituitary hypoplasia | Recessive (murine): recessive or dominant (human) |
|  | Pituitary hypoplasia |  |  |
| PROP1 | GH, TSH, Prl deficiency | GH, TSH, Prl, LH/FSH deficiencies; inconstant ACTH deficiency. Inconstant transient pituitary hyperplasia and then hypoplasia | Recessive (murine and human) |
| HESX1 | Variable phenotype, midline anomalies. Eye anomalies. Pituitary hypoplasia or hyperplasia | Variable pituitary deficiencies (from isolated GH deficiency to panhypopituitarism); normal or hypoplasic pituitary. Septo-optic dysplasia | Recessive (murine): recessive or dominant (human) |
| OTX2 | Severe anomalies of anterior brain structures, pituitary dysmorphology | Variable pituitary deficiencies (from isolated GH deficiency to panhypopituitarism). Normal or hypoplasic pituitary, normal or ectopic posterior pituitary. Inconstant brain anomalies | Recessive (murine and human) |
| LHX3 | Pituitary aplasia | GH, TSH, LH/FSH deficiencies; inconstant ACTH deficiency. Hypoplasic or hyperplasic pituitary. Neck rotation anomalies; deafness | Recessive (murine and human) |
| LHX4 | Hypoplasic pituitary | Pituitary deficiencies, extrapituitary anomalies | Recessive (murine), dominant (human) |

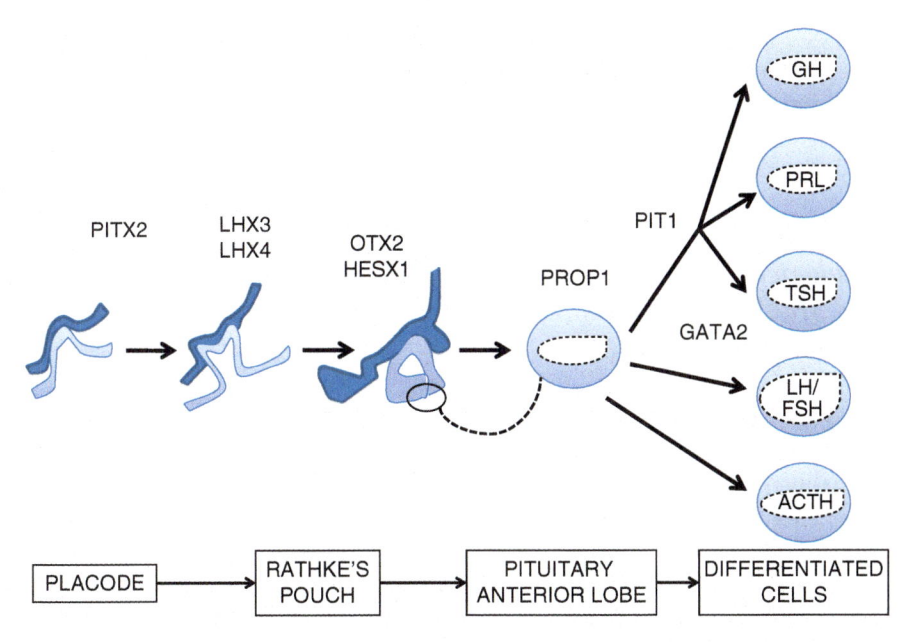

**Fig. 12.1** Simplified scheme representing the main transcription factor expression during pituitary development. Note that early transcription factor dysfunction is associated with pituitary and extrapituitary anomalies, whereas late transcription factor (PIT-1, PROP1) dysfunction is associated with pure pituitary phenotype

(e14.5, intermediate lobe), growth hormone (GH) and prolactin (Prl) (e15.5) [10], luteinizing hormone (Lh)β (e16.5), and finally follicle-stimulating hormone (Fsh)β (e17.5). Precise mechanisms leading to this differentiation and the formation of pituitary cell networks remain incompletely understood. Pituitary specific or nonspecific transcription factors are involved in a timely manner during these steps of differentiation, early acting such as LIM homeobox (Lhx)3, Lhx4, paired-like homeodomain transcription factor (Pitx)2, Hesx1 (also known as Rpx), or ARNT2 [11] or late-acting such as prophet of Pit-1 (Prop1) and Pou1f1 (Pit-1). Early acting transcription factors are also involved in the development of other organs (e.g., the eye, inner ear), and their defects lead to extrapituitary anomalies, whereas alterations of late-acting transcription factors usually lead to a pure pituitary phenotype. A summarized scheme of the timing of expression of the transcription factors known to be involved in CPHD is given in Fig. 12.1.

# Early Acting Transcription Factors: The Pituitary Phenotype Is Usually Not Alone

Anomalies of these transcription factors are characterized by a wide range of phenotypes, usually including anterior pituitary hormone deficiencies, extrapituitary abnormalities, and malformations such as pituitary stalk interruption syndrome

(PSIS) or midline defects. These complex phenotypes are due to the non-pituitary-specific expression of these transcription factors, which are also involved in the development of the forebrain and related midline structures such as the hypothalamus. To make the description easier, we focused on the phenotypic traits that should guide the clinician to certain transcription factors.

## Etiological Possibilities in Patients Carrying Pituitary Deficiency and Midline Anomalies: HESX1, GLI2, FGF8 and FGFR1, PROK2, and PROKR2

What do we call midline anomalies? It is a large group of diseases from pituitary stalk interruption syndrome to septo-optic dysplasia (SOD) and holoprosencephaly. Pituitary stalk interruption syndrome is defined on brain MRI by the association of an absent or thin pituitary stalk, pituitary hypoplasia, and/or ectopic posterior pituitary [12]. As only 30 % of patients with PSIS have a history of traumatic event, it is likely that a high number of cases are actually due to genetic anomalies. Septo-optic dysplasia is defined by at least two of the following criteria: septum or corpus callosum agenesis, optic nerve hypoplasia, and pituitary deficiencies [13]. Holoprosencephaly is a complex brain malformation, affecting both the brain and face (cyclopia, median or bilateral labial and/or palatal cleft, hypotelorism or a single median incisor in milder cases) due to an abnormal division of the prosencephalon between days 18 and 28. Intellectual disability is frequently associated. Recent studies emphasize the continuum between these different genetic causes leading to phenotypes of variable severity depending on the degree of abnormal development of the anterior brain [14–16]. This likely explains why, for any given pathway or transcription factor, the phenotype can be highly variable from mild to extremely severe. This group mainly includes anomalies of the paired transcription factor HESX1, and few novelties less well known such as GLI2, or pathways previously thought to be only involved in isolated hypogonadotropic hypogonadism. We will see, however, in the next paragraph that other transcription factors, more likely involved in eye development, can also lead to midline anomalies, which makes this classification difficult to perform.

### HESX1

Hesx1 is a paired homeodomain transcription factor that has been well characterized over the last 15 years. It is a major actor in pituitary development as its expression and then inhibition are crucial at given time points to allow the formation of a mature Rathke's pouch. The expression profile of Hesx1 perfectly illustrates the complexity of pituitary development. For instance, decreased expression of Hesx1 at e13 in mice is necessary for Prop1 and secondarily Pou1f1 expression, two late transcription factors necessary for proper differentiation of GH-, TSH-, and Prl-secreting cells [17–20]. Appropriate expression of other early acting transcription factors such as Lhx1, Lhx3, or Six3 (some being involved in human disease) is also necessary for early proper Hesx1 expression [21]: the lack of Hesx1 in mice (homozygous inactivation $Hesx1^{-/-}$) indeed leads to a very severe phenotype with corpus callosum aplasia and ectopic posterior pituitary. In humans, HESX1 mutations can lead to a wide range of phenotypes: 16 *HESX1* mutations have been reported [17, 22–30], the homozygous anomalies (40 % cases) usually leading to a more severe phenotype [31]. GH deficiency is constant; other pituitary deficiencies are reported in 50 % cases. Optic nerve anomalies are the other major phenotypic sign, observed in 30 % cases. One should not consider, however, that SOD is always due to *HESX1* mutations, as only 1 % cases have actually been linked to this genotype [31–34]. Brain MRI usually reveals pituitary hypoplasia (80 % cases) and midline anomalies such as ectopic or non-visible posterior pituitary in 50–60 % cases and corpus callosum agenesis or hypoplasia in 25 % cases.

## Sonic Hedgehog and GLI2

Sonic hedgehog (SHH) signaling pathway is involved in the early steps of pituitary development: *SHH* mutations have been reported in patients with severe forms of isolated holoprosencephaly [35]. SHH targets, GLI transcription factors, have also been involved in CPHD: *GLI2* heterozygous mutations have been reported in patients with holoprosencephaly or with pituitary hormone deficits and less severe midline craniofacial anomalies and pituitary hypoplasia, corpus callosum agenesis, or ectopic posterior pituitary on brain MRI; some individuals also have polydactyly.

## Pathways Known to Be Involved in Hypogonadotropic Hypogonadism

### FGF8 and FGFR1

*FGFR1* and *FGF8* heterozygous mutations were first reported in 10 % of Kallmann syndrome and 7 % of normosmic hypogonadism [36]. Pituitary MRI showed normal or hypoplastic anterior pituitary and inconstant ectopic posterior pituitary. Penetrance was incomplete [37, 38]. However, the expression of Fgf8 and Fgfr1 in the ventral diencephalon is necessary for proper Rathke's pouch formation, temporospatial pattern of pituitary cell lineages, and the development of extrapituitary structures [39]. This explains why other anomalies were then reported such as ear hypoplasia, dental agenesis, cleft palate, and distal limb malformations. Finally, *FGFR1* and *FGF8* mutations have also been reported in patients with SOD, with about 4 % prevalence [14].

PROK2 and PROKR2

Prokineticin pathway is known to be involved in portal angiogenesis and neuronal development and migration [40]: this suggested its potential involvement in pituitary stalk development. *PROK2* and *PROKR2* mutations have recently been reported in a cohort of patients with pituitary deficiencies, anterior pituitary hypoplasia or aplasia, and PSIS [15]. Mutations in these genes were also reported thereafter in patients with SOD, and inconstant additional brain abnormalities, such as cerebellar hypoplasia, Dandy-Walker cyst, or focal abnormality of mesial frontal cortex [16].

## *Etiological Possibilities in Patients Carrying Pituitary Deficiency and Eye Anomalies: OTX2, SOX2, PITX2, ARNT2*

Whereas *OTX2* mutations seem to play an important role in CPHD, the other factors reported here have been recently described or do not seem to be involved in a large number of patients. This explains why they are usually not screened in patients, except in case of a specific phenotypic sign associated to CPHD.

### OTX2

Otx2 is a paired homeodomain transcription factor involved in the early steps of brain development. In mice, Otx2 is expressed from e10.5 to e14.5 in the ventral diencephalon, where it likely interacts with Hesx1, and from e10.5 to e12.5 in Rathke's pouch. Otx2 is also involved in gonadotropin-releasing hormone (GnRH) neuronal development [41]. In mice, homozygous inactivation of *Otx2* ($Otx2^{-/-}$) leads to a severe brain phenotype; heterozygous inactivation leads to a wide range of phenotype, with eye anomalies, inconstant holoprosencephaly, and usually pituitary hypoplasia. This phenotype is close to the one observed in humans: 25 heterozygous de novo *OTX2* mutations have been reported, including nine in patients with congenital hypopituitarism; the remaining 16 mutations were reported in patients with ophthalmic diseases and no mention of pituitary deficiency. Individuals can either present with isolated GH deficiency or panhypopituitarism and inconstant hypoplastic pituitary, ectopic posterior pituitary, and Chiari syndrome. There is no genotype/phenotype correlation [42–46].

### SOX2

Sox2 is an "HMG DNA-binding domain" (similar to SRY gene) transcription factor. At e9.5, Sox2 expression is observed in the brain, the neural tube, the oral endoderm, the sensorial placodes, and the branchial arcs. At e11.5, Sox2 is expressed in Rathke's pouch and the future hypothalamus. Sox2 is then expressed in the periluminal proliferative zone where it could be involved in the maintenance and function of pituitary progenitors [47]. At adult age, Sox2 is expressed in the periventricular zone of the lateral ventricles and in the dentate gyrus, but its precise role (promoting the differentiation of stem cells in injured pituitary?) is unknown. Homozygous inactivation is lethal in mice; heterozygous inactivation leads to increased perinatal death, epilepsy, and almost complete panhypopituitarism (corticotroph axis is usually functional); in contrast, eye anomalies are inconstant. The phenotype is different in humans: heterozygous de novo *SOX2* mutations have been observed in six patients with hypogonadotropic hypogonadism, bilateral microphthalmia, corpus callosum hypoplasia, and inconstant intellectual disability. Pituitary phenotypes included inconstant GH, TSH, or ACTH deficiencies, and pituitary hypoplasia in 80 % cases. Surprisingly, corpus callosum anomaly has been reported in one case [47].

## PITX2

PITX2 is not the perfect example of a transcription factor to think about in patients with CPHD. Despite its obvious roles in pituitary development, only three patients have been reported as having GH deficiency and pituitary hypoplasia [48–50]. As shown in mice, it is probably because of compensatory mechanisms, at least in the pituitary, likely due to a close transcription factor, Pitx1. Pitx2 is a paired homeodomain transcription factor expressed in Rathke's pouch at e10.5 [51, 52] and pituitary anterior and intermediate lobes at e12.5. At adult age, Pitx2 is expressed in thyrotrophs and gonadotrophs [53]. Pitx2 expression is ubiquitous, as it has also been observed in the adult brain, eye, kidney, lungs, testis, and tongue [51, 54]. In humans, *PITX2* mutations have been reported in patients with Axenfeld-Rieger syndrome, which is characterized by anomalies in the ocular anterior compartment and systemic malformations (craniofacial dysmorphy, dental, and umbilical anomalies) [55, 56]. *PITX2* mutations should thus be screened in patients with this phenotype, keeping in mind that some pituitary deficiencies might be associated. It does not make sense to routinely screen for *PITX2* mutations in patients with CPHD.

## ARNT2

A recent report described a large consanguineous family with eye abnormalities, congenital hypopituitarism, diabetes insipidus, and renal and central nervous system (CNS) anomalies, related to a defect in the helix-loop-helix transcription factor ARNT2. ARNT2 is known to be involved in the development of the hypothalamus, other CNS structures, the kidneys, and the eyes. All patients presented with a thin pituitary stalk, hypoplastic anterior pituitary, ectopic or nonvisualized posterior pituitary, hypoplastic frontal and temporal lobes, thin corpus callosum, and delay in brain myelination [11]. Precise roles of ARNT2 during pituitary and extrapituitary structure development are, however, imperfectly determined, and the search for other mutations in patients with CPHD has been negative to date.

## Etiological Possibilities in Patients Carrying Pituitary Deficiency and Neurogenesis Anomalies: The LIM Domain Transcription Factors

LHX4 and LHX3 are two close transcription factors belonging to a large family of transcription factors known to be involved in the development of several structures. Several mutations of LHX4 and LHX3 have been reported for the last 10 years in patients with CPHD. In contrast, up to now, no mutation has been identified in patients with a pituitary phenotype in the other LIM domain transcription factors.

### LHX4

Lhx4 is involved in the early steps of pituitary ontogenesis. In mice, Lhx4 expression has been reported in Rathke's pouch at e9.5 and in the anterior part of the pituitary at e12.5. A low expression is still observed at adult age [57, 58]. The phenotype of homozygous inactivation of Lhx4 in mice is lethal due to respiratory distress, whereas heterozygous inactivation is not symptomatic. The main difference with humans is actually the transmission mode of inheritance, as all human *LHX4* mutations are in a heterozygous state: 11 sporadic or familial *LHX4* mutations have been reported in 17 patients [59], with a wide intra- and interfamilial phenotypic variability in terms of pituitary phenotype (ranging from isolated GH deficiency to complete panhypopituitarism) [60, 61] and brain MRI (pituitary hypoplasia, inconstant ectopic posterior pituitary and sellar hypoplasia, corpus callosum hypoplasia, or Chiari syndrome). Of note, one patient carrying a 1q25 microdeletion (including *LHX4* deletion) also presented with a cardiac defect (but it was likely multifactorial).

### LHX3

Lhx3 is the perfect example of how extrapolating a human phenotype from a mouse phenotype is complex: while homozygous *Lhx3* inactivation in mice is lethal, heterozygous inactivation does not lead to any particular phenotype. In contrast, in humans, all described *LHX3* mutations were homozygous, and even if the phenotype was complex, it was never lethal. This discrepancy might be explained by the different weight of compensatory mechanisms performed by Lhx4 in both species, but this remains highly hypothetical [57]. The role of Lhx3 during pituitary development is crucial, as it is necessary for proper expression of several other transcription factors or receptors such as Hesx1 [62], forkhead box (fox)l2, Notch2, splicing factor (SF) 1, T-box (tbx)19 (involved in corticotroph differentiation), GnRH receptor and FSHβ [63–65], and Pou1f1 [66]. In addition to its role during pituitary development, Lhx3 is involved in the development of extrapituitary structures, such as medullar motoneurons [67, 68] (which likely explains neck rotation anomalies in humans with *LHX3* mutations) and inner ear [69, 70] (which explains hearing trouble in humans with *LHX3* mutations). In humans, 12 homozygous *LHX3* mutations have been reported [71–77]. Pituitary phenotype usually includes GH, TSH, and LH/FSH deficiencies, while ACTH deficiency is inconstant (roughly half of the cases). On MRI, pituitary aplasia or hypoplasia is observed in 60 % cases, whereas hyperplasia is observed in 30 % cases. The mechanisms for hyperplasia are unknown but may be close to the ones reported for *PROP1* mutations (detailed later in the text). As previously mentioned, extrapituitary phenotype can include abnormal head and neck rotation (70 % cases), vertebral abnormalities (50 % cases), and mild to severe hearing deficits (50 % cases).

## Late-Acting Transcription Factors: The Pituitary Phenotype Is Alone

If we only focus on transcription factors with anomalies reported in CPHD, then the list is short: PROP1 and POU1F1 are the only major actors known to be involved in pure pituitary phenotype. It does not mean that the final differentiation of thyrotrophs, for instance, or their function does not require other transcription factors such as GATA2 or maybe ISL1; it only means that no mutation of these genes has been reported so far in humans. Patients with *PROP1* or *POU1F1* mutations thus present anterior pituitary hormone deficiencies (progressive or not), normal hypothalamo-pituitary morphology at MRI (regardless of the size of the pituitary gland), and no extrapituitary malformations. In such a context, *PROP1* mutations remain the most frequently reported genetic defect.

### *PROP1*

Prop1 is a pituitary-specific paired domain transcription factor. In mice, its expression is observed from e10 to e15.5, with a peak around e12 [78]. Prop1 is necessary for proper Pou1f1 expression, leading to somato-lactotroph and thyrotroph cell differentiation [55, 79]. In mice, the phenotype is close to the one reported in humans, except for the lack of ACTH deficiency. The reason why humans might have corticotroph deficiency (seen in about 50 % of cases) remains a mystery, and the large period of appearance (from young age to 40 years old) is another intriguing fact. In humans, at least 25 *PROP1* mutations have been reported [80–101]. Homozygous or compound heterozygous *PROP1* mutations, transmitted in an autosomal recessive manner, currently represent the most frequently identified etiologies of CPHD [1, 102, 103]. Pituitary phenotype includes GH, TSH, LH/FSH, ACTH, and PRL deficiencies, diagnosed from childhood to adulthood [104]. Pituitary MRI can show transient pituitary hyperplasia and normal or hypoplastic pituitary; pituitary hyperplasia sometimes precedes spontaneous hypoplasia [82, 105–109]. A hypothesis that may account for this phenomenon is that pituitary progenitors might not differentiate in the absence of Prop1, thus accumulating in the intermediate lobe causing hyperplasia, with apoptosis then resulting in final hypoplasia [110].

## *PIT-1/POU1F 1*

Pit-1 was the first pituitary-specific transcription factor identified in *Snell* mice and then in humans (POU1F1, human ortholog of Pit-1) [111]. Pou1f1 expression is first observed at e13.5 during pituitary development. Pou1f1 is necessary for thyrotroph, somatotroph, and lactotroph differentiation and remains expressed in these cell lineages at adult age. In humans, *POU1F1* mutations can be transmitted as an autosomal recessive or dominant trait. Complete TSH and GH deficiencies are usually observed during childhood, whereas gonadotroph and corticotroph axes remain functional. Brain MRI can be normal or show pituitary hypoplasia.

## Conclusions and Perspectives

The identification of almost all genes identified to date in CPHD was based on the murine model. Even if it is clear that having a close animal model is crucial, the discrepancy between mice and humans might explain why only 10 % of the etiologies of CPHD have been identified today. This is an issue, as identifying the etiologies of congenital hypopituitarism is of major importance to better diagnose and treat the patients, in particular in the differential diagnosis of a pituitary mass on MRI, or to identify the patients at risk of developing delayed corticotroph deficiency and as a prenatal diagnosis to decrease the risk of early death (undiagnosed corticotroph deficiency, for instance).

Another possibility to explain this poor rate of identification is the limits in the detection techniques that we have: classical Sanger sequencing has, for instance, inherent limits with the impossibility to identify large deletions or insertions or intronic alterations leading to splicing anomalies. The development of new techniques in the recent years should dramatically improve the rate of identification of etiologies of congenital hypopituitarism: array comparative genomic hybridization (aCGH) has been created for identifying segmental genomic copy number variations (gain or loss) such as structural rearrangements (deletions, duplications, insertions, translocations) or complex chromosomal aneuploidies; it can be designed in a whole genome approach, where the array targets are equally spaced with coverage of 100 to 1000 kb. Another promising approach is whole-exome sequencing, which is based on the assumption that 85 % of mutations are located in coding regions of the genome. This technique should be of great interest in highly penetrant Mendelian diseases. However, reporting new variants in a single patient does not mean pathogenicity and requires confirmation by a similar finding in other persons presenting with similar phenotypes. Moreover, confirmatory steps by bioinformatics analysis after a usually large dataset of results can be highly challenging.

To summarize, in one sentence, huge progress has been made over the last 20 years, but we are only at the beginning of the path. Thinking differently might likely help explaining the majority of yet unknown causes of CPHD.

**Acknowledgments** This work was supported by grants from the "Agence Nationale de la Recherche" (ANR), # 08-GENOPAT-026 and from the "Association pour le Développement de la Recherche au centre hospitalier de Marseille" (A.DE.RE.M). For inquiries on genetic screening strategies for individual patients, contact defhy@ap-hm.fr and visit the website www.ap-hm.fr/defhy/ for information on withdrawal and shipment guidelines.

# References

1. Kelberman D, Rizzoti K, Lovell-Badge R, Robinson IC, Dattani MT. Genetic regulation of pituitary gland development in human and mouse. Endocr Rev. 2009;30(7):790–829. doi:10.1210/er.2009-0008.
2. Castinetti F, Reynaud R, Saveanu A, Quentien MH, Albarel F, Barlier A, Enjalbert A, Brue T. Clinical and genetic aspects of combined pituitary hormone deficiencies. Ann Endocrinol. 2008;69(1):7–17. doi:10.1016/j.ando.2008.01.001.
3. Schlosser G. Induction and specification of cranial placodes. Dev Biol. 2006;294(2):303–51. doi:10.1016/j.ydbio.2006.03.009.
4. Rizzoti K, Lovell-Badge R. Early development of the pituitary gland: induction and shaping of Rathke's pouch. Rev Endocr Metab Disord. 2005;6(3):161–72. doi:10.1007/s11154-005-3047-7.
5. Fauquier T, Rizzoti K, Dattani M, Lovell-Badge R, Robinson IC. SOX2-expressing progenitor cells generate all of the major cell types in the adult mouse pituitary gland. Proc Natl Acad Sci U S A. 2008;105(8):2907–12. doi:10.1073/pnas.0707886105.
6. Gleiberman AS, Michurina T, Encinas JM, Roig JL, Krasnov P, Balordi F, Fishell G, Rosenfeld MG, Enikolopov G. Genetic approaches identify adult pituitary stem cells. Proc Natl Acad Sci U S A. 2008;105(17):6332–7. doi:10.1073/pnas.0801644105.
7. Garcia-Lavandeira M, Quereda V, Flores I, Saez C, Diaz-Rodriguez E, Japon MA, Ryan AK, Blasco MA, Dieguez C, Malumbres M, Alvarez CV. A GRFa2/Prop1/stem (GPS) cell niche in the pituitary. PLoS One. 2009;4(3), e4815. doi:10.1371/journal.pone.0004815.
8. Gleiberman AS, Fedtsova NG, Rosenfeld MG. Tissue interactions in the induction of anterior pituitary: role of the ventral diencephalon, mesenchyme, and notochord. Dev Biol. 1999;213(2):340–53.
9. Japon MA, Rubinstein M, Low MJ. In situ hybridization analysis of anterior pituitary hormone gene expression during fetal mouse development. J Histochem Cytochem. 1994;42(8):1117–25.
10. Lamolet B, Pulichino AM, Lamonerie T, Gauthier Y, Brue T, Enjalbert A, Drouin J. A pituitary cell-restricted T box factor, Tpit, activates POMC transcription in cooperation with Pitx homeoproteins. Cell. 2001;104(6):849–59.
11. Webb EA, AlMutair A, Kelberman D, Bacchelli C, Chanudet E, Lescai F, Andoniadou CL, Banyan A, Alsawaid A, Alrifai MT, Alahmesh MA, Balwi M, Mousavy-Gharavy SN, Lukovic B, Burke D, McCabe MJ, Kasia T, Kleta R, Stupka E, Beales PL, Thompson DA, Chong WK, Alkuraya FS, Martinez-Barbera JP, Sowden JC, Dattani MT. ARNT2 mutation causes hypopituitarism, post-natal microcephaly, visual and renal anomalies. Brain. 2013;136(Pt 10):3096–105. doi:10.1093/brain/awt218.
12. Di Iorgi N, Allegri AE, Napoli F, Bertelli E, Olivieri I, Rossi A, Maghnie M. The use of neuroimaging for assessing disorders of pituitary development. Clin Endocrinol. 2012;76(2):161–76. doi:10.1111/j.1365-2265.2011.04238.x.

13. Kelberman D, Dattani MT. Genetics of septo-optic dysplasia. Pituitary. 2007;10(4):393–407. doi:10.1007/s11102-007-0055-5.
14. Raivio T, Avbelj M, McCabe MJ, Romero CJ, Dwyer AA, Tommiska J, Sykiotis GP, Gregory LC, Diaczok D, Tziaferi V, Elting MW, Padidela R, Plummer L, Martin C, Feng B, Zhang C, Zhou QY, Chen H, Mohammadi M, Quinton R, Sidis Y, Radovick S, Dattani MT, Pitteloud N. Genetic overlap in Kallmann syndrome, combined pituitary hormone deficiency, and septo-optic dysplasia. J Clin Endocrinol Metab. 2012;97(4):E694–9. doi:10.1210/jc.2011-2938.
15. Reynaud R, Jayakody SA, Monnier C, Saveanu A, Bouligand J, Guedj AM, Simonin G, Lecomte P, Barlier A, Rondard P, Martinez-Barbera JP, Guiochon-Mantel A, Brue T. PROKR2 variants in multiple hypopituitarism with pituitary stalk interruption. J Clin Endocrinol Metab. 2012;97(6):E1068–73. doi:10.1210/jc.2011-3056.
16. McCabe MJ, Gaston-Massuet C, Gregory LC, Alatzoglou KS, Tziaferi V, Sbai O, Rondard P, Masumoto KH, Nagano M, Shigeyoshi Y, Pfeifer M, Hulse T, Buchanan CR, Pitteloud N, Martinez-Barbera JP, Dattani MT. Variations in PROKR2, but not PROK2, are associated with hypopituitarism and septo-optic dysplasia. J Clin Endocrinol Metab. 2013;98(3):E547–57. doi:10.1210/jc.2012-3067.
17. Dattani MT, Martinez-Barbera JP, Thomas PQ, Brickman JM, Gupta R, Martensson IL, Toresson H, Fox M, Wales JK, Hindmarsh PC, Krauss S, Beddington RS, Robinson IC. Mutations in the homeobox gene HESX1/Hesx1 associated with septo-optic dysplasia in human and mouse. Nat Genet. 1998;19(2):125–33. doi:10.1038/477.
18. Martinez-Barbera JP, Rodriguez TA, Beddington RS. The homeobox gene Hesx1 is required in the anterior neural ectoderm for normal forebrain formation. Dev Biol. 2000;223(2):422–30. doi:10.1006/dbio.2000.9757.
19. Thomas PQ, Johnson BV, Rathjen J, Rathjen PD. Sequence, genomic organization, and expression of the novel homeobox gene Hesx1. J Biol Chem. 1995;270(8):3869–75.
20. Webb GC, Thomas PQ, Ford JH, Rathjen PD. Hesx1, a homeobox gene expressed by murine embryonic stem cells, maps to mouse chromosome 14, bands A3-B. Genomics. 1993;18(2):464–6. doi:10.1006/geno.1993.1505.
21. Gaston-Massuet C, Andoniadou CL, Signore M, Sajedi E, Bird S, Turner JM, Martinez-Barbera JP. Genetic interaction between the homeobox transcription factors HESX1 and SIX3 is required for normal pituitary development. Dev Biol. 2008;324(2):322–33. doi:10.1016/j.ydbio.2008.08.008.
22. Corneli G, Vivenza D, Prodam F, Di Dio G, Vottero A, Rapa A, Bellone S, Bernasconi S, Bona G. Heterozygous mutation of HESX1 causing hypopituitarism and multiple anatomical malformations without features of septo-optic dysplasia. J Endocrinol Invest. 2008;31(8):689–93.
23. Sobrier ML, Maghnie M, Vie-Luton MP, Secco A, di Iorgi N, Lorini R, Amselem S. Novel HESX1 mutations associated with a life-threatening neonatal phenotype, pituitary aplasia, but normally located posterior pituitary and no optic nerve abnormalities. J Clin Endocrinol Metab. 2006;91(11):4528–36. doi:10.1210/jc.2006-0426.
24. Sobrier ML, Netchine I, Heinrichs C, Thibaud N, Vie-Luton MP, Van Vliet G, Amselem S. Alu-element insertion in the homeodomain of HESX1 and aplasia of the anterior pituitary. Hum Mutat. 2005;25(5):503. doi:10.1002/humu.9332.
25. Tajima T, Hattorri T, Nakajima T, Okuhara K, Sato K, Abe S, Nakae J, Fujieda K. Sporadic heterozygous frameshift mutation of HESX1 causing pituitary and optic nerve hypoplasia and combined pituitary hormone deficiency in a Japanese patient. J Clin Endocrinol Metab. 2003;88(1):45–50. doi:10.1210/jc.2002-020818.
26. Cohen RN, Cohen LE, Botero D, Yu C, Sagar A, Jurkiewicz M, Radovick S. Enhanced repression by HESX1 as a cause of hypopituitarism and septooptic dysplasia. J Clin Endocrinol Metab. 2003;88(10):4832–9. doi:10.1210/jc.2002-021868.
27. Carvalho LR, Woods KS, Mendonca BB, Marcal N, Zamparini AL, Stifani S, Brickman JM, Arnhold IJ, Dattani MT. A homozygous mutation in HESX1 is associated with evolving hypopituitarism due to impaired repressor-corepressor interaction. J Clin Invest. 2003;112(8):1192–201. doi:10.1172/JCI18589.

28. Mitchell LA, Thomas PQ, Zacharin MR, Scheffer IE. Ectopic posterior pituitary lobe and periventricular heterotopia: cerebral malformations with the same underlying mechanism? Am J Neuroradiol. 2002;23(9):1475–81.
29. Thomas PQ, Dattani MT, Brickman JM, McNay D, Warne G, Zacharin M, Cameron F, Hurst J, Woods K, Dunger D, Stanhope R, Forrest S, Robinson IC, Beddington RS. Heterozygous HESX1 mutations associated with isolated congenital pituitary hypoplasia and septo-optic dysplasia. Hum Mol Genet. 2001;10(1):39–45.
30. Brickman JM, Clements M, Tyrell R, McNay D, Woods K, Warner J, Stewart A, Beddington RS, Dattani M. Molecular effects of novel mutations in Hesx1/HESX1 associated with human pituitary disorders. Development. 2001;128(24):5189–99.
31. Kelberman D, Dattani MT. Septo-optic dysplasia – novel insights into the aetiology. Horm Res. 2008;69(5):257–65. doi:10.1159/000114856.
32. McNay DE, Turton JP, Kelberman D, Woods KS, Brauner R, Papadimitriou A, Keller E, Keller A, Haufs N, Krude H, Shalet SM, Dattani MT. HESX1 mutations are an uncommon cause of septooptic dysplasia and hypopituitarism. J Clin Endocrinol Metab. 2007;92(2):691–7. doi:10.1210/jc.2006-1609.
33. Reynaud R, Gueydan M, Saveanu A, Vallette-Kasic S, Enjalbert A, Brue T, Barlier A. Genetic screening of combined pituitary hormone deficiency: experience in 195 patients. J Clin Endocrinol Metab. 2006;91(9):3329–36. doi:10.1210/jc.2005-2173.
34. Webb EA, Dattani MT. Septo-optic dysplasia. Eur J Hum Genet. 2009;18(4):393–7. doi:10.1038/ejhg.2009.125.
35. Dubourg C, Bendavid C, Pasquier L, Henry C, Odent S, David V. Holoprosencephaly. Orphanet J Rare Dis. 2007;2:8. doi:10.1186/1750-1172-2-8.
36. Raivio T, Sidis Y, Plummer L, Chen H, Ma J, Mukherjee A, Jacobson-Dickman E, Quinton R, Van Vliet G, Lavoie H, Hughes VA, Dwyer A, Hayes FJ, Xu S, Sparks S, Kaiser UB, Mohammadi M, Pitteloud N. Impaired fibroblast growth factor receptor 1 signaling as a cause of normosmic idiopathic hypogonadotropic hypogonadism. J Clin Endocrinol Metab. 2009;94(11):4380–90. doi:10.1210/jc.2009-0179.
37. Dode C, Levilliers J, Dupont JM, De Paepe A, Le Du N, Soussi-Yanicostas N, Coimbra RS, Delmaghani S, Compain-Nouaille S, Baverel F, Pecheux C, Le Tessier D, Cruaud C, Delpech M, Speleman F, Vermeulen S, Amalfitano A, Bachelot Y, Bouchard P, Cabrol S, Carel JC, Delemarre-van de Waal H, Goulet-Salmon B, Kottler ML, Richard O, Sanchez-Franco F, Saura R, Young J, Petit C, Hardelin JP. Loss-of-function mutations in FGFR1 cause autosomal dominant Kallmann syndrome. Nat Genet. 2003;33(4):463–5. doi:10.1038/ng1122.
38. Falardeau J, Chung WC, Beenken A, Raivio T, Plummer L, Sidis Y, Jacobson-Dickman EE, Eliseenkova AV, Ma J, Dwyer A, Quinton R, Na S, Hall JE, Huot C, Alois N, Pearce SH, Cole LW, Hughes V, Mohammadi M, Tsai P, Pitteloud N. Decreased FGF8 signaling causes deficiency of gonadotropin-releasing hormone in humans and mice. J Clin Invest. 2008;118(8):2822–31. doi:10.1172/JCI34538.
39. Treier M, Gleiberman AS, O'Connell SM, Szeto DP, McMahon JA, McMahon AP, Rosenfeld MG. Multistep signaling requirements for pituitary organogenesis in vivo. Genes Dev. 1998;12(11):1691–704.
40. Martin C, Balasubramanian R, Dwyer AA, Au MG, Sidis Y, Kaiser UB, Seminara SB, Pitteloud N, Zhou QY, Crowley Jr WF. The role of the prokineticin 2 pathway in human reproduction: evidence from the study of human and murine gene mutations. Endocr Rev. 2011;32(2):225–46. doi:10.1210/er.2010-0007.
41. Larder R, Mellon PL. Otx2 induction of the gonadotropin-releasing hormone promoter is modulated by direct interactions with Grg co-repressors. J Biol Chem. 2009;284(25):16966–78. doi:10.1074/jbc.M109.002485.
42. Diaczok D, Romero C, Zunich J, Marshall I, Radovick S. A novel dominant negative mutation of OTX2 associated with combined pituitary hormone deficiency. J Clin Endocrinol Metab. 2008;93(11):4351–9. doi:10.1210/jc.2008-1189.
43. Dateki S, Fukami M, Sato N, Muroya K, Adachi M, Ogata T. OTX2 mutation in a patient with anophthalmia, short stature, and partial growth hormone deficiency: functional studies

using the IRBP, HESX1, and POU1F1 promoters. J Clin Endocrinol Metab. 2008;93(10):3697–702. doi:10.1210/jc.2008-0720.
44. Tajima T, Ohtake A, Hoshino M, Amemiya S, Sasaki N, Ishizu K, Fujieda K. OTX2 loss of function mutation causes anophthalmia and combined pituitary hormone deficiency with a small anterior and ectopic posterior pituitary. J Clin Endocrinol Metab. 2009;94(1):314–9. doi:10.1210/jc.2008-1219.
45. Dateki S, Kosaka K, Hasegawa K, Tanaka H, Azuma N, Yokoya S, Muroya K, Adachi M, Tajima T, Motomura K, Kinoshita E, Moriuchi H, Sato N, Fukami M, Ogata T. Heterozygous orthodenticle homeobox 2 mutations are associated with variable pituitary phenotype. J Clin Endocrinol Metab. 2009;95(2):756–64.
46. Henderson RH, Williamson KA, Kennedy JS, Webster AR, Holder GE, Robson AG, FitzPatrick DR, van Heyningen V, Moore AT. A rare de novo nonsense mutation in OTX2 causes early onset retinal dystrophy and pituitary dysfunction. Mol Vis. 2009;15:2442–7.
47. Kelberman D, Rizzoti K, Avilion A, Bitner-Glindzicz M, Cianfarani S, Collins J, Chong WK, Kirk JM, Achermann JC, Ross R, Carmignac D, Lovell-Badge R, Robinson IC, Dattani MT. Mutations within Sox2/SOX2 are associated with abnormalities in the hypothalamo-pituitary-gonadal axis in mice and humans. J Clin Invest. 2006;116(9):2442–55. doi:10.1172/JCI28658.
48. Sadeghi-Nejad A, Senior B. A familial syndrome of isolated "aplasia" of the anterior pituitary. Diagnostic studies and treatment in the neonatal period. J Pediatr. 1974;84(1):79–84.
49. Feingold M, Shiere F, Fogels HR, Donaldson D. Rieger's syndrome. Pediatrics. 1969;44(4):564–9.
50. Mammi I, De Giorgio P, Clementi M, Tenconi R. Cardiovascular anomaly in Rieger syndrome: heterogeneity or contiguity? Acta Ophthalmol Scand. 1998;76(4):509–12.
51. Hjalt TA, Semina EV, Amendt BA, Murray JC. The Pitx2 protein in mouse development. Dev Dyn. 2000;218(1):195–200.
52. Lin CR, Kioussi C, O'Connell S, Briata P, Szeto D, Liu F, Izpisua-Belmonte JC, Rosenfeld MG. Pitx2 regulates lung asymmetry, cardiac positioning and pituitary and tooth morphogenesis. Nature. 1999;401(6750):279–82. doi:10.1038/45803.
53. Charles MA, Suh H, Hjalt TA, Drouin J, Camper SA, Gage PJ. PITX genes are required for cell survival and Lhx3 activation. Mol Endocrinol. 2005;19(7):1893–903. doi:10.1210/me.2005-0052.
54. Gage PJ, Camper SA. Pituitary homeobox 2, a novel member of the bicoid-related family of homeobox genes, is a potential regulator of anterior structure formation. Hum Mol Genet. 1997;6(3):457–64.
55. Tumer Z, Bach-Holm D. Axenfeld-Rieger syndrome and spectrum of PITX2 and FOXC1 mutations. Eur J Hum Genet. 2009;17(12):1527–39. doi:10.1038/ejhg.2009.93.
56. Semina EV, Reiter R, Leysens NJ, Alward WL, Small KW, Datson NA, Siegel-Bartelt J, Bierke-Nelson D, Bitoun P, Zabel BU, Carey JC, Murray JC. Cloning and characterization of a novel bicoid-related homeobox transcription factor gene, RIEG, involved in Rieger syndrome. Nat Genet. 1996;14(4):392–9. doi:10.1038/ng1296-392.
57. Raetzman LT, Ward R, Camper SA. Lhx4 and Prop1 are required for cell survival and expansion of the pituitary primordia. Development. 2002;129(18):4229–39.
58. Sheng HZ, Moriyama K, Yamashita T, Li H, Potter SS, Mahon KA, Westphal H. Multistep control of pituitary organogenesis. Science. 1997;278(5344):1809–12.
59. Tajima T, Ishizu K, Nakamura A. Molecular and clinical findings in patients with LHX4 and OTX2 mutations. Clin Pediatr Endocrinol. 2013;22(2):15–23. doi:10.1292/cpe.22.15.
60. Castinetti F, Saveanu A, Reynaud R, Quentien MH, Buffin A, Brauner R, Kaffel N, Albarel F, Guedj AM, El Kholy M, Amin M, Enjalbert A, Barlier A, Brue T. A novel dysfunctional LHX4 mutation with high phenotypical variability in patients with hypopituitarism. J Clin Endocrinol Metab. 2008;93(7):2790–9. doi:10.1210/jc.2007-2389.
61. Pfaeffle RW, Hunter CS, Savage JJ, Duran-Prado M, Mullen RD, Neeb ZP, Eiholzer U, Hesse V, Haddad NG, Stobbe HM, Blum WF, Weigel JF, Rhodes SJ. Three novel missense mutations within the LHX4 gene are associated with variable pituitary hormone deficiencies. J Clin Endocrinol Metab. 2008;93(3):1062–71. doi:10.1210/jc.2007-1525.

62. Chou SJ, Hermesz E, Hatta T, Feltner D, El-Hodiri HM, Jamrich M, Mahon K. Conserved regulatory elements establish the dynamic expression of Rpx/HesxI in early vertebrate development. Dev Biol. 2006;292(2):533–45. doi:10.1016/j.ydbio.2005.12.053.
63. McGillivray SM, Bailey JS, Ramezani R, Kirkwood BJ, Mellon PL. Mouse GnRH receptor gene expression is mediated by the LHX3 homeodomain protein. Endocrinology. 2005;146(5):2180–5. doi:10.1210/en.2004-1566.
64. Granger A, Bleux C, Kottler ML, Rhodes SJ, Counis R, Laverriere JN. The LIM-homeodomain proteins Isl-1 and Lhx3 act with steroidogenic factor 1 to enhance gonadotrope-specific activity of the gonadotropin-releasing hormone receptor gene promoter. Mol Endocrinol. 2006;20(9):2093–108. doi:10.1210/me.2005-0184.
65. West BE, Parker GE, Savage JJ, Kiratipranon P, Toomey KS, Beach LR, Colvin SC, Sloop KW, Rhodes SJ. Regulation of the follicle-stimulating hormone beta gene by the LHX3 LIM-homeodomain transcription factor. Endocrinology. 2004;145(11):4866–79. doi:10.1210/en.2004-0598.
66. Girardin SE, Benjannet S, Barale JC, Chretien M, Seidah NG. The LIM homeobox protein mLIM3/Lhx3 induces expression of the prolactin gene by a Pit-1/GHF-1-independent pathway in corticotroph AtT20 cells. FEBS Lett. 1998;431(3):333–8.
67. Thaler JP, Lee SK, Jurata LW, Gill GN, Pfaff SL. LIM factor Lhx3 contributes to the specification of motor neuron and interneuron identity through cell-type-specific protein-protein interactions. Cell. 2002;110(2):237–49.
68. Sharma K, Sheng HZ, Lettieri K, Li H, Karavanov A, Potter S, Westphal H, Pfaff SL. LIM homeodomain factors Lhx3 and Lhx4 assign subtype identities for motor neurons. Cell. 1998;95(6):817–28.
69. Huang M, Sage C, Li H, Xiang M, Heller S, Chen ZY. Diverse expression patterns of LIM-homeodomain transcription factors (LIM-HDs) in mammalian inner ear development. Dev Dyn. 2008;237(11):3305–12. doi:10.1002/dvdy.21735.
70. Hume CR, Bratt DL, Oesterle EC. Expression of LHX3 and SOX2 during mouse inner ear development. Gene Expr Patterns. 2007;7(7):798–807. doi:10.1016/j.modgep.2007.05.002.
71. Pfaeffle RW, Savage JJ, Hunter CS, Palme C, Ahlmann M, Kumar P, Bellone J, Schoenau E, Korsch E, Bramswig JH, Stobbe HM, Blum WF, Rhodes SJ. Four novel mutations of the LHX3 gene cause combined pituitary hormone deficiencies with or without limited neck rotation. J Clin Endocrinol Metab. 2007;92(5):1909–19. doi:10.1210/jc.2006-2177.
72. Savage JJ, Hunter CS, Clark-Sturm SL, Jacob TM, Pfaeffle RW, Rhodes SJ. Mutations in the LHX3 gene cause dysregulation of pituitary and neural target genes that reflect patient phenotypes. Gene. 2007;400(1–2):44–51. doi:10.1016/j.gene.2007.05.017.
73. Bhangoo AP, Hunter CS, Savage JJ, Anhalt H, Pavlakis S, Walvoord EC, Ten S, Rhodes SJ. Clinical case seminar: a novel LHX3 mutation presenting as combined pituitary hormonal deficiency. J Clin Endocrinol Metab. 2006;91(3):747–53. doi:10.1210/jc.2005-2360.
74. Sloop KW, Parker GE, Hanna KR, Wright HA, Rhodes SJ. LHX3 transcription factor mutations associated with combined pituitary hormone deficiency impair the activation of pituitary target genes. Gene. 2001;265(1-2):61–9.
75. Howard PW, Maurer RA. A point mutation in the LIM domain of Lhx3 reduces activation of the glycoprotein hormone alpha-subunit promoter. J Biol Chem. 2001;276(22):19020–6. doi:10.1074/jbc.M101782200.
76. Netchine I, Sobrier ML, Krude H, Schnabel D, Maghnie M, Marcos E, Duriez B, Cacheux V, Moers A, Goossens M, Gruters A, Amselem S. Mutations in LHX3 result in a new syndrome revealed by combined pituitary hormone deficiency. Nat Genet. 2000;25(2):182–6. doi:10.1038/76041.
77. Kristrom B, Zdunek AM, Rydh A, Jonsson H, Sehlin P, Escher SA. A novel mutation in the LIM homeobox 3 gene is responsible for combined pituitary hormone deficiency, hearing impairment, and vertebral malformations. J Clin Endocrinol Metab. 2009;94(4):1154–61. doi:10.1210/jc.2008-0325.
78. Sornson MW, Wu W, Dasen JS, Flynn SE, Norman DJ, O'Connell SM, Gukovsky I, Carriere C, Ryan AK, Miller AP, Zuo L, Gleiberman AS, Andersen B, Beamer WG, Rosenfeld

MG. Pituitary lineage determination by the Prophet of Pit-1 homeodomain factor defective in Ames dwarfism. Nature. 1996;384(6607):327–33. doi:10.1038/384327a0.
79. Ikeshita N, Kawagishi M, Shibahara H, Toda K, Yamashita T, Yamamoto D, Sugiyama Y, Iguchi G, Iida K, Takahashi Y, Kaji H, Chihara K, Okimura Y. Identification and analysis of prophet of Pit-1-binding sites in human Pit-1 gene. Endocrinology. 2008;149(11):5491–9. doi:10.1210/en.2008-0030.
80. Kelberman D, Turton JP, Woods KS, Mehta A, Al-Khawari M, Greening J, Swift PG, Otonkoski T, Rhodes SJ, Dattani MT. Molecular analysis of novel PROP1 mutations associated with combined pituitary hormone deficiency (CPHD). Clin Endocrinol. 2009;70(1):96–103. doi:10.1111/j.1365-2265.2008.03326.x.
81. Zimmermann A, Schenk JP, Grigorescu Sido P, Pfaffle R, Lazea C, Zimmermann T, Heinrich U, Weber MM, Bettendorf M. MRI findings and genotype analysis in patients with childhood onset growth hormone deficiency–correlation with severity of hypopituitarism. J Pediatr Endocrinol Metab. 2007;20(5):587–96.
82. Vieira TC, da Silva MR, Abucham J. The natural history of the R120C PROP1 mutation reveals a wide phenotypic variability in two untreated adult brothers with combined pituitary hormone deficiency. Endocrine. 2006;30(3):365–9.
83. Nose O, Tatsumi K, Nakano Y, Amino N. Congenital combined pituitary hormone deficiency attributable to a novel PROP1 mutation (467insT). J Pediatr Endocrinol Metab. 2006;19(4):491–8.
84. Lemos MC, Gomes L, Bastos M, Leite V, Limbert E, Carvalho D, Bacelar C, Monteiro M, Fonseca F, Agapito A, Castro JJ, Regateiro FJ, Carvalheiro M. PROP1 gene analysis in Portuguese patients with combined pituitary hormone deficiency. Clin Endocrinol. 2006;65(4):479–85. doi:10.1111/j.1365-2265.2006.02617.x.
85. Abrao MG, Leite MV, Carvalho LR, Billerbeck AE, Nishi MY, Barbosa AS, Martin RM, Arnhold IJ, Mendonca BB. Combined pituitary hormone deficiency (CPHD) due to a complete PROP1 deletion. Clin Endocrinol. 2006;65(3):294–300. doi:10.1111/j.1365-2265. 2006.02592.x.
86. Reynaud R, Barlier A, Vallette-Kasic S, Saveanu A, Guillet MP, Simonin G, Enjalbert A, Valensi P, Brue T. An uncommon phenotype with familial central hypogonadism caused by a novel PROP1 gene mutant truncated in the transactivation domain. J Clin Endocrinol Metab. 2005;90(8):4880–7. doi:10.1210/jc.2005-0119.
87. Lebl J, Vosahlo J, Pfaeffle RW, Stobbe H, Cerna J, Novotna D, Zapletalova J, Kalvachova B, Hana V, Weiss V, Blum WF. Auxological and endocrine phenotype in a population-based cohort of patients with PROP1 gene defects. Eur J Endocrinol. 2005;153(3):389–96. doi:10.1530/eje.1.01989.
88. Voutetakis A, Maniati-Christidi M, Kanaka-Gantenbein C, Dracopoulou M, Argyropoulou M, Livadas S, Dacou-Voutetakis C, Sertedaki A. Prolonged jaundice and hypothyroidism as the presenting symptoms in a neonate with a novel Prop1 gene mutation (Q83X). Eur J Endocrinol. 2004;150(3):257–64.
89. Tatsumi KI, Kikuchi K, Tsumura K, Amino N. A novel PROP1 gene mutation (157delA) in Japanese siblings with combined anterior pituitary hormone deficiency. Clin Endocrinol. 2004;61(5):635–40. doi:10.1111/j.1365-2265.2004.02147.x.
90. Reynaud R, Chadli-Chaieb M, Vallette-Kasic S, Barlier A, Sarles J, Pellegrini-Bouiller I, Enjalbert A, Chaieb L, Brue T. A familial form of congenital hypopituitarism due to a PROP1 mutation in a large kindred: phenotypic and in vitro functional studies. J Clin Endocrinol Metab. 2004;89(11):5779–86. doi:10.1210/jc.2003-032124.
91. Bottner A, Keller E, Kratzsch J, Stobbe H, Weigel JF, Keller A, Hirsch W, Kiess W, Blum WF, Pfaffle RW. PROP1 mutations cause progressive deterioration of anterior pituitary function including adrenal insufficiency: a longitudinal analysis. J Clin Endocrinol Metab. 2004;89(10):5256–65. doi:10.1210/jc.2004-0661.
92. Paracchini R, Giordano M, Corrias A, Mellone S, Matarazzo P, Bellone J, Momigliano-Richiardi P, Bona G. Two new PROP1 gene mutations responsible for compound pituitary hormone deficiency. Clin Genet. 2003;64(2):142–7.

93. Arroyo A, Pernasetti F, Vasilyev VV, Amato P, Yen SS, Mellon PL. A unique case of combined pituitary hormone deficiency caused by a PROP1 gene mutation (R120C) associated with normal height and absent puberty. Clin Endocrinol. 2002;57(2):283–91.
94. Vallette-Kasic S, Barlier A, Teinturier C, Diaz A, Manavela M, Berthezene F, Bouchard P, Chaussain JL, Brauner R, Pellegrini-Bouiller I, Jaquet P, Enjalbert A, Brue T. PROP1 gene screening in patients with multiple pituitary hormone deficiency reveals two sites of hypermutability and a high incidence of corticotroph deficiency. J Clin Endocrinol Metab. 2001;86(9):4529–35. doi:10.1210/jcem.86.9.7811.
95. Pernasetti F, Toledo SP, Vasilyev VV, Hayashida CY, Cogan JD, Ferrari C, Lourenco Jr DM, Mellon PL. Impaired adrenocorticotropin-adrenal axis in combined pituitary hormone deficiency caused by a two-base pair deletion (301-302delAG) in the prophet of Pit-1 gene. J Clin Endocrinol Metab. 2000;85(1):390–7. doi:10.1210/jcem.85.1.6324.
96. Agarwal G, Bhatia V, Cook S, Thomas PQ. Adrenocorticotropin deficiency in combined pituitary hormone deficiency patients homozygous for a novel PROP1 deletion. J Clin Endocrinol Metab. 2000;85(12):4556–61. doi:10.1210/jcem.85.12.7013.
97. Rosenbloom AL, Almonte AS, Brown MR, Fisher DA, Baumbach L, Parks JS. Clinical and biochemical phenotype of familial anterior hypopituitarism from mutation of the PROP1 gene. J Clin Endocrinol Metab. 1999;84(1):50–7. doi:10.1210/jcem.84.1.5366.
98. Deladoey J, Fluck C, Buyukgebiz A, Kuhlmann BV, Eble A, Hindmarsh PC, Wu W, Mullis PE. "Hot spot" in the PROP1 gene responsible for combined pituitary hormone deficiency. J Clin Endocrinol Metab. 1999;84(5):1645–50. doi:10.1210/jcem.84.5.5681.
99. Wu W, Cogan JD, Pfaffle RW, Dasen JS, Frisch H, O'Connell SM, Flynn SE, Brown MR, Mullis PE, Parks JS, Phillips 3rd JA, Rosenfeld MG. Mutations in PROP1 cause familial combined pituitary hormone deficiency. Nat Genet. 1998;18(2):147–9. doi:10.1038/ng0298-147.
100. Fofanova O, Takamura N, Kinoshita E, Parks JS, Brown MR, Peterkova VA, Evgrafov OV, Goncharov NP, Bulatov AA, Dedov II, Yamashita S. Compound heterozygous deletion of the PROP-1 gene in children with combined pituitary hormone deficiency. J Clin Endocrinol Metab. 1998;83(7):2601–4. doi:10.1210/jcem.83.7.5094.
101. Cogan JD, Wu W, Phillips 3rd JA, Arnhold IJ, Agapito A, Fofanova OV, Osorio MG, Bircan I, Moreno A, Mendonca BB. The PROP1 2-base pair deletion is a common cause of combined pituitary hormone deficiency. J Clin Endocrinol Metab. 1998;83(9):3346–9. doi:10.1210/jcem.83.9.5142.
102. Vieira TC, Boldarine VT, Abucham J. Molecular analysis of PROP1, PIT1, HESX1, LHX3, and LHX4 shows high frequency of PROP1 mutations in patients with familial forms of combined pituitary hormone deficiency. Arq Bras Endocrinol Metabol. 2007;51(7):1097–103.
103. Halasz Z, Toke J, Patocs A, Bertalan R, Tombol Z, Sallai A, Hosszu E, Muzsnai A, Kovacs L, Solyom J, Fekete G, Racz K. High prevalence of PROP1 gene mutations in Hungarian patients with childhood-onset combined anterior pituitary hormone deficiency. Endocrine. 2006;30(3):255–60. doi:10.1007/s12020-006-0002-7.
104. Fluck C, Deladoey J, Rutishauser K, Eble A, Marti U, Wu W, Mullis PE. Phenotypic variability in familial combined pituitary hormone deficiency caused by a PROP1 gene mutation resulting in the substitution of Arg→Cys at codon 120 (R120C). J Clin Endocrinol Metab. 1998;83(10):3727–34. doi:10.1210/jcem.83.10.5172.
105. Voutetakis A, Sertedaki A, Livadas S, Xekouki P, Bossis I, Dacou-Voutetakis C, Argyropoulou MI. Pituitary size fluctuation in long-term MR studies of PROP1 deficient patients: a persistent pathophysiological mechanism? J Endocrinol Investig. 2006;29(5):462–6.
106. Voutetakis A, Argyropoulou M, Sertedaki A, Livadas S, Xekouki P, Maniati-Christidi M, Bossis I, Thalassinos N, Patronas N, Dacou-Voutetakis C. Pituitary magnetic resonance imaging in 15 patients with Prop1 gene mutations: pituitary enlargement may originate from the intermediate lobe. J Clin Endocrinol Metab. 2004;89(5):2200–6. doi:10.1210/jc.2003-031765.
107. Riepe FG, Partsch CJ, Blankenstein O, Monig H, Pfaffle RW, Sippell WG. Longitudinal imaging reveals pituitary enlargement preceding hypoplasia in two brothers with combined pituitary hormone deficiency attributable to PROP1 mutation. J Clin Endocrinol Metab. 2001;86(9):4353–7. doi:10.1210/jcem.86.9.7828.

108. Fofanova O, Takamura N, Kinoshita E, Vorontsov A, Vladimirova V, Dedov I, Peterkova V, Yamashita S. MR imaging of the pituitary gland in children and young adults with congenital combined pituitary hormone deficiency associated with PROP1 mutations. AJR Am J Roentgenol. 2000;174(2):555–9. doi:10.2214/ajr.174.2.1740555.
109. Mendonca BB, Osorio MG, Latronico AC, Estefan V, Lo LS, Arnhold IJ. Longitudinal hormonal and pituitary imaging changes in two females with combined pituitary hormone deficiency due to deletion of A301, G302 in the PROP1 gene. J Clin Endocrinol Metab. 1999;84(3):942–5. doi:10.1210/jcem.84.3.5537.
110. Himes AD, Raetzman LT. Premature differentiation and aberrant movement of pituitary cells lacking both Hes1 and Prop1. Dev Biol. 2009;325(1):151–61. doi:10.1016/j.ydbio.2008.10.010.
111. Bodner M, Castrillo JL, Theill LE, Deerinck T, Ellisman M, Karin M. The pituitary-specific transcription factor GHF-1 is a homeobox-containing protein. Cell. 1988;55(3):505–18.

# Chapter 13
# Cranial Radiation and Growth Hormone Deficiency

**Wassim Chemaitilly**

## Introduction

Endocrine complications affect between 20 and 50 % of childhood cancer survivors and often occur as therapy-related late effects [1, 2]. Individuals with central nervous system (CNS) tumors and those whose hypothalamus and/or pituitary were exposed to surgery or radiotherapy are at risk of hypothalamic/pituitary deficits, including growth hormone deficiency (GHD) [3]. When caused by tumoral expansion in close proximity to the sellar region and/or by surgical treatments involving this area, GHD tends to be associated from the outset with other hypothalamic/pituitary deficits and to become clinically evident fairly quickly following the primary diagnosis or surgery. In contrast, GHD following the exposure of the hypothalamus/pituitary to direct or scatter radiation may not become evident for many years; it may not be associated with other hormonal deficiencies from the outset as the radiation threshold dose and the time course of hormone dysfunctions vary for the different anterior pituitary hormones [4, 5]. Nevertheless, GHD is the most common, and often the only, pituitary deficiency observed in survivors of childhood brain tumors and those with a history of exposure to cranial radiotherapy (CRT) or total body irradiation (TBI) [4, 6–9]. The present chapter aims at summarizing current knowledge regarding the occurrence of GHD as a complication of radiotherapy with a focus on the diagnostic and management challenges that are specific to survivors of childhood neoplasia with a history of hypothalamic/pituitary radiation exposure.

---

W. Chemaitilly (✉)
Division of Endocrinology, Department of Pediatric Medicine, MS-737, St. Jude Children's Research Hospital, 262 Danny Thomas Place, Memphis, TN 38105, USA
e-mail: wassim.chemaitilly@stjude.org

## Pathophysiology

The site and precise mechanism through which radiotherapy causes neuroendocrinopathies (purely neuronal vs. neurovascular, hypothalamic vs. pituitary) are unknown [10]. In a study using single-photon emission computed tomography (CT) imaging, hypothalamic blood flow was significantly lower in a group of 34 individuals (aged 30–65 years) treated with radiotherapy (46–56 Gy to the hypothalamic/pituitary area via a fractionated regimen) for nasopharyngeal carcinoma when compared to a group of four healthy controls [11]. There were no significant differences among patients treated with radiotherapy when they were grouped according to follow-up duration (6 months vs. 1 year vs. 5 years) [11]. The apparent contradiction between this finding and the well-described trend of time and dose-dependent worsening of hypothalamic pituitary dysfunctions after exposure to radiotherapy [12] led the authors to favor direct insult to the neurons (vs. vascular injury) as the primary mechanism of hypothalamic damage without completely ruling out a possible role for chronic ischemic changes [11]. The most likely site of radiation-induced GHD seems to be the hypothalamus rather than the pituitary given the observation of better preserved GH response to exogenous GH-releasing hormone (GHRH) in comparison to other GH secretagogues in individuals exposed to CRT [13].

## Prevalence and Risk Factors

Radiation-induced GHD occurs in a time- and dose-dependent fashion (Fig. 13.1) [12]. The risk increases at higher doses of radiation and with longer durations of follow-up [12, 14]. Growth hormone deficiency can be observed within 5 years when the dose exceeds 30 Gy [9]. Following lower doses, such as 18–24 Gy, GHD may not become evident for 10 or more years [15]. In a recent study of 748 adult survivors (mean age 34.2 years) of childhood cancers and brain tumors treated with CRT and followed for a mean 27.3 years, GHD was shown to continue to appear during adulthood and middle age; a trend that was significantly more pronounced but not unique to GHD among anterior pituitary hormone deficiencies (Fig. 13.2) [4]. In this study, the point prevalence of GHD, diagnosed using plasma insulin-like growth factor-1 (IGF-I) levels <-2 $z$-score for age and sex in lieu of dynamic testing, was estimated at 46.5 % (95% CI 42.9–50.2 %) overall, 47.5 % (95% CI 43.8–51.3 %) at doses of CRT ≥18 Gy, and 30.2 % (95% CI 17.2–46.1 %) at doses <18 Gy ($p=0.03$) [4]. Up to 60.9 % of suspected cases of GHD appeared during adulthood and were detected through the risk-based assessments offered through participation in the St. Jude Lifetime cohort study [4]. The occurrence of GHD in a both dose- and time-dependent fashion was further demonstrated in this study as comparable risks were found among individuals treated with doses <22 Gy, most likely to

13 Cranial Radiation and Growth Hormone Deficiency 197

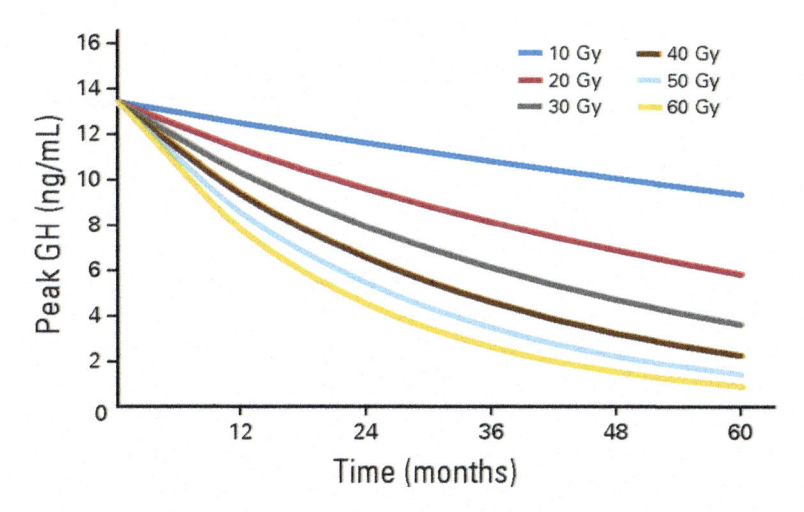

**Fig. 13.1** Growth hormone secretion after irradiation of the hypothalamus/pituitary. Reproduced with permission from [12]. © 2011 by American Society of Clinical Oncology

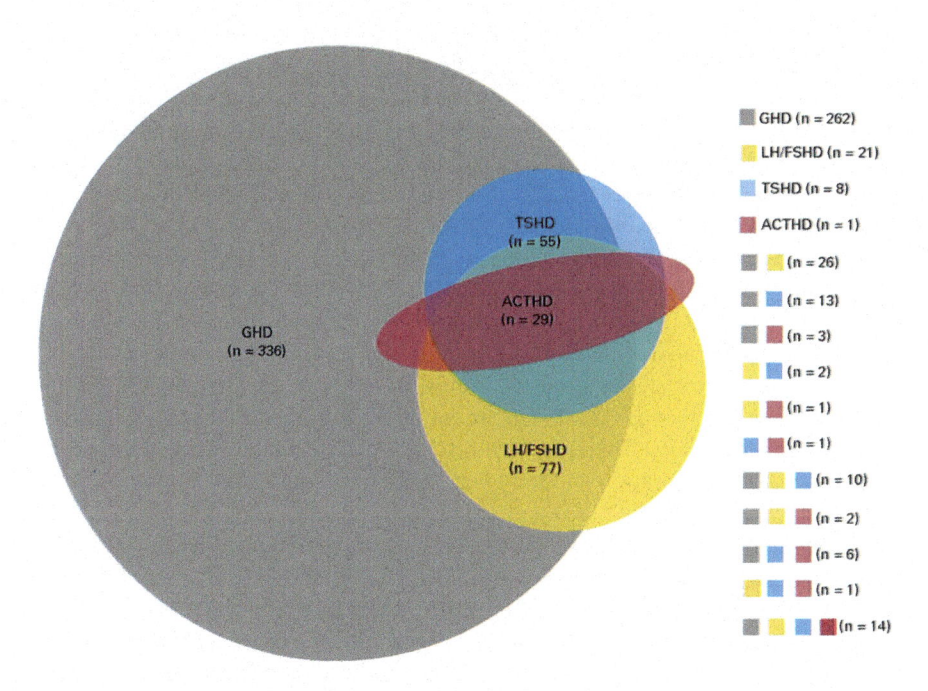

**Fig. 13.2** Relative proportions and overlap among anterior pituitary hormone deficiencies following cranial radiotherapy. Reproduced with permission from [4]. © 2015 by American Society of Clinical Oncology

represent an older group of acute lymphoblastic leukemia survivors treated with prophylactic CRT in past decades, and individuals exposed to doses ≥30 Gy and who are by majority a much younger group of survivors of childhood brain tumors followed for a significantly shorter period of time [4]. Young age at exposure to CRT has been described as an additional risk factor for GHD by some, but not all, authors [16, 17].

## Diagnosis

The diagnosis of radiation-induced GHD follows the same process and relies on the same diagnostic criteria as in patients not treated with radiotherapy [1]. There are, however, several factors that deserve special attention in individuals with a history of past exposure to direct or scatter radiotherapy to the hypothalamus and/or pituitary. Endocrine and non-endocrine treatment-related factors could affect linear growth in children independently of GH and need to be recognized and identified in advance for both diagnostic and prognostic considerations. Patients with a history of spinal exposure to radiotherapy may incur direct damage to the vertebral growth plates leading to a form of skeletal dysplasia where the growth of the spine is more affected than that of the legs [18–21]. This can be identified by measuring the patient's sitting height, plotting the value on a specific growth chart and comparing the sitting height, expressed in standard deviation (SD) for age and sex, to the standing height SD. A discrepancy between these values would be suggestive of radiation-induced skeletal dysplasia. Individuals with severe obesity can continue to grow despite having GHD; insulin resistance and/or hypersecretion has been cited as possible mechanisms of this poorly understood phenomenon [22, 23]. Central precocious puberty, which is fairly common in individuals with tumors near the hypothalamus or optic pathways and those treated with CRT, is an additional confounding factor [8]. Owing to the effect of sex steroids, patients may experience a relatively accelerated linear growth rate that can mask concurrent GHD with seemingly normal, prepubertal, growth velocity. This is unfortunately occurring at the expense of rapidly advancing bone maturation and may lead to an irreversible loss in growth prospects if the association of GHD and precocious puberty is not quickly identified [8]. Conversely, rising levels of sex steroids during puberty are necessary for the generation of a pubertal growth spurt and for sustaining adequate growth rates during teenage years because of their effect on GH secretion and on local growth factors in the growth plates [24]. These observations further emphasize the need for a close monitoring of pubertal status in children assessed for growth disorders. It is also important to note that testicular volume should not be used in assessing pubertal onset and progress in males exposed to direct testicular radiotherapy and/or gonadotoxic chemotherapy regimens (such as alkylating agents) given the effect of these treatments on testicular size [1]. Other markers such as pubarche, penile size, and scrotal thinning should be carefully assessed, and practitioners should not hesitate to obtain confirmatory plasma testosterone level measurements when pubertal changes are suspected [1].

There are special considerations regarding the choice and interpretation of laboratory tests used for the assessment of individuals for radiation-induced GHD. While failing two dynamic tests using different secretagogues is necessary for the diagnosis of GHD in the general population, the consensus guidelines of the GH Research Society have deemed that in individuals with a history of a CNS insult affecting the hypothalamic/pituitary axis such as tumors and CRT, one test is generally sufficient for the diagnosis [25]. The contribution of radiation-induced GHD to poor growth and short stature should also be weighed against the contribution of other factors such as a history of exposure to aggressive multi-agent chemotherapy or medications directly affecting the growth plates (such as *cis*-retinoic acid and imatinib) in the context of severe or relapsing malignancy, as in patients with neuroblastoma [26, 27]. Given the likely hypothalamic origin of GHD, the combination of GHRH and arginine (GHRH-Arg), which is the most widely used test in adults assessed for GHD, should be avoided in individuals with a history of hypothalamic/pituitary exposure to radiotherapy; [28, 29]. Additionally, GHRH is presently not available for use in the United States. The gold standard test in adults remains the insulin tolerance test (ITT), but because of the risks associated with the hypoglycemia induced by insulin, dynamic testing using glucagon has been suggested as an alternative [30]. Priming with sex steroids prior to GH testing in children with pubertal delay and adjustment of the GH peak to body mass index (BMI) have been suggested as untreated hypogonadism and obesity are known to blunt the GH response in non-GH-deficient individuals [31, 32]. Surrogate markers for GH secretion, such as plasma IGF-I and IGF-binding protein-3 (IGFBP-3) levels, may not be reliable in individuals with a history of exposure to CRT and may result in the underdiagnosis of GHD [33, 34]. Hence, GH dynamic tests should still be offered when clinical suspicion is present.

## Treatment

Adult height prospects can be significantly improved in children with radiation-induced GHD by the use of human recombinant GH (hGH) replacement therapy [35–44]. Better height outcomes were described when treatment with hGH was initiated at a younger age and higher doses [35]. Children treated with spinal radiotherapy and those exposed to TBI may not completely recover the loss in their growth potential, but it is possible that their height outcomes would be even worse without replacement with hGH [37–44].

Given the pro-mitogenic and proliferative effects of GH and IGF-I in vitro, the safety of hGH in individuals with a history of malignancy or neoplasia has been a source of concern for patients, families, and prescribing physicians for many years [45]. Large-scale studies conducted in long-term survivors of childhood cancers have not demonstrated higher risks of disease recurrence of death in individuals treated with hGH during childhood when compared to those who did not receive replacement therapy [46–48]. However, there are data to suggest a small increase in the risk of a secondary solid tumor [48, 49]. In a report on a cohort of 13,222 participants, including 361 patients treated with hGH from the Childhood Cancer Survivor Study (CCSS), 15 patients with a history of treatment with hGH developed second neoplasms [48]. Exposure to hGH was significantly associated with the development of second neoplasms (RR 3.21, 95 % CI 1.88–5.46, $p<0.0001$) even after adjustment for age at diagnosis, sex, and cancer treatment modalities [48]. A second CCSS report, specifically dedicated to the study of the association between hGH and second neoplasms, confirmed this association (RR 2.15, 95 % CI 1.3–3.5) using data from an additional 3 years of follow-up [49]. The 20 cases of reported second neoplasms in individuals treated with hGH included a majority with a subsequent diagnosis of meningioma ($n=9$), all of whom had been exposed to CRT, which is a known risk factor for this type of neoplasia [49, 50]. Neither the dose of hGH nor the duration of therapy were significant factors in this association [49]. In a third report from the CCSS dedicated to the study of the risk of second CNS neoplasms following treatment with hGH and allowing for an even longer duration of follow-up, individuals treated with hGH during childhood were not found to be at a higher risk of developing second CNS neoplasms when compared to others [51]. These findings were consistent with those of a previous study comparing 110 survivors of childhood and adult cancers treated with hGH to 110 matched non-hGH-treated controls followed for a median of 14.5 years [52]. In summary, treatment with hGH can be offered to GH-deficient children who achieve remission (for at least 1 year per expert opinion) after completing therapy for a malignancy or brain tumor if they are cleared to receive hGH after the critical, individualized, and multidisciplinary assessment of their predisposition to recurrence and/or complications and provided they can be closely monitored for these risks during therapy [53].

Over the past two decades, the use of hGH has been extended to adults with hypopituitarism given potential beneficial effects on body composition, plasma lipids, bone mass, and quality of life [40, 54–57]. In the report on anterior hypopituitarism from the St. Jude Lifetime cohort, untreated radiation-induced GHD was associated with increased waist-to-height ratio, low muscle mass, low energy expenditure, low handgrip strength, and poor exercise tolerance, which are all components of frailty, a phenotype that has been shown to be associated with early mortality [4]. There are, however, no studies specifically assessing the effects of hGH in adult survivors of childhood cancers or brain tumors with radiation-induced GHD. Whether hGH is safe and whether it provides sustainable improvements in overall states of health are questions that need to be specifically addressed in this population given the patients' complex medical history, possible exposure to several other cancer treatment modalities and drug toxicities, and markedly increased risk of developing life-threatening chronic health conditions [4, 55, 58–60].

## Conclusions

Growth hormone deficiency is the most common, and often only, anterior pituitary dysfunction in individuals with a history of direct or scatter radiotherapy to the hypothalamus and/or pituitary. Radiation-induced GHD poises specific challenges when compared to other forms of GHD because of its dose- and time-dependent relationship with radiation exposure; its frequent association with other, endocrine and non-endocrine, comorbidities; and its continued appearance through childhood, adulthood, and middle age. Individuals with a history of hypothalamic/pituitary exposure to radiotherapy should be offered lifelong follow-up for potential endocrine dysfunctions, including GHD. The amplitude and sustainability of improvements on overall health brought about by hGH in adult survivors of childhood cancers and brain tumors deserve further investigation.

## References

1. Barnes N, Chemaitilly W. Endocrinopathies in survivors of childhood neoplasia. Front Pediatr. 2014;2:101.
2. Chemaitilly W, Sklar CA. Endocrine complications in long-term survivors of childhood cancers. Endocr Relat Cancer. 2010;17(3):R141–59.
3. Gurney JG, Kadan-Lottick NS, Packer RJ, Neglia JP, Sklar CA, Punyko JA, et al. Endocrine and cardiovascular late effects among adult survivors of childhood brain tumors: Childhood Cancer Survivor Study. Cancer. 2003;97(3):663–73.
4. Chemaitilly W, Li Z, Huang S, Ness KK, Clark KL, Green DM, et al. Anterior hypopituitarism in adult survivors of childhood cancers treated with cranial radiotherapy: a report from the St Jude Lifetime Cohort Study. J Clin Oncol. 2015;33(5):492–500.
5. Constine LS, Woolf PD, Cann D, Mick G, McCormick K, Raubertas RF, et al. Hypothalamic-pituitary dysfunction after radiation for brain tumors. N Engl J Med. 1993;328(2):87–94.
6. Heikens J, Michiels EM, Behrendt H, Endert E, Bakker PJ, Fliers E. Long-term neuro-endocrine sequelae after treatment for childhood medulloblastoma. Eur J Cancer. 1998;34(10):1592–7.
7. Chrousos GP, Poplack D, Brown T, O'Neill D, Schwade J, Bercu BB. Effects of cranial radiation on hypothalamic-adenohypophyseal function: abnormal growth hormone secretory dynamics. J Clin Endocrinol Metab. 1982;54(6):1135–9.
8. Sklar CA, Constine LS. Chronic neuroendocrinological sequelae of radiation therapy. Int J Radiat Oncol Biol Phys. 1995;31(5):1113–21.
9. Laughton SJ, Merchant TE, Sklar CA, Kun LE, Fouladi M, Broniscer A, et al. Endocrine outcomes for children with embryonal brain tumors after risk-adapted craniospinal and conformal primary-site irradiation and high-dose chemotherapy with stem-cell rescue on the SJMB-96 trial. J Clin Oncol. 2008;26(7):1112–8.
10. Spoudeas HA. Growth and endocrine function after chemotherapy and radiotherapy in childhood. Eur J Cancer. 2002;38(13):1748–59.

11. Chieng PU, Huang TS, Chang CC, Chong PN, Tien RD, Su CT. Reduced hypothalamic blood flow after radiation treatment of nasopharyngeal cancer: SPECT studies in 34 patients. AJNR Am J Neuroradiol. 1991;12(4):661–5.
12. Merchant TE, Rose SR, Bosley C, Wu S, Xiong X, Lustig RH. Growth hormone secretion after conformal radiation therapy in pediatric patients with localized brain tumors. J Clin Oncol. 2011;29(36):4776–80.
13. Schriock EA, Lustig RH, Rosenthal SM, Kaplan SL, Grumbach MM. Effect of growth hormone (GH)-releasing hormone (GRH) on plasma GH in relation to magnitude and duration of GH deficiency in 26 children and adults with isolated GH deficiency or multiple pituitary hormone deficiencies: evidence for hypothalamic GRH deficiency. J Clin Endocrinol Metab. 1984;58(6):1043–9.
14. Clayton PE, Shalet SM. Dose dependency of time of onset of radiation-induced growth hormone deficiency. J Pediatr. 1991;118(2):226–8.
15. Brennan BM, Rahim A, Mackie EM, Eden OB, Shalet SM. Growth hormone status in adults treated for acute lymphoblastic leukaemia in childhood. Clin Endocrinol (Oxf). 1998;48(6):777–83.
16. Schmiegelow M, Lassen S, Poulsen HS, Feldt-Rasmussen U, Schmiegelow K, Hertz H, et al. Cranial radiotherapy of childhood brain tumours: growth hormone deficiency and its relation to the biological effective dose of irradiation in a large population based study. Clin Endocrinol (Oxf). 2000;53(2):191–7.
17. Brauner R, Czernichow P, Rappaport R. Greater susceptibility to hypothalamopituitary irradiation in younger children with acute lymphoblastic leukemia. J Pediatr. 1986;108(2):332.
18. Shalet SM, Gibson B, Swindell R, Pearson D. Effect of spinal irradiation on growth. Arch Dis Child. 1987;62(5):461–4.
19. Brauner R, Fontoura M, Zucker JM, Devergie A, Souberbielle JC, Prevot-Saucet C, et al. Growth and growth hormone secretion after bone marrow transplantation. Arch Dis Child. 1993;68(4):458–63.
20. Thomas BC, Stanhope R, Plowman PN, Leiper AD. Growth following single fraction and fractionated total body irradiation for bone marrow transplantation. Eur J Pediatr. 1993;152(11):888–92.
21. Clayton PE, Shalet SM. The evolution of spinal growth after irradiation. Clin Oncol (R Coll Radiol). 1991;3(4):220–2.
22. Iwayama H, Kamijo T, Ueda N. Hyperinsulinemia may promote growth without GH in children after resection of suprasellar brain tumors. Endocrine. 2011;40(1):130–3.
23. Lustig RH, Post SR, Srivannaboon K, Rose SR, Danish RK, Burghen GA, et al. Risk factors for the development of obesity in children surviving brain tumors. J Clin Endocrinol Metab. 2003;88(2):611–6.
24. Cole TJ, Ahmed ML, Preece MA, Hindmarsh P, Dunger DB. The relationship between Insulin-like Growth Factor 1, sex steroids and timing of the pubertal growth spurt. Clin Endocrinol (Oxf). 2014;82:862–9.
25. GH Research Society. Consensus guidelines for the diagnosis and treatment of growth hormone (GH) deficiency in childhood and adolescence: summary statement of the GH Research Society. J Clin Endocrinol Metab. 2000;85(11):3990–3.
26. Cohen LE, Gordon JH, Popovsky EY, Gunawardene S, Duffey-Lind E, Lehmann LE, et al. Late effects in children treated with intensive multimodal therapy for high-risk neuroblastoma: high incidence of endocrine and growth problems. Bone Marrow Transplant. 2014;49(4):502–8.
27. Rastogi MV, Stork L, Druker B, Blasdel C, Nguyen T, Boston BA. Imatinib mesylate causes growth deceleration in pediatric patients with chronic myelogenous leukemia. Pediatr Blood Cancer. 2012;59(5):840–5.
28. Ham JN, Ginsberg JP, Hendell CD, Moshang Jr T. Growth hormone releasing hormone plus arginine stimulation testing in young adults treated in childhood with cranio-spinal radiation therapy. Clin Endocrinol (Oxf). 2005;62(5):628–32.
29. Darzy KH, Aimaretti G, Wieringa G, Gattamaneni HR, Ghigo E, Shalet SM. The usefulness of the combined growth hormone (GH)-releasing hormone and arginine stimulation test in the

diagnosis of radiation-induced GH deficiency is dependent on the post-irradiation time interval. J Clin Endocrinol Metab. 2003;88(1):95–102.
30. Conceicao FL, da Costa e Silva A, Leal Costa AJ, Vaisman M. Glucagon stimulation test for the diagnosis of GH deficiency in adults. J Endocrinol Invest. 2003;26(11):1065–70.
31. Ghigo E, Aimaretti G, Corneli G. Diagnosis of adult GH deficiency. Growth Horm IGF Res. 2008;18(1):1–16.
32. De Sanctis V, Soliman AT, Yassin M, Di Maio S. Is priming with sex steroids useful for defining patients who will benefit from GH treatment? Pediatr Endocrinol Rev. 2014;11(3):284–7.
33. Sklar C, Sarafoglou K, Whittam E. Efficacy of insulin-like growth factor binding protein 3 in predicting the growth hormone response to provocative testing in children treated with cranial irradiation. Acta Endocrinol (Copenh). 1993;129(6):511–5.
34. Weinzimer SA, Homan SA, Ferry RJ, Moshang T. Serum IGF-I and IGFBP-3 concentrations do not accurately predict growth hormone deficiency in children with brain tumours. Clin Endocrinol (Oxf). 1999;51(3):339–45.
35. Leung W, Rose SR, Zhou Y, Hancock ML, Burstein S, Schriock EA, et al. Outcomes of growth hormone replacement therapy in survivors of childhood acute lymphoblastic leukemia. J Clin Oncol. 2002;20(13):2959–64.
36. Gleeson HK, Stoeter R, Ogilvy-Stuart AL, Gattamaneni HR, Brennan BM, Shalet SM. Improvements in final height over 25 years in growth hormone (GH)-deficient childhood survivors of brain tumors receiving GH replacement. J Clin Endocrinol Metab. 2003;88(8):3682–9.
37. Brownstein CM, Mertens AC, Mitby PA, Stovall M, Qin J, Heller G, et al. Factors that affect final height and change in height standard deviation scores in survivors of childhood cancer treated with growth hormone: a report from the Childhood Cancer Survivor Study. J Clin Endocrinol Metab. 2004;89(9):4422–7.
38. Dai QY, Souillet G, Bertrand Y, Galambrun C, Bleyzac N, Manel AM, et al. Antileukemic and long-term effects of two regimens with or without TBI in allogeneic bone marrow transplantation for childhood acute lymphoblastic leukemia. Bone Marrow Transplant. 2004;34(8):667–73.
39. Sanders JE, Guthrie KA, Hoffmeister PA, Woolfrey AE, Carpenter PA, Appelbaum FR. Final adult height of patients who received hematopoietic cell transplantation in childhood. Blood. 2005;105(3):1348–54.
40. Bakker B, Oostdijk W, Geskus RB, Stokvis-Brantsma WH, Vossen JM, Wit JM. Growth hormone (GH) secretion and response to GH therapy after total body irradiation and haematopoietic stem cell transplantation during childhood. Clin Endocrinol (Oxf). 2007;67(4):589–97.
41. Chemaitilly W, Boulad F, Heller G, Kernan NA, Small TN, O'Reilly RJ, et al. Final height in pediatric patients after hyperfractionated total body irradiation and stem cell transplantation. Bone Marrow Transplant. 2007;40(1):29–35.
42. Ciaccio M, Gil S, Guercio G, Vaiani E, Alderete D, Palladino M, et al. Effectiveness of rhGH treatment on adult height in GH-deficient childhood survivors of medulloblastoma. Horm Res Paediatr. 2010;73(4):281–6.
43. Beckers D, Thomas M, Jamart J, Francois I, Maes M, Lebrethon MC, et al. Adult final height after GH therapy for irradiation-induced GH deficiency in childhood survivors of brain tumors: the Belgian experience. Eur J Endocrinol. 2010;162(3):483–90.
44. Isfan F, Kanold J, Merlin E, Contet A, Sirvent N, Rochette E, et al. Growth hormone treatment impact on growth rate and final height of patients who received HSCT with TBI or/and cranial irradiation in childhood: a report from the French Leukaemia Long-Term Follow-Up Study (LEA). Bone Marrow Transplant. 2012;47(5):684–93.
45. Chemaitilly W, Robison LL. Safety of growth hormone treatment in patients previously treated for cancer. Endocrinol Metab Clin North Am. 2012;41(4):785–92.
46. Swerdlow AJ, Reddingius RE, Higgins CD, Spoudeas HA, Phipps K, Qiao Z, et al. Growth hormone treatment of children with brain tumors and risk of tumor recurrence. J Clin Endocrinol Metab. 2000;85(12):4444–9.

47. Packer RJ, Boyett JM, Janss AJ, Stavrou T, Kun L, Wisoff J, et al. Growth hormone replacement therapy in children with medulloblastoma: use and effect on tumor control. J Clin Oncol. 2001;19(2):480–7.
48. Sklar CA, Mertens AC, Mitby P, Occhiogrosso G, Qin J, Heller G, et al. Risk of disease recurrence and second neoplasms in survivors of childhood cancer treated with growth hormone: a report from the Childhood Cancer Survivor Study. J Clin Endocrinol Metab. 2002;87(7):3136–41.
49. Ergun-Longmire B, Mertens AC, Mitby P, Qin J, Heller G, Shi W, et al. Growth hormone treatment and risk of second neoplasms in the childhood cancer survivor. J Clin Endocrinol Metab. 2006;91(9):3494–8.
50. Paulino AC, Ahmed IM, Mai WY, Teh BS. The influence of pretreatment characteristics and radiotherapy parameters on time interval to development of radiation-associated meningioma. Int J Radiat Oncol Biol Phys. 2009;75(5):1408–14.
51. Patterson BC, Chen Y, Sklar CA, Neglia J, Yasui Y, Mertens A, et al. Growth hormone exposure as a risk factor for the development of subsequent neoplasms of the central nervous system: a report from the Childhood Cancer Survivor Study. J Clin Endocrinol Metab. 2014;99(6):2030–7.
52. Mackenzie S, Craven T, Gattamaneni HR, Swindell R, Shalet SM, Brabant G. Long-term safety of growth hormone replacement after CNS irradiation. J Clin Endocrinol Metab. 2011;96(9):2756–61.
53. Raman S, Grimberg A, Waguespack SG, Miller BS, Sklar CA, Meacham LR, et al. Risk of neoplasia in pediatric patients receiving growth hormone therapy - a report from the Pediatric Endocrine Society Drug and Therapeutics Committee. J Clin Endocrinol Metab. 2015;100:2192–203. jc20151002.
54. Link K, Moell C, Garwicz S, Cavallin-Stahl E, Bjork J, Thilen U, et al. Growth hormone deficiency predicts cardiovascular risk in young adults treated for acute lymphoblastic leukemia in childhood. J Clin Endocrinol Metab. 2004;89(10):5003–12.
55. van den Heijkant S, Hoorweg-Nijman G, Huisman J, Drent M, van der Pal H, Kaspers GJ, et al. Effects of growth hormone therapy on bone mass, metabolic balance, and well-being in young adult survivors of childhood acute lymphoblastic leukemia. J Pediatr Hematol Oncol. 2011;33(6):e231–8.
56. Elbornsson M, Gotherstrom G, Bosaeus I, Bengtsson BA, Johannsson G, Svensson J. Fifteen years of GH replacement increases bone mineral density in hypopituitary patients with adult-onset GH deficiency. Eur J Endocrinol. 2012;166(5):787–95.
57. Elbornsson M, Gotherstrom G, Bosaeus I, Bengtsson BA, Johannsson G, Svensson J. Fifteen years of GH replacement improves body composition and cardiovascular risk factors. Eur J Endocrinol. 2013;168(5):745–53.
58. Mukherjee A, Tolhurst-Cleaver S, Ryder WD, Smethurst L, Shalet SM. The characteristics of quality of life impairment in adult growth hormone (GH)-deficient survivors of cancer and their response to GH replacement therapy. J Clin Endocrinol Metab. 2005;90(3):1542–9.
59. Murray RD, Darzy KH, Gleeson HK, Shalet SM. GH-deficient survivors of childhood cancer: GH replacement during adult life. J Clin Endocrinol Metab. 2002;87(1):129–35.
60. Follin C, Thilen U, Ahren B, Erfurth EM. Improvement in cardiac systolic function and reduced prevalence of metabolic syndrome after two years of growth hormone (GH) treatment in GH-deficient adult survivors of childhood-onset acute lymphoblastic leukemia. J Clin Endocrinol Metab. 2006;91(5):1872–5.

# Chapter 14
# Traumatic Brain Injury and Growth Hormone Deficiency

**Erick Richmond and Alan D. Rogol**

## Introduction

Traumatic brain injury (TBI) is a common cause of death and disability in young adults with consequences ranging from physical disabilities to long-term cognitive, behavioral, psychological, and social deficits. It is considered a significant public health problem worldwide. The most common causes of TBI are falls, child abuse, violence, and sports injuries.

The pathophysiology of TBI involves not only the primary mechanical event, but also secondary insults such as hypotension, hypoxia, increased intracranial pressure, and changes in cerebral blood flow and metabolism. The most common isolated hormonal deficiency after TBI in both children and adults is growth hormone deficiency (GHD), although some studies note an almost equal incidence of gonadotropin deficiency in adults.

Pituitary function after TBI undergoes remarkable variation over time; dissimilar methodologies could account for marked variations in prevalence of GHD, and the lack of a gold standard test for GHD raises questions regarding the true incidence of GHD after TBI. Endocrine surveillance, in particular, height velocity in children, is recommended to ensure early intervention and diminish long-term sequelae. All patients with documented severe GHD are candidates for growth hormone (GH) replacement therapy.

---

E. Richmond
Pediatric Endocrinology, National Children's Hospital, San José, Costa Rica
e-mail: erickrichmond@hotmail.com

A.D. Rogol (✉)
Pediatric Endocrinology, University of Virginia,
685 Explorers Road, Charlottesville, VA 22911-8441, USA
e-mail: adrogol@comcast.net

## Epidemiology

TBI is increasingly common and the leading cause of death in industrialized countries for individuals between the ages of 1 and 45 [1]. Rates of TBI are highest in early childhood (0–4 years), young adults (15–24 years), and the elderly (>65 years). The most common causes of TBI are motor vehicle accidents (including pedestrian-car and bicycle-car encounters), falls, child abuse, violence, and sports injuries. Younger children are more likely to have TBI due to falls, while teenagers have more TBI than any other population from motor vehicle accidents. Many survivors live with significant physical and psychological sequelae [2]. Despite the high prevalence of TBI in the general population, posttraumatic hypopituitarism remains largely underdiagnosed. Until recently, evidence for pituitary insufficiency secondary to TBI was limited to anecdotal case reports. The first report of a patient with hypopituitarism after TBI was published in 1918, and subsequent to this, autopsy series showed high rates of pituitary damage following fatal TBI [3]. A meta-analysis including more than 1000 patients with TBI reported a pooled prevalence of hypopituitarism of 27.5 %; pituitary evaluation was performed in a range of 3 months to 7 years after the head trauma [4]. GHD is the most common hormonal deficiency reported after TBI; the prevalence varies widely among published studies depending on the population evaluated, the severity of the head injury, the time interval between head injury and assessment, and the testing methods used to evaluate the endocrine function.

## Pathophysiology

The pathophysiology of TBI is not completely understood. It involves not only the primary mechanical event, but also secondary insults such as hypotension, hypoxia, increased intracranial pressure, and changes in cerebral blood flow and metabolism. Skull fracture, edema, and acute hemorrhage can lead to increased intracranial pressure [5]. Direct mechanical damage through axonal shearing injury can also lead to hypothalamic-pituitary injury [6, 7].

Anterior pituitary dysfunction in survivors of TBI is more common than posterior lobe dysfunction, because the blood supply to the anterior lobe is derived from the long hypophyseal vessels and the portal capillaries in the pituitary stalk, which are more susceptible to damage than the short hypophyseal vessels that supply the posterior lobe. Located in the lateral regions of the anterior pituitary gland, somatotrophic and gonadotrophic cells are more vulnerable due to their location and blood supply. Distributed more centrally, corticotrophic and thyrotrophic cells may be somewhat less vulnerable.

Recent research suggests a possible role of autoimmunity in the development of hypopituitarism following TBI. Antipituitary antibodies are present in patients with TBI-induced pituitary dysfunction and persist even 3 years after diagnosis [8].

Predictors of poor outcome after TBI include altered systemic and cerebral hemodynamics. Three phases of change in cerebral blood flow following TBI have been documented: in the first 6–12 h after injury, the brain may suffer poor perfusion and cerebral ischemia. A second phase includes hyperemia and increased intracranial pressure. Finally, vasospasm and poor perfusion may follow [9].

## Diagnosis and Clinical Presentation

In childhood and adolescence, diminished height velocity represents the hallmark of GHD. Adults frequently report diminished exercise tolerance, develop central body fat distribution and dyslipidemia, and complain of fatigue and difficulty initiating activities.

For the somatotrophic axis evaluation after TBI, determination of IGF-I levels, plus dynamic testing with one or more GH secretagogues (e.g., GHRH + arginine, GHRH + GHRP-6, or glucagon), is indicated. Insulin-induced hypoglycemia (ITT) testing can be used when not contraindicated and experienced personnel performing this test are available. The choice of one test rather than another one often depends on the preference and familiarity with it of the endocrinology team, as well as the availability of the individual agents, a number of which are unavailable in the USA [10].

The time interval between TBI and pituitary function evaluation is one of the major factors responsible for the reported variations in the prevalence of GHD. Studies evaluating patients after TBI reported very high rates of GHD soon after initial trauma with a diminished rate in the first year of follow-up [11]. A recent study of 20 male patients who suffered mild combat-related TBI found a high prevalence (25 %) of GHD. Patients were evaluated >3 months after mild TBI, and GHD was defined by a GH peak <3 µg/L after glucagon stimulation test [12]. A multicenter study among 112 patients followed over 4 years, starting 1 year after a TBI, found a 2.7 % prevalence of patients meeting severe GHD criteria. A strict methodology included GHRH stimulation test to replace insulin tolerance test (ITT) only when the latter was formally contraindicated [13]. A large Danish registry illustrates in more detail how the testing modality can influence the prevalence of GHD. Four hundred and thirty-nine patients and 124 healthy controls underwent dynamic assessment of GH secretion 2.5 years after TBI. The authors found significant discordance among the tests, with GHRH-arginine assigning more GHD to patients than ITT [14]. Another study of 70 children who experienced TBI at a mean age of 8.1 years assessed pituitary function at least 1 year after head injury. Patients with mild, moderate, and severe TBI were included. All children underwent auxological evaluation at baseline and 6 months after the first evaluation. A GH stimulation test was performed only in those with slow growth velocity at 12 months of follow-up. A combined test using GHRH + arginine was used to stimulate peak GH secretion, and GHD was defined if GH peak was <20 µg/L. Thirteen patients with slow growth underwent GH stimulation and four (5.7 %) were diagnosed with GHD [15].

A prospective study argued in favor of systemic hormonal assessment in children and adolescents after severe TBI. In this study, 87 children and adolescents, median age 6.7 years, 9.5 months after severe TBI were recruited for basal and dynamic GH testing. The diagnosis of GHD was based on the association of two GH peaks <5 µg/L to stimulation and low IGF-I levels. The results indicated a 6 % prevalence of GHD [16]. In this study, the interval between the assessments was too short to calculate growth velocity accurately, and a longer follow-up is necessary to better analyze the GH/IGF-I axis.

A recent study in early childhood after structural TBI evaluated 156 children injured when less than 5 years of age but an average of 6.5 years after injury. Intracerebral hemorrhage, cerebral injury, and skull fracture occurred in most as an isolated event or in combination. The diagnosis of GHD was based on an integrated assessment of stimulated GH peak (<5 µg/L), IGF-I level, and growth pattern. In this study, 80 % of low GH responses to stimulation tests became normal when the tests were repeated, and the remainder had normal IGF-I levels and linear growth. The authors found no children with GHD and concluded that invasive assessment should be reserved for selected patients with slow growth and/or other clinical suspicion of GHD [17]. Another study in childhood evaluated patients 4.3 years after TBI. Mean age at injury was 9.5 years and included minor, moderate, and severe TBI. GHD was based on a peak GH <5 µg/L after ITT or glucagon test. A total of 33 patients underwent either ITT or glucagon test: while seven subjects (21 %) had suboptimal peak GH responses, all had height SDS within the normal range and six had normal height velocity; only one who had slow growth and suboptimal GH response was treated with GH despite findings consistent with constitutional delay of growth and puberty. It should be noted that priming with testosterone prior to the stimulation test was not performed. The authors concluded that their findings do not justify routine GH stimulation after TBI [18]. A recent study after TBI evaluated 36 children with mean age at injury of 3.8 years and meantime interval between head trauma and endocrine assessment of 3.3 years. All children had skull fractures or intracranial hemorrhage. Four had low IGF-I levels and were reassessed 1 year later. They all show spontaneous increase of IGF-I levels and normal height velocity. In this study, no subjects with GHD after TBI were found, and the authors argued in favor of monitoring growth in this population and against routine stimulation tests [19].

These studies exemplify some of the most important factors that may explain the marked variations in the prevalence of GHD reported after TBI, which include different populations, diverse severity of head trauma, various time intervals between head trauma and hormonal measurements, and different diagnostic testing protocols.

## Effects of GH Therapy in GH-Deficient Subjects Following TBI

Growth hormone has several targets in the central nervous system (CNS) including the limbic structures related to well-being and hypothalamic centers associated with pituitary hormone regulation [20]. Growth hormone deficiency, whether caused by TBI or other mechanisms, may lead to a syndrome of mental health-related problems including a decreased sense of well-being and loss of memory and cognitive capabilities [21]. In fact, it is the diminished sense of well-being that became a major factor in the approval process for GH therapy in GH-deficient adults in the USA. Beyond the reversal of some of the metabolic abnormalities, GH treatment of GH-deficient adults enhances energy, motivation, and sense of well-being.

There are objective findings for improved memory and cognitive capabilities following GH therapy [21, 22]. GH is permeable to the brain, and there are receptors for both GH and IGF-I in areas associated with cognitive function and behavior (reviewed in [21]). Some patients with GH deficiency following TBI experience improvements in motor and/or cognitive difficulties in response to therapy with GH [23, 24]. Whether the salutary effects of GH work directly through the GH receptor or indirectly through IGF-I production and then the IGF-I receptor is at present unknown; this issue is actively being researched.

## Conclusion

How and when to evaluate the GH axis after TBI in children and adults is evolving. Despite the inherent limitations to this field of research, available data depict the importance of evaluating patients with TBI for GHD. GHD affects not only linear growth, but may influence patients' overall well-being and cognition as manifested clinically through symptoms such as fatigue and memory problems. Growth hormone is a metabolic regulator as well, and there are profound effects on body composition and the regional distribution of body fat in those deficient. Replacement therapy may ameliorate these abnormalities [25, 26].

Pituitary function after TBI undergoes remarkable variation over time. Dissimilar methodologies could account for marked variations in prevalence of GHD, and the lack of a gold standard test for GHD raises questions regarding the true incidence of GHD after TBI. Although somewhat controversial, most recent well-designed studies in children argue in favor of performing dynamic GH tests only in those with slow growth after appropriate follow-up. All patients with documented severe GHD are candidates for GH replacement.

A note of caution is appropriate when encountering patients with severe TBI. It may very well be that prolongation of the acute stress response (see [27]) for approximately 3 months, at least in adults, is responsible for early abnormalities rather than brain damage itself. Early responses include increases of some stress hormones (cortisol and prolactin) with decreased gonadal and thyroid function. This is considered an adaptive response. Additionally, concomitant medications (e.g., antidepressants, antipsychotics, and antiemetics) may affect the evaluation. Most of the deficits defined at 3 months resolve by 12 months [27].

# References

1. Rutland-Brown W, Langlois JA, Xi YL. Incidence of traumatic brain injury in the United States, 2003. J Head Trauma Rehabil. 2006;21:544–8.
2. Zaloshnja E, Miller T, Langlois JA, Selassie AW. Prevalence of long-term disability from traumatic brain injury in the civilian population of the United States, 2005. J Head Trauma Rehabil. 2008;23:394–400.
3. Cyran E. Hypophysenschadigung durch Schadelbasisfraktur. Dtsch Med Wschr. 1918;44:1261.
4. Schneider HJ, Schneider M, Saller B, Petersenn S, Uhr M, et al. Prevalence of anterior pituitary insufficiency 3 and 12 months after traumatic brain injury. Eur J Endocrinol. 2006;154:259–65.
5. Wachter D, Gündling K, Oertel MF, Stracke H, Böker DK. Pituitary insufficiency after traumatic brain injury. J Clin Neurosci. 2009;16:202–8.
6. Salehi F, Kovacs K, Scheithauer BW, Pfeifer EA, Cusimano M. Histologic study of the human pituitary gland in acute traumatic brain injury. Brain Inj. 2007;21:651–6.
7. Benvenga S, Campenni A, Ruggeri RM, Trimarchi F. Clinical review 113: hypopituitarism secondary to head trauma. J Clin Endocrinol Metab. 2000;85:1353–61.
8. Tanriverdi F, De Bellis A, Battaglia M, Bellastella G, Bizzarro A, et al. Investigation of antihypothalamus and antipituitary antibodies in amateur boxers: is chronic repetitive head trauma-induced pituitary dysfunction associated with autoimmunity? Eur J Endocrinol. 2010;162:861–7.
9. White JR, Farukhi Z, Bull C, Christensen J, Gordon T, Paidas C, Nichols DG. Predictors of outcome in severely head-injured children. Crit Care Med. 2001;29:534–40.
10. Gasco V, Prodam F, Pagano L, Grottoli S, Belcastro S, et al. Hypopituitarism following brain injury: when does it occur and how best to test? Pituitary. 2012;15:20–4.
11. Schneider HJ, Kreitschmann-Andermahr I, Ghigo E, Stalla GK, Agha A. Hypothalamopituitary dysfunction following traumatic brain injury and aneurysmal subarachnoid hemorrhage: a systematic review. JAMA. 2007;298:1429–38.
12. Ioachimescu AG, Hampstead BM, Moore A, Burgess E, Phillips LS. Growth hormone deficiency after mild combat-related traumatic brain injury. Pituitary. 2014. doi:10.1007/s11102-014-0606-5.
13. Kokshoorn NE, Smit JW, Nieuwlaat WA, Tiemensma J, Bisschop PH, Groote Veldman R, et al. Low prevalence of hypopituitarism after traumatic brain injury: a multicenter study. Eur J Endocrinol. 2011;165:225–31.
14. Klose M, Stochholm K, Janukonyte J, Lehman Christensen L, Frystyk J, Andersen M, et al. Prevalence of posttraumatic growth hormone deficiency is highly dependent on the diagnostic set-up: results from The Danish National Study on Posttraumatic Hypopituitarism. J Clin Endocrinol Metab. 2014;99:101–10.
15. Bellone S, Einaudi S, Caputo M, Prodam F, Busti A, Belcastro S, et al. Measurement of height velocity is a useful marker for monitoring pituitary function in patients who had traumatic brain injury. Pituitary. 2013;16:499–506.
16. Personnier C, Crosnier H, Meyer P, Chevignard M, Flechtner I, Boddaert N, et al. Prevalence of pituitary dysfunction after severe traumatic brain injury in children and adolescents: a large prospective study. J Clin Endocrinol Metab. 2014;99:2052–60.
17. Heather NL, Jefferies C, Hofman PL, Derraik JG, Brennan C, Kelly P, et al. Permanent hypopituitarism is rare after structural traumatic brain injury in early childhood. J Clin Endocrinol Metab. 2012;97:599–604.
18. Khadr SN, Crofton PM, Jones PA, Wardhaugh B, Roach J, Drake AJ, et al. Evaluation of pituitary function after traumatic brain injury in childhood. Clin Endocrinol (Oxf). 2010;73:637–43.
19. Salomon-Estebanez MA, Grau G, Vela A, Rodriguez A, Morteruel E, Castaño L, et al. Is routine endocrine evaluation necessary after paediatric traumatic brain injury? J Endocrinol Invest. 2014;37:143–8.

20. Nyberg F. The role of the somatotropic axis in neuroprotection and neuroregeneration of the addictive brain. Int Rev Neurobiol. 2009;88:399–427.
21. Nyberg F. Growth hormone and cognitive function. Nat Rev Endocrinol. 2013;9:357–65.
22. Deijen JB, de Boer H, van der Veen EA. Cognitive changes during growth hormone replacement in adult men. Psychoneuroendocrinology. 1998;23:45–55.
23. Maric NP, Doknic M, Pavlovic D, Pekic S, Stojanovic M, et al. Psychiatric and neuropsychological changes in growth hormone-deficient patients after traumatic brain injury in response to growth hormone therapy. J Endocrinol Invest. 2010;33:770–5.
24. Devesa J, Reimunde P, Devesa P, Barbera M, Arce V. Growth hormone (GH) and brain trauma. Horm Behav. 2013;63:331–44.
25. Birzniece V, Khaw CH, Nelson AE, Meinhardt U, Ho KK. A critical evaluation of bioimpedance spectroscopy analysis in estimating body composition during GH treatment: comparison with bromide dilution and dual X-ray absorptiometry. Eur J Endocrinol. 2015;172:21–8.
26. Molitch ME, Clemmons DR, Malozowski S, Merriam GR, Vance ML, Endocrine Society. Evaluation and treatment of adult growth hormone deficiency: an Endocrine Society clinical practice guideline. J Clin Endocrinol Metab. 2011;96:1587–609.
27. Marina D, Klose M, Nordenbo A, Liebach A, Feldt-Rasmussen U. Early endocrine alterations reflect prolonged stress and relate to one year functional outcome in patients with severe brain injury. Eur J Endocrinol. 2015;172:813–22.

# Chapter 15
# Syndromes Associated with Growth Hormone Deficiency

Sara A. DiVall

Normal pituitary development is a prerequisite for normal growth hormone (GH) synthesis and secretion. Pituitary development involves a cascade of events that begin at week 4 in the fetus with formation of Rathke's pouch, culminating in a fully differentiated adenohypophysis by week 16. Significant cerebral, heart, and limb maturation also occurs during this developmental window. Therefore, growth hormone deficiency (GHD) is often seen as one feature of a syndrome with multiple defects in various organs.

This chapter will discuss some major syndromes in which GH deficiency is a major feature. Many syndromes that feature GHD also feature other cranial defects. Polygenetic, single-gene, or deletion syndromes will be discussed. The current level of knowledge regarding underlying genetic and pathophysiologic mechanisms is presented. Single-gene defects implicated in combined pituitary hormone deficiency (CPHD), pituitary stalk formation, or isolated GH deficiency will not be discussed as they are covered elsewhere in this book (Chaps. 11 and 12).

*Septo-optic Dysplasia* A syndrome commonly encountered in modern pediatric endocrine practice is septo-optic dysplasia (SOD) present in 0.8–1 in 10,000 births [1, 2]. Previously called de Morsier syndrome, it classically entails the absence of the septum pellucidum, optic nerve hypoplasia/abnormalities, and hypopituitarism. However, it encompasses a wide spectrum of severity and manifestations, so diagnosis is made clinically if two of the three features are present [3]. Absence of the corpus callosum, whether in the absence or presence of the septum pellucidum, is considered by some to meet diagnostic criteria [4]. In case series [2, 5], 25–30 % of SOD cases have all three features, while 62–80 % have pituitary hormone deficiencies and 60–65 % have an absent septum pellucidum. The pituitary dysfunction can range from isolated GH deficiency (11 % of SOD cases) to variable degrees

---

S.A. DiVall (✉)
Pediatric Endocrinology, Seattle Children's Hospital, Seattle, WA 98105, USA
e-mail: sara.divall@seattlechildrens.org

of anterior hypopituitarism (55 %), and 18 % have additional neurohypophysis dysfunction with diabetes insipidus [2]. Rarely, isolated neurohypophysis dysfunction is described.

Children with SOD commonly present at birth in the context of midline abnormalities or clinical signs/symptoms of neonatal hypopituitarism. Children can also present later in infancy upon investigation of visual disturbances and subsequent diagnosis of optic nerve hypoplasia or even later with growth delay [3]. Upon initial diagnosis of optic nerve hypoplasia, up to 80 % have some pituitary dysfunction [6], leading to recommendations that children diagnosed with optic nerve hypoplasia have a thorough endocrine and neurological evaluation. In multiple series [5, 6], it was observed that the degree of hypopituitarism can evolve in some children with SOD, prompting recommendations to regularly evaluate diagnosed children for additional pituitary hormone deficiencies. There is also heterogeneity in neurological manifestations and the degree of ophthalmological and neurological dysfunction [7].

Considering the associated brain abnormalities, it is widely accepted that SOD is a developmental abnormality of the early forebrain. However, underlying genetic abnormalities are found in <1 % of patients with SOD [8]. *HESX1* mutations have been reported, with affected patients exhibiting variable phenotypes [8]. *HESX1* is a member of the homeobox gene family. It is expressed in the ectoderm very early in development in the area that gives rise to the ventral prosencephalon (that later becomes Rathke's pouch) and forebrain. Gene expression diminishes after 4–5 days. It is a transcriptional repressor; the diminution of its expression is thought to be important for the increase in transcription of other genes important for pituitary development such as *PROP1*. Thirteen separate mutations (homozygous and heterozygous) have been described thus far. In general, mutations result in proteins with altered binding of HESX1 to DNA [8]. However, one described mutation in a patient with classic SOD resulted in a HESX1 that exhibited enhanced DNA binding [9]. Theoretically, enhanced repression may also prevent subsequent expression of pituitary development genes. The mouse model of targeted disruption of *Hesx1* exhibits a phenotype that resembles SOD in humans [8].

Risk factors for SOD include young maternal age and primiparity [2]. It has been suggested that antenatal smoking or alcohol use are also risk factors [2, 8]. Given the varied presentation, risk factors, and low incidence of causal mutations, it has been hypothesized that SOD may result from a vascular disruption sequence [10].

Ten separate SOX2 mutations have been described in patients with anophthalmia and various degrees of hypogonadotropic hypogonadism and anterior pituitary hypoplasia [8]. Interestingly, in only one mutation has the phenotype included GH deficiency [11].

*Holoprosencephaly Sequence*: The holoprosencephaly (HPE) sequence is also a developmental defect in forebrain development. It occurs in approximately 1/10,000 births. The forebrain does not separate at all or to varying degrees, resulting in a spectrum of clinical phenotypes. Complete absence of forebrain results in cyclopia, whereas near-complete separation leads to mild signs of incomplete midline facial development such as cleft lip and palate, hypotelorism, and single central incisor.

Extracranial defects are also seen. HPE is thought to result from chromosomal abnormalities, teratogenic exposure (e.g., gestational diabetes), or secondary to genetic mutations, with mutations in 12 genes described [12].

Diabetes insipidus is common, with anterior pituitary deficiencies variably described [12]. Mutation in either of four genes (*SHH*, *ZIC2*, *SIX3*, and *TGIF*) underlies about 25–30 % of nonchromosomal, nonsyndromic HPE [12, 13]. The presence of anterior hypopituitarism with accompanying GH deficiency was reported in <5 % of patients with *SHH* mutation [14].

Mutations in *GLI2* were found in patients with HPE associated with hypopituitarism [15]. However, a later study found pathogenic *GLI2* mutations in persons with congenital hypopituitarism but without HPE [16]. Later analysis of 400 persons with HPE-like disorders or craniofacial anomalies clarified that of the 112 patients identified with variants in *GLI2*, only 3 % had HPE with clear lobar abnormalities [17]. Of the persons with *GLI2* variants that could potentially lead to GLI2 malfunction (such as truncating mutations), over 80 % had reported pituitary insufficiencies with 90 % having polydactyly [17]. For persons with truncating mutations, common facial features included midface hypoplasia, cleft lip/palate, or hypotelorism. Thus, pathologic *GLI2* mutations may exhibit a phenotype that is distinct from HPE.

GLI2 is a zinc-finger transcription factor that is downstream from SHH signaling. Global deletion of the Gli2 gene in mice is embryonically lethal with loss of the pituitary in half of embryos [18]. Mice with targeted disruption of *Gli2* in neural ridge cells that later invaginate into Rathke's pouch exhibit a small pituitary due to diminished cell proliferation, but not alteration in cell patterning/fate [19]. *Gli2* disrupted cells cannot express Bmp4 or Fgf8, genes involved in the proper formation and closure of Rathke's pouch [19].

*Pallister-Hall Syndrome*: Minimal diagnostic criteria for Pallister-Hall syndrome (PHS) include hypothalamic hamartoma and polydactyly with the polydactyly seemingly inherited in an autosomal dominant manner. Affected patients may also have variable pituitary hormone deficiencies, intracranial defects, genital abnormalities, imperforate anus, or renal abnormalities. There is a range of severity; severe cases can result in multiple organ malformation and large hypothalamic hamartomas with neonatal lethality. Affected family members can have a milder phenotype of isolated polydactyly. Persons with a severe phenotype of PHS have phenotypic features that overlap with syndromes such as Greig cephalopolysyndactyly or Smith-Lemli-Opitz. However, unlike Smith-Lemli-Opitz, persons with PHS do not have evidence of a defect in cholesterol biosynthesis.

PHS is a rare disorder; molecular characterization was carried out in 52 patients from 26 families in the USA [20] and 21 patients from 17 families in Europe [21]. Severe and mild phenotypes of PHS are correlated to heterozygous mutations in *GLI3* [20, 21]. Patients with PHS have mutations that cause a truncated form of the GLI3 protein with the pathologic mutations occurring in the middle third of the gene, in regions that translate into a proteolytic cleavage site, or in a transactivation domain. The zinc-finger DNA-binding domain is not affected. Interestingly, patients with Greig cephalopolysyndactyly (who do not have pituitary insufficiency but have other deformities similar to PHS) have mutations in other regions of *GLI3* that do not result in a truncated protein. Like GLI2, GLI3 is a zinc-finger protein of the SHH pathway. It functions as a transcriptional activator in the presence of SHH and repressor in the absence of SHH. Global *Gli3* gene deletion is embryonically lethal in mice [22], but the global knockout has normal proliferation late in pituitary development after closure of Rathke's pouch [19]. The combined *Gli2/Gli3* disrupted embryo, however, has no pituitary development in all embryos. This suggests overlapping roles for *Gli2* and *Gli3* in mice. Thus, the mechanism underlying the pituitary malformation in persons with a truncated GLI3 protein (with presumably normal GLI2 function) is not fully elucidated.

*CHARGE Syndrome*: CHARGE syndrome is comprised of **c**oloboma, **h**eart anomaly, **c**hoanal atresia, (growth) **r**etardation, **g**enital, and **e**ar anomalies. It is present in 1–2/10,000 births and is clinically diagnosed according to specified four major and seven minor criteria [23]. Up to 80 % of persons have poor postnatal growth with height less than-2SD commonly seen. Hypogonadotropic hypogonadism is seen in approximately 90 % of patients, often accompanied by anosmia. In case series varying from 15 to 32 patients, 5–10 % of patients clinically diagnosed with CHARGE syndrome have GHD based upon auxologic criteria, insulin-like growth factor-I (IGF-I) levels, and GH stimulation tests [24–26]. In all series, pituitary anatomy was reported as normal. In at least one series, the persons with GHD were found to be a height of -3SD [24]. Of the three patients treated in one study, the mean change in height standard deviation score (SDS) was 1.33 with an average duration of GH therapy of 2 years. Thus, given the high baseline incidence of postnatal growth failure, it is unclear whether patients with CHARGE syndrome and GH deficiency have similar growth response to GH therapy as other children with GH deficiency.

Up to 90 % of patients who meet strict clinical criteria of CHARGE syndrome have heterozygous mutations or deletions in CHD7 (chromodomain helicase DNA-binding protein) [27]. A minority of persons who meet some, but not all, of the clinical criteria for CHARGE syndrome have *CHD7* mutations; conversely, *CHD7* mutations have been found in relatives of probands with very mild ear abnormalities. CHD7 is a transcriptional regulator that interacts with the gene *PBAF* to affect neural crest formation [28]. It is expressed in the pituitary. Homozygous *Chd7* deletion in mice is embryonically lethal; hypoplasia of Rathke's pouch and the olfactory pit is noted [29]. Gregory et al. described two patients with CHARGE syndrome, GHD, and ectopic posterior pituitary with *CHD7* gene variations that resulted in a splice variation that were carried by a seemingly unaffected parent [30]. Thus, the role of CHD7 in the pituitary malformation of these patients is unclear.

*Axenfeld-Rieger Syndrome* Axenfeld-Rieger syndrome (ARS) refers to overlapping conditions that all feature dysgenesis of the anterior segment of the eye including iris hypoplasia, corneal abnormalities, and changes in the chamber angle. These features cause glaucoma in the majority of patients. Some persons also have hypodontia/microdontia, redundant umbilical skin, cardiac defects, anal stenosis, hypospadias, and GHD. It is estimated to affect about 1/200,000 live births. ARS has been associated with deletion in the *PITX2* or *FOXC2* gene in 40 % of cases [31]. In general, persons with *PITX2* gene deletion have the extraocular features, while those with FOXC2 mutations do not [32]. The incidence of GHD in ARS syndrome has not been reported.

Given the rarity of the disorder, the relative incidence of *PITX2* vs. *FOXC2* mutations in persons with ARS has not been determined. *PITX2* encodes for the pituitary homeobox 2 gene, while *FOXC2* encodes for forkhead box C2 gene. Both are transcription factors expressed early in embryonic development. In animal studies, Pitx2 is an early transcription factor expressed in oral ectoderm from which Rathke's pouch emerges. It is regulated by NF1 and TCF/LEF in early ectoderm [33]. Pitx2 is both a transcriptional repressor and activator; the Wnt/Dvl/beta-catenin pathway induces *Pitx2* expression and also serves to induce the switch from transcriptional repressor to activator [34]. In the pituitary, *Pitx2* induces transcription of genes important in pituitary development including *Pou1f1* (*Pit1*), *Plod-1*, *Lef-1*, and possibly *Hesx1* [32]. In other tissues, Pitx2 induces cyclin D2 activity and therefore cell proliferation [34]. In this way, Pitx2 plays a broad role in tissue development including dental and cardiac tissue. Homozygous null deletion of *Pitx2* in mice leads to absence of pituitary development, as well as ventral wall and heart defects. Heterozygous null mice exhibit eye defects [35] implying a gene dosage effect.

In ARS families, the same mutation may result in different phenotypes. Height within the normal range has been described in the majority of persons with ARS. The phenotypic variability and mild pituitary phenotype imply redundancy to the molecular actions of Pitx2 in tissues.

*Prader-Willi Syndrome*: Prader-Willi syndrome (PWS) features hypotonia, poor feeding during infancy, hyperphagia after age 3 causing obesity, hypogonadotropic hypogonadism, short stature, and cognitive delay with behavioral difficulties. The estimated prevalence of the disease is 1/10,000 to 1/25,000. Age-specific diagnostic criteria were developed in 1993 before the advent of diagnostic testing [36]. Some have advocated loosening the diagnostic criteria, since an estimated 15–20 % of persons with molecular alterations consistent with PWS do not meet the strict clinical diagnostic criteria [37]. Guidelines for the care of children with PWS have been published [38, 39] which include information on clinical diagnosis and criteria for molecular testing as well as health maintenance.

Some features of PWS are also features in persons with untreated classic GHD (low muscle tone, short stature despite obesity, altered body composition, low IGF-I levels). Many children also fail GH-provocative testing, although interpretation of GH stimulation testing in the setting of obesity is problematic (see Chap. 6). The similarities between PWS and classic GHD led to trials testing the effectiveness of GH in PWS. Multiple trials have shown improvement in growth velocity and body composition in children with PWS (for review, see 40) treated with GH. This led to a PWS-specific indication for GH therapy by the FDA in 2000. Cases of sudden death in PWS after initiation of GH have been reported. The deaths were thought to be due to worsening of baseline obstructive sleep apnea by GH-induced increase in lymphoid tissue. For this reason, baseline polysomnography and treatment of sleep apnea is recommended prior to initiating GH in PWS patients [40]. Clinical outcome goals and consideration for discontinuation of GH in adolescents and adults who have reached adult height have not been firmly established. Guidelines specific to the use of GH in PWS have been developed [40].

PWS is present when genes of the paternal allele in the chromosomal region 15q11-q13 are not expressed. Non-expression of the paternally inherited genes in this region may be due to the deletion of the paternally inherited allele (70 % of cases) or inheritance and thus expression of the maternal allele only (uniparental disomy; 20 % of cases). This chromosomal region contains many genes that are subject to imprinting, which leads to silencing of gene expression on a particular allele. About 5 % of cases are due to altered imprinting of genes in this region, effectively silencing the paternal allele. Less than 5 % of cases are due to chromosomal translocation. The 15q11-q13 region is flanked by regions of DNA that are duplicated, which predisposes the whole region to deletion events. Altered methylation genes to silence it (imprinting defect) are a heritable trait; thus, it is important to identify these children and counsel the parents on heritability in future offspring.

Recommendations for molecular diagnosis in individuals exhibiting features of PWS have been published [38, 39]. It is recommended that methylation analysis occur first to document the absence of the paternal allele, as there are methylation patterns unique to the maternal or paternal allele. If the paternal allele is absent, then analysis progresses to in site fluorescence hybridization (FISH) to investigate for allelic deletions. If normal, then investigation for uniparental disomy ensues. If both maternal and paternal alleles are present (independent of the methylation pattern), then a methylation defect is the cause.

The genes in the 15q11-q13 region include genes that encode for polypeptides (*MKRN3*, *MAGEL2*, *NECDIN*, *SNURF-SNRPN*) and six small nucleolar RNA (snoRNA) genes [41]. *SNURF-SNRPN* regulates the expression of the snoRNA genes. To date, there is not convincing evidence that absence of a single gene in the region leads to the PWS phenotype. Persons with truncating mutations in *MKRN3* have precocious puberty without PWS features [42]. Isolated truncating mutations in *MAGEL2* have been implicated in four persons with PWS-like features [43] and the *Magel2* null mouse has some features of PWS [44]. Yet, persons with PWS and intact *MAGEL2* have been described [45]. Additionally, reports of individuals with microdeletions in the snoRNA region (specifically in the region of *SNORD116*) also exhibit features of PWS [46]. Mice with deletion of *Snord116* exhibit growth retardation with and deficiencies in motor learning with moderate hyperphagia [47].

*Other Syndromes*: Case reports or series in which GHD has been described in other genetic syndromes are listed in Table 15.1. In many of the cases, the etiology of the GH secretion abnormality is unclear, either because the underlying genetic defect is not known or the gene defect described does not clearly involve GH synthesis or secretion. In other cases, such as mitochondrial disorders, general cellular dysfunction may lead to both poor GH secretion and cellular response to GH. Table 15.1 is divided into syndromes associated with cranial defects and those that are not associated with cranial defects, as well as mitochondrial disorders.

Table 15.1 Other syndromes with reported Growth hormone Deficiency

| Sub-category | Syndrome | Reference |
| --- | --- | --- |
| With craniofacial abnormalities | DiGeorge | [48] |
| | Robinow | [49] |
| | Craniofaciocutaneous | [50] |
| | Costello | [51] |
| | Joubert | [52] |
| | Kabuki | [53] |
| | Peters plus | [54] |
| Without craniofacial abnormalities | IMAGe | [55] |
| Mitochondrial diseases | Kearns-Sayre | [56] |
| | MELAS | [57] |

# References

1. Patel L, McNally RJQ, Harrison E, Lloyd IC, Clayton PE. Geographical distribution of optic nerve hypoplasia and septo-optic dysplasia in Northwest England. J Pediatr. 2006;148(1):85–8.
2. Atapattu N, Ainsworth J, Willshaw H, Parulekar M, MacPherson L, Miller C, et al. Septo-optic dysplasia: antenatal risk factors and clinical features in a regional study. Horm Res Paediatr. 2012;78(2):81–7.
3. Webb EA, Dattani MT. Septo-optic dysplasia. Eur J Hum Genet. 2010;18(4):393–7.
4. Barkovich AJ, Fram EK, Norman D. Septo-optic dysplasia: MR imaging. Radiology. 1989;171(1):189–92.
5. Morishima A, Aranoff GS. Syndrome of septo-optic-pituitary dysplasia: the clinical spectrum. Brain Dev. 1986;8(3):233–9.
6. Haddad NG, Eugster EA. Hypopituitarism and neurodevelopmental abnormalities in relation to central nervous system structural defects in children with optic nerve hypoplasia. J Pediatr Endocrinol Metab. 2005;18(9):853–8.
7. Garcia ML, Ty EB, Taban M, David Rothner A, Rogers D, Traboulsi EI. Systemic and ocular findings in 100 patients with optic nerve hypoplasia. J Child Neurol. 2006;21(11):949–56.
8. McCabe MJ, Alatzoglou KS, Dattani MT. Septo-optic dysplasia and other midline defects: the role of transcription factors: HESX1 and beyond. Best Pract Res Clin Endocrinol Metab. 2011;25(1):115–24.
9. Cohen RN, Cohen LE, Botero D, Yu C, Sagar A, Jurkiewicz M, et al. Enhanced repression by HESX1 as a cause of hypopituitarism and septooptic dysplasia. J Clin Endocrinol Metab. 2003;88(10):4832–9.
10. Stevens CA, Dobyns WB. Septo-optic dysplasia and amniotic bands: further evidence for a vascular pathogenesis. Am J Med Genet A. 2004;125A(1):12–6.
11. Macchiaroli A, Kelberman D, Auriemma RS, Drury S, Islam L, Giangiobbe S, et al. A novel heterozygous SOX2 mutation causing congenital bilateral anophthalmia, hypogonadotropic hypogonadism and growth hormone deficiency. Gene. 2014;534(2):282–5.
12. Solomon BD, Mercier S, Velez JI, Pineda-Alvarez DE, Wyllie A, Zhou N, et al. Analysis of genotype-phenotype correlations in human holoprosencephaly. Am J Med Genet C Semin Med Genet. 2010;154C(1):133–41.
13. Mercier S, Dubourg C, Garcelon N, Campillo-Gimenez B, Gicquel I, Belleguic M, et al. New findings for phenotype-genotype correlations in a large European series of holoprosencephaly cases. J Med Genet. 2011;48(11):752–60.
14. Solomon BD, Bear KA, Wyllie A, Keaton AA, Dubourg C, David V, et al. Genotypic and phenotypic analysis of 396 individuals with mutations in Sonic Hedgehog. J Med Genet. 2012;49(7):473–9.

15. Roessler E, Du Y, Mullor JL, Casas E, Allen WP, Gillessen-Kaesbach G, et al. Loss-of-function mutations in the human GLI2 gene are associated with pituitary anomalies and holoprosencephaly-like features. Proc Natl Acad Sci. 2003;100(23):13424–9.
16. Franca MM, Jorge AA, Carvalho LR, Costalonga EF, Vasques GA, Leite CC, et al. Novel heterozygous nonsense GLI2 mutations in patients with hypopituitarism and ectopic posterior pituitary lobe without holoprosencephaly. J Clin Endocrinol Metab. 2010;95(11):E384–91.
17. Bear KA, Solomon BD, Antonini S, Arnhold IJ, Franca MM, Gerkes EH, et al. Pathogenic mutations in GLI2 cause a specific phenotype that is distinct from holoprosencephaly. J Med Genet. 2014;51(6):413–8.
18. Park HL, Bai C, Platt KA, Matise MP, Beeghly A, Hui CC, et al. Mouse Gli1 mutants are viable but have defects in SHH signaling in combination with a Gli2 mutation. Development. 2000;127(8):1593–605.
19. Wang Y, Martin JF, Bai CB. Direct and indirect requirements of Shh/Gli signaling in early pituitary development. Dev Biol. 2010;348(2):199–209.
20. Johnston JJ, Olivos-Glander I, Killoran C, Elson E, Turner JT, Peters KF, et al. Molecular and clinical analyses of Greig cephalopolysyndactyly and Pallister-Hall syndromes: robust phenotype prediction from the type and position of GLI3 mutations. Am J Hum Genet. 2005;76(4):609–22.
21. Demurger F, Ichkou A, Mougou-Zerelli S, Le Merrer M, Goudefroye G, Delezoide AL, et al. New insights into genotype-phenotype correlation for GLI3 mutations. Eur J Hum Genet. 2015;23(1):92–102.
22. Aoto K, Nishimura T, Eto K, Motoyama J. Mouse GLI3 regulates Fgf8 expression and apoptosis in the developing neural tube, face, and limb bud. Dev Biol. 2002;251(2):320–32.
23. Hsu P, Ma A, Wilson M, Williams G, Curotta J, Munns CF, et al. CHARGE syndrome: a review. J Paediatr Child Health. 2014;50(7):504–11.
24. Pinto G, Abadie V, Mesnage R, Blustajn J, Cabrol S, Amiel J, et al. CHARGE syndrome includes hypogonadotropic hypogonadism and abnormal olfactory bulb development. J Clin Endocrinol Metab. 2005;90(10):5621–6.
25. Asakura Y, Toyota Y, Muroya K, Kurosawa K, Fujita K, Aida N, et al. Endocrine and radiological studies in patients with molecularly confirmed CHARGE syndrome. J Clin Endocrinol Metab. 2008;93(3):920–4.
26. Shoji Y, Ida S, Etani Y, Yamada H, Kayatani F, Suzuki Y, et al. Endocrinological characteristics of 25 Japanese patients with CHARGE syndrome. Clin Pediatr Endocrinol. 2014;23(2):45–51.
27. Bergman JE, Janssen N, Hoefsloot LH, Jongmans MC, Hofstra RM, van Ravenswaaij-Arts CM. CHD7 mutations and CHARGE syndrome: the clinical implications of an expanding phenotype. J Med Genet. 2011;48(5):334–42.
28. Bajpai R, Chen DA, Rada-Iglesias A, Zhang J, Xiong Y, Helms J, et al. CHD7 cooperates with PBAF to control multipotent neural crest formation. Nature. 2010;463(7283):958–62.
29. Hurd EA, Capers PL, Blauwkamp MN, Adams ME, Raphael Y, Poucher HK, et al. Loss of Chd7 function in gene-trapped reporter mice is embryonic lethal and associated with severe defects in multiple developing tissues. Mamm Genome. 2007;18(2):94–104.
30. Gregory LC, Gevers EF, Baker J, Kasia T, Chong K, Josifova DJ, et al. Structural pituitary abnormalities associated with CHARGE syndrome. J Clin Endocrinol Metab. 2013;98(4):E737–43.
31. Titheradge H, Togneri F, McMullan D, Brueton L, Lim D, Williams D. Axenfeld-Rieger syndrome: further clinical and array delineation of four unrelated patients with a 4q25 microdeletion. Am J Med Genet A. 2014;164(7):1695–701.
32. Tumer Z, Bach-Holm D. Axenfeld-Rieger syndrome and spectrum of PITX2 and FOXC1 mutations. Eur J Hum Genet. 2009;17(12):1527–39.
33. Ai D, Wang J, Amen M, Lu M, Amendt BA, Martin JF. Nuclear factor 1 and T-cell factor/LEF recognition elements regulate Pitx2 transcription in pituitary development. Mol Cell Biol. 2007;27(16):5765–75.

34. Kioussi C, Briata P, Baek SH, Rose DW, Hamblet NS, Herman T, et al. Identification of a Wnt/Dvl/β-Catenin → Pitx2 pathway mediating cell-type-specific proliferation during development. Cell. 2002;111(5):673–85.
35. Gage PJ, Suh H, Camper SA. Dosage requirement of Pitx2 for development of multiple organs. Development. 1999;126(20):4643–51.
36. Holm VA, Cassidy SB, Butler MG, Hanchett JM, Greenswag LR, Whitman BY, et al. Prader-Willi syndrome: consensus diagnostic criteria. Pediatrics. 1993;91(2):398–402.
37. Gunay-Aygun M, Schwartz S, Heeger S, O'Riordan MA, Cassidy SB. The changing purpose of Prader-Willi syndrome clinical diagnostic criteria and proposed revised criteria. Pediatrics. 2001;108(5):e92.
38. Goldstone AP, Holland AJ, Hauffa BP, Hokken-Koelega A, Tauber M. Recommendations for the diagnosis and management of Prader-Willi syndrome. J Clin Endocrinol Metab. 2008;93(11):4183–97.
39. The Committee on Genetics. Health supervision for children with Prader-Willi syndrome. Pediatrics. 2011;127(1):195–204.
40. Deal CL, Tony M, Höybye C, Allen DB, Tauber M, Christiansen JS, et al. Growth Hormone Research Society workshop summary: consensus guidelines for recombinant human growth hormone therapy in Prader-Willi syndrome. J Clin Endocrinol Metab. 2013;98(6):E1072–87.
41. Cassidy SB, Schwartz S, Miller JL, Driscoll DJ. Prader-Willi syndrome. Genet Med. 2012;14(1):10–26.
42. Abreu AP, Dauber A, Macedo DB, Noel SD, Brito VN, Gill JC, et al. Central precocious puberty caused by mutations in the imprinted gene MKRN3. N Engl J Med. 2013;368(26):2467–75.
43. Schaaf CP, Gonzalez-Garay ML, Xia F, Potocki L, Gripp KW, Zhang B, et al. Truncating mutations of MAGEL2 cause Prader-Willi phenotypes and autism. Nat Genet. 2013;45(11):1405–8.
44. Bischof JM, Stewart CL, Wevrick R. Inactivation of the mouse Magel2 gene results in growth abnormalities similar to Prader-Willi syndrome. Hum Mol Genet. 2007;16(22):2713–9.
45. Kanber D, Giltay J, Wieczorek D, Zogel C, Hochstenbach R, Caliebe A, et al. A paternal deletion of MKRN3, MAGEL2 and NDN does not result in Prader-Willi syndrome. Eur J Hum Genet. 2009;17(5):582–90.
46. Bieth E, Eddiry S, Gaston V, Lorenzini F, Buffet A, Conte Auriol F, et al. Highly restricted deletion of the SNORD116 region is implicated in Prader-Willi syndrome. Eur J Hum Genet. 2015;23(2):252–5.
47. Ding F, Li HH, Zhang S, Solomon NM, Camper SA, Cohen P, et al. SnoRNA Snord116 (Pwcr1/MBII-85) deletion causes growth deficiency and hyperphagia in mice. PLoS One. 2008;3(3):e1709.
48. Weinzimer SA, McDonald-McGinn DM, Driscoll DA, Emanuel BS, Zackai EH, Moshang T. Growth hormone deficiency in patients with a 22q11.2 deletion: expanding the phenotype. Pediatrics. 1998;101(5):929–32.
49. Castells S, Chakurkar A, Qazi Q, Bastian W. Robinow syndrome with growth hormone deficiency: treatment with growth hormone. J Pediatr Endocrinol Metab. 1999;12(4):565–71.
50. Schulz AL, Albrecht B, Arici C, van der Burgt I, Buske A, Gillessen-Kaesbach G, et al. Mutation and phenotypic spectrum in patients with cardio-facio-cutaneous and Costello syndrome. Clin Genet. 2008;73(1):62–70.
51. Stein RI, Legault L, Daneman D, Weksberg R, Hamilton J. Growth hormone deficiency in Costello syndrome. Am J Med Genet A. 2004;129A(2):166–70.
52. Valente EM, Brancati F, Boltshauser E, Dallapiccola B. Clinical utility gene card for: Joubert syndrome--update 2013. Eur J Hum Genet 2013;21(10). doi:10.1038/ejhg.2013.10. Epub 2013 Feb 13.
53. Schrander-Stumpel CT, Spruyt L, Curfs LM, Defloor T, Schrander JJ. Kabuki syndrome: clinical data in 20 patients, literature review, and further guidelines for preventive management. Am J Med Genet A. 2005;132A(3):234–43.
54. Lee KW, Lee PD. Growth hormone deficiency (GHD): a new association in Peters' Plus Syndrome (PPS). Am J Med Genet A. 2004;124A(4):388–91.

55. Pedreira CC, Savarirayan R, Zacharin MR. IMAGe syndrome: a complex disorder affecting growth, adrenal and gonadal function, and skeletal development. J Pediatr. 2004;144(2):274–7.
56. Berio A, Piazzi A. Multiple endocrinopathies (growth hormone deficiency, autoimmune hypothyroidism and diabetes mellitus) in Kearns-Sayre syndrome. Pediatr Med Chir. 2013;35(3):137–40.
57. Matsuzaki M, Izumi T, Shishikura K, Suzuki H, Hirayama Y. Hypothalamic growth hormone deficiency and supplementary GH therapy in two patients with mitochondrial myopathy, encephalopathy, lactic acidosis and stroke-like episodes. Neuropediatrics. 2002;33(5):271–3.

# Index

**A**
Adiponectin, 85–86
Adiposity, 63–64, 68, 69, 72, 79, 83, 85, 153
Adrenocorticotropin (ACTH), 141, 142, 178, 183, 185
Adult GHD
  arginine test, 115, 116
  diagnosis, 110–111
  GH secretion, 109
  ghrelin mimetics, 116–118
  GHRH-arginine test, 114–115
  GST, 113, 114, 118
  IGF-I, 109
  ITT, 111, 112, 118
  laboratory testing, 118
  medical conditions, 109
  multicenter study, 117
  stimulation tests, 110
  weight-based dosing regimen, 117
Anorexia nervosa (AN)
  body composition and glycemia, 54
  bone, 54
  cholinergic drugs, 53
  cluster and deconvolutional analyses, 51, 52
  eating disorder, 51
  ghrelin, 53
  hypothalamus, 53
  liver, 53
  low body weight, 51
  pituitary, 53
  rhGH, 53
Apparent diffusion coefficient (ADC), 126
Arginine, 96, 97, 99, 100
Arginine test, 115, 116
ARNT2, 177, 179, 183

Array comparative genomic hybridization (aCGH), 186
Autosomal dominant GHD, 160–162, 165–166
Auxological parameters, 100
Axenfeld-Rieger syndrome (ARS), 183, 216, 217

**B**
Bioactive GH syndrome, 166–167
Bone morphogenetic protein 4 (Bmp4), 178, 215
Brain MRI, 139, 180, 181, 184, 186

**C**
Cachexia, 54–55
Cardiac mass and function, 86–87
Central nervous system (CNS), 195, 208
CHARGE syndrome, 216
Chiasmatic–hypothalamic gliomas, 140
Childhood cancer survivors, 195, 200
Children/adolescents, 205, 207, 208
Clonidine, 97, 100
Coffin–Siris syndrome, 131
Coloboma, heart anomaly, choanal atresia, retardation, genital, and ear anomalies (CHARGE) syndrome, 131, 132
Combined pituitary hormone deficiency (CPHD), 213
Computerized tomography (CT), 124
Congenital pituitary gland absence (aplasia), 136
Constructive interference in steady state (CISS), 124

Cortisol, 209
Craniofacial abnormalities, 218, 219
Craniopharyngiomas, 139

## D
de Morsier syndrome, 213
Diffusion tensor imaging (DTI), 126
Diffusion-weighted imaging (DWI), 125
Driven equilibrium (DRIVE), 124
Dwarfism, 151

## E
Ectopic posterior pituitary (EPP), 130
Empty sella, 137–138
Endoplasmic reticulum (ER), 165
Endothelial adhesion molecules, 84–85
Endothelial dysfunction, 83–85
Estradiol, 22–24

## F
Fast imaging employing steady-state acquisition (FIESTA), 124
*FGF8* heterozygous mutation, 181
Fibroblast growth factor 8 (Fgf8), 178
Fluid attenuation inversion recovery (FLAIR), 125
Follicle-stimulating hormone (Fsh)β, 179
Free fatty acids (FFA), 65

## G
GH receptor (GHR), 8, 50, 51, 53, 55–58, 84, 96, 166, 209
GH replacement therapy, 39, 80, 84, 88, 199
GH1
  abnormalities, 167
  autosomal recessive concentrations, 158–159
  circulating GH (classical type IA), 156–157
  height variation, 167
  mutations, 155–159
GH-binding protein (GHBP), 96
Ghrelin mimetics, 116–117
GHRH-arginine test, 114–115
GHRHR mutations
  autosomal recessive. Haploinsufficiency, 151
  CpG hotspots, 151
  dwarf mouse model, 151
  GH-IGF axis, 154
  ghrelin analogues, 154
  microcephaly, 154
  pathogenicity, 152
  postnatal growth retardation, 153
  POU1F1-binding sites, 151
  somatostatin, 153
  somatotroph tumors, 154
  volumetric bone density, 153
Glucagon, 97
Glucagon stimulation test (GST), 111, 113, 114
Growth hormone (GH), 21, 40, 95
  bioinactive GH syndrome, 163–164
  cadaveric human, 3
  cytokines and GH-IGF-I axis, 56–58
  definition, dwarfs, 1
  diagnosis, 95
  FDA approval therapy, 3
  GHD (*see* Growth hormone deficiency (GHD))
  hypothalamus, 55
  implications, 17
  inflammatory conditions, 56–57
  JAK STAT pathway, 48
  liver, 55
  metabolic functions, 47
  neuroendocrine secretion, 47
  pituitary, 55
  recombinant human GH, 1
  regulation, pituitary gland, 1
  sex steroids (*see* Sex steroids and GH secretion)
  SRIH, 48
  testing
    analytical, 96–97
    consistency, 97
    GHD, 98–99
    health problems, 102
    interpretation, 97
    obesity, 101–102
    provocative, 101
    provocative tests, 97
    pubertal delay, 102
  TH (*see* Thyroid hormone (TH))
  therapy, 2, 3
Growth hormone deficiency (GHD), 205. *See also* Adult GHD
  in children
    decision-making, 103–104
    diagnosis, 98–99, 103
    growth velocity, 98, 99, 101–104
    immunometric assay, 96
    normative data, 99–100
    outcome-based estimation, 100
    peak response, 98–99
  cranial radiotherapy, 197
  diagnosis, 198, 199

Index

vs. GH-sufficient groups, 96
hypothalamic/pituitary deficits, 195
hypothalamus/pituitary, 197
limbic structures, 208
memory and cognitive capabilities, 209
pathophysiology, 196
prevalence and risk factors, 196–198
treatment, 199–200
Growth hormone-releasing hormone (GHRH), 21–22, 48
Growth hormone-releasing hormone receptor (GHRHR)
autosomal recessive inheritance, 149
definition, 162
detectable GH Concentra, 165
heterozygous mutations, 162
mutations, 149
pathogenic mutations, 152
phenotype, 149
Growth Research Society (GRS), 110
Growth velocity
auxological criteria, 104
GHD, 103
hypothesis, 101
measured GH, 99
normative data, 101
pituitary deficiencies, 103
prepubertal, 102
zero/near-zero, 98

## H
Head trauma, 206
Hesx1, 180, 181
Holoprosencephaly (HPE), 180, 214, 215
Homocysteine, 83
Hormone-sensitive lipase (HSL), 68
HPE. *See* Holoprosencephaly (HPE)
Human Gene Mutation Database (HGMD), 162
Human growth hormone
GHR biological activities, 9
Pegvisomant, 9
rhGH therapy, 9–10
Hypopituitarism, 206, 207, 214
Hypothyroidism
adult height, 39
congenital, 39
gene transcription, 38
standard deviation score (SDS), 38–39

## I
Idiopathic short stature (ISS), 130
Immunometric assays, 96
Inflammatory bowel disease (IBD), 56

Infundibulum, 178
Insulin, 97
Insulin tolerance test (ITT), 111, 112
Insulin-induced hypoglycemia testing, 207
Insulin-like growth factor-I (IGF-I), 109
regulation, GH secretion, 16
and sex steroids
actions of estrogen, 24
concentrations, 23
estrogen and hepatic IGF-I production, 24
GH secretion, 23
hypopituitarism, 24
International Cooperative Growth Study (ICGS), 100
Intima-media thickness (IMT), 87–88
Intracerebral hemorrhage, 208
Isolated GHD (IGHD), 130
Isolated growth hormone deficiency (IGHD)
autosomal dominant inheritance, 150
genetic studies, 150
X-linked type, 150

## J
Janus kinase (JAK) signal transduction and activators of transcription (STAT) pathway, 48
Juvenile idiopathic arthritis, 56

## K
Kallmann syndrome, 131

## L
Langerhans cell histiocytosis (LCH), 139
L-dopa, 97
LEPROT-like 1 (LEPROTL1), 51
Leptin receptor overlapping transcript (LEPROT), 51
Lhx3, 184, 185
Lhx4, 184
Lipoprotein(a), 82
Locus control regions (LCRs), 155
Lymphocytic hypophysitis, 139, 140

## M
Magnetic resonance imaging (MRI)
phenotypes
agenesis, pituitary gland, 136–137
and pituitary genes, 140
anterior pituitary gland aplasia and Chiari I malformation, 137

Magnetic resonance imaging (MRI)
  phenotypes (cont.)
  empty sella, 137–138
  Endocrine/pituitary phenotypes, 140–142
  idiopathic GHD, 133, 136
  ISS and SGA, 131
  pituitary dystopia, 131–135
  pituitary hypoplasia, 131
  posterior lobe ectopia, 132, 134
  secondary GHD, 139–140
  sellar suprasellar mass lesions, 139
Metabolic abnormalities
  adiponectin, 85–86
  body composition, 79–80
  cardiac dimensions and volumes, GHD, 87
  cardiac mass and function, 86–87
  cardiovascular risk factors, 79
  cholesterol and triglycerides levels, 80, 89
  coagulation factors, 82–83
  endothelial dysfunction, 83–85
  fasting and postprandial lipids, 80–82
  fasting and postprandial triglycerides, 82
  growth hormone therapy, 81
  homocysteine, 83
  IMT and vascular reactivity, 87–88
  insulin resistance, 88–89
  lipoprotein(a), 82
  on and off GH replacement, 88
  treated and untreated GHD adolescents and
    healthy controls, 81, 86
Midline defects, 124
Mitochondrial diseases, 218, 219
MR spectroscopy (MRS), 126
Multiple pituitary hormone deficits
  (MPHD), 130
Murine phenotypes, 178
Murine pituitary development, 177–179

## N
National Cooperative Growth Study (NCGS), 100
Neuroimaging
  childhood, 126–129
  hypothalamic–pituitary axis MRI, 129
  normal pituitary size, 129–130
  normal sellar region, 125, 126
  pubertal hyperplasia, 127, 128
  T1-weighted images, 126, 128
Neurosecretory dysfunction, 101
Nutrition, GH secretion
  fasting vs. fed conditions, 15
  hyperglycemia, 15
  hypoglycemia, 15
  obesity, 16

## O
Obesity
  abdominal adiposity, 63–64
  altered growth hormone secretion,
    64–65
  BMI, 63
  body composition and metabolic
    parameters, 71, 72
  dyslipidemia, 68
  GH testing, 101–102
  GHD, 67
  GHRH-arginine stimulation testing, 63, 64
  glucose homeostasis, 69, 73
  IGF-I and IGF-binding proteins, 65–67
  insulin/FFA, 65
  interpretation GH-IGF-I axis testing, 70–71
  intrahepatic and intramyocellular lipid, 68
  lean and fat mass, 71
  meta-analysis, 68
  metabolic and cardiovascular risk, 68, 69
  percentage of patients testing, 70
  premenopausal women, 69
  self-reinforcing cycle, 68
  short-term nutritional status, 65
  visceral fat, 68
Otx2, 182

## P
p.Glu72* mutation, 152
Pallister–Hall syndrome (PHS), 131, 215
Physiology, growth hormone, 7–17
  biochemistry, 9
    human (see Human growth hormone)
    recombinant human GH, 7
    somatotropin, 7
    structure, 8–9
  neurotransmitters and neuropeptides, 14
  regulation, 15
    GH secretion, 11
    ghrelin and GH secretagogues, 13
    GHRH, 12
    GHRH receptor, 11
    IGF-I, 16
    neurotransmitters and neuropeptides, 13
    nongrowth-related biological
      processes, 10
    nutrition (see Nutrition, GH secretion)
    secretion, 10
    sex steroids, 16–17
    sleep, 15
    SRIF, 14
  structure, 8
Pituitary development, 213

Pituitary dwarfism, 98
Pituitary dwarfs, 98
Pituitary dystopia, 131–135
Pituitary function, 205, 207, 209
  auxological evaluation, 207
  IGF-1 levels, 208
Pituitary gland imaging
  anterior and posterior pituitary lobes, 123
  GHD, 123
  hypothalamic–pituitary abnormalities, 124
  imaging techniques, 124–126
  MRI, 123, 124, 126, 127
Pituitary gland morphology, 140
Pituitary hypoplasia, 131
Pituitary stalk, 124, 129, 134, 135, 138
Pituitary stalk interruption syndrome (PSIS), 179–180
PITX2, 183
Polyclonal radioimmunoassays, 96
Post-marketing surveys, 100
POU1F1 (Pit-1), 155, 186
Prader–Willi Syndrome (PWS), 71, 217, 218
Progenitors, 178
Prokineticin pathway, 182
Prolactin, 209
Prop1, 185, 186
Prosencephalon, 180
Provocative testing, 97, 101
Puberty
  administration of testosterone, 23
  delay and GH testing, 102
  estrogen effects, 23
  GH and gonadal steroids, 23
  GH secretion, 22
  growth spurt, 22
  Laron syndrome, 23
  testosterone and changes, 22
  treatment, prepubertal boys, 23

**R**
Randomized control trial (RCT), 98
Receiver-operator characteristic (ROC) curve, 99
Recombinant human growth hormone (rhGH), 53
Resistance to thyroid hormone (RTH), 37, 38

**S**
Septo-optic dysplasia (SOD), 132, 135, 180, 213, 214
Sex steroids and GH secretion, 22–23
  bone and epiphyseal fusion, 24–25
  child to adulthood, 21
  childhood growth and gender influences, 22
  GHRH, 21, 22
  IGF-I, 23–24
  mechanisms, 21
  puberty (*see* Puberty)
  regulation, 17
  variation in height, 25
Sirtuin1 (SIRT1), 51
Sleep on GH secretion, 15
Small for gestational age (SGA), 71, 72, 130
SOD. *See* Septo-optic dysplasia (SOD)
Somatotropin-inhibiting factor (SRIF), 14
Sonic hedgehog (SHH) signaling pathway, 181
Sox2, 182, 183
Suprasellar germinomas, 139

**T**
Thyroid hormone (TH)
  and GH stimulators
    acute illness, 37
    exercise, 36
    food restriction and obesity, 36
    type 1 diabetes mellitus, 37
  children, 40
  deficiencies, 29
  early diagnosis, 40
  GH replacement therapy, 39
  GH secretion and action, 29
  IGF-I, 29
  in vitro and animal models
    GH and bone development, 36
    regulation of GH secretion, 33–34
    stimulation, GH secretion, 34, 35
  normal growth, 29
  nuclear action, 31
  regulation, GH, 33
    in humans, 40
    in vitro and animals
    secretion and action, 33
  regulation, GH expression
    metabolism and transport, 32–33
    receptor, 30–32
  RTH, 37, 38
  treatment, hypothyroidism
    (*see* Hypothyroidism)
Thyrotropin-releasing hormone (TRH), 30
Total body irradiation, 195
Traumatic brain injury (TBI)
  children and adults, 209
  diagnosis and clinical presentation, 207–208
  epidemiology, 206
  pathophysiology, 206, 207

Traumatic brain injury (TBI) (*cont.*)
   pituitary function, 205
   young adults, 205
Triglyceride-rich lipoprotein particles
   (TRP), 81
Tumor necrosis factor-alpha (TNF-alpha), 84
Turner syndrome, 71

## U
Undernutrition, 51–54
   AN (*see* Anorexia nervosa (AN))
   decreased energy availability
     acute and chronic malnutrition, 49
     caloric replenishment, 49
     FGF21, 51
     hypoglycemia and stress, 49
     hypothalamus, GHRH and
       somatostatin, 49
     LEPROT and LEPROTL1, 51
     liver, receptor and post-receptor
       modifications, 50, 51
     mechanism, 50
     pituitary, 50
     protein-energy malnutrition, 49
     SIRT1, 51
     weight gain, 49

## V
Vascular reactivity, 87–88
Very low-density lipoproteins (VLDL), 81